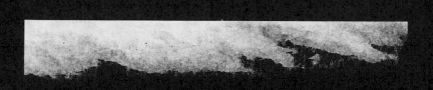

THE MIRACLE OF THE EMPTY BEDS:
A HISTORY OF TUBERCULOSIS IN CANADA

GEORGE JASPER WHERRETT

The Miracle of the Empty Beds: A History of Tuberculosis in Canada

UNIVERSITY OF TORONTO PRESS

Toronto and Buffalo

Canadian Cataloguing in Publication Data

Wherrett, George Jasper, 1896–
The miracle of the empty beds

Bibliography: p.
Includes index.
ISBN 0-8020-2269-3

1.Tuberculosis – Canada – History. 2. Tuberculosis – Prevention – History. I. Title
RA644.T7W54   614.5'42'0971   C77-001162-4

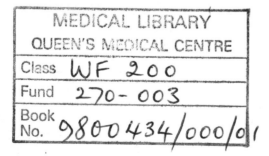
This book has been published during the
Sesquicentennial year of the University of Toronto

This book is dedicated to the tens of thousands
who were victims of tuberculosis,
and to the men and women, both volunteers and professionals,
who with vision and determination initiated the
programs for diagnosis, treatment, and prevention
and carried them through so successfully.

Contents

Photographs

Tables

Foreword

When the author invited me to write an introduction to his monumental work I was well aware that no contribution of mine to the conquest of tuberculosis in Canada was inferred. Rather, I represent the once-typical segment of our society with a bad family history and a personal experience with the disease – in other words, a horrible example.

When I was six my father died at home in his early forties of a malady known to us as galloping consumption. His brother, also a victim, adopted the geographic-climatic approach and went to Kamloops where he soon succumbed. My only brother, thoroughly exposed to the infection, died at the age of two from tuberculous meningitis. During my puny childhood every cough and sniffle was regarded with suspicion, but it was not until the final year of residency training at the Hospital for Sick Children that I stained the bloody sputum and found it swarming with acid-fast bacilli. There followed a period of only three months' duration at Calydor Sanatorium and my respiratory function has been normal for fifty years.

The real reason for my intervention is that Dr George Jasper Wherrett and I, in our professional lives, have witnessed a revolution which is unprecedented. Not so dramatic, perhaps, as the elimination of poliomyelitis, but much more substantial in terms of life and health, and one which involved the participation of the public to a degree that was remarkable. Lacking specific therapeutic resources, the emergence of the sanatorium, the preventorium, and the dispensary represented our approach to diagnosis, rest, and isolation and there were no empty beds in my day.

The development of collapse therapy represented a significant advance in pulmonary surgery, though the mortality statistics were not remarkably improved. Bovine tuberculosis, which affects bones, joints, and other structures, was virtually eliminated by the pasteurization of milk and the gradual elimination of infected cattle from the herds. It is salutary to be reminded of this miracle as well, because it emptied the beds of our hospitals where child patients were undergoing prolonged orthopaedic treatment.

Tuberculin testing, mass surveys, enlistment films, and above all routine chest x-rays on every hospital admission were all aids to the earlier diagnosis of pulmonary tuberculosis. Although immunization with BCG was a great aid in protecting previously uninfected individuals, we remained woefully lacking in our therapeutic armamentarium. The measures which might be classified as 'expectant treatment,' faithfully applied, are reflected in the slowly declining death rates in Canada.

The painful progress may be gauged by comparing the rate of 87.7 tuberculous deaths in Canada per 100,000 population in 1921 with the rate of 53 twenty years later. This is in sharp contrast to the decline in mortality after the introduction of the newer drugs in the late forties. Not being statistically minded, I prefer Dr Wherrett's quote from Dr George Porter's memoirs: 'In 1908 it was true that every time the clock struck the hour in the daytime one Canadian died from tuberculosis and every time during the night, two Canadians died of the same disease.' In 1971 the death rate was 2.1 per 100,000.

The dawning of the new day occurred in 1944 with Waksman's discovery of streptomycin, the first specific antibiotic which proved lethal to the mycobacterium. Isoniazid and PAS quickly followed, and their prompt adoption for treatment and the prevention of recurrences produced the miraculous consequences which are the subject of this book.

The account of the endeavours of dedicated and unselfish professional workers as well as the army of voluntary lay workers is a tribute to the quality of the Canadian people, and it is good that their story is here recorded. It has been a pleasure for me to be reminded of Canadian friends and acquaintances who were leaders in the long, drawn-out campaign. To realize that most of them got into the field because they themselves had been victims is to admire their contribution to public health.

Early in this superficial appraisal I used the word *conquest* to describe the current position in Canada. No conquest has ever been so absolute that pockets of resistance and insurrection do not remain. Tuberculosis is still a major problem among our Indian and Eskimo fellow citizens, and our immigrant population has a higher risk than the native born. Eternal vigilance is the price of health and we should never forget that in many parts of the world the scourge has not been eliminated. With our tuberculin-negative young population natural immunity no longer applies and sporadic cases will erupt. So let us not be complacent with our current mortality statistics, even though we may be justifiably proud of the miracle which has been achieved.

Dr George Jasper Wherrett's personal contribution to the miracle has been impressive. No living Canadian has been so deeply involved, and few could have expended the effort required in research and writing to produce a work which is an absorbing story as well as a reference text which will endure.

A. D. KELLY, MB

Preface

One hundred years ago the word *consumption* (as tuberculosis was then called) struck terror in human hearts. Only the intrepid could face diagnosis of the disease with equanimity. Today, in the western world, it barely evokes any emotion save a too easy surprise that it still exists.

So appalling was the ever present spectre a century ago that it intruded into the work of great novelists, poets, musicians, and artists. Dramatists and the composers of opera wove plots around the slow, pitiless course of the disease. Heroines of grand opera sang their beautiful but tragic arias and collapsed. The great Molière actually haemorrhaged on stage and died within a few hours.

Fictional distress portrayed in novels and drama was but a reflection of what readers and audience could see in life around them, and moved dedicated men and women to take the first steps toward succour of mankind from so much misery.

This book presents the story of how one country, Canada, successfully attacked and controlled tuberculosis and became a model which less fortunate countries could emulate. The programs which were developed not only reduced the death rate year after year until hope replaced despair and lethargy, but created the environment which, once the drugs for specific treatment were developed, made it possible to use them so widely and with such dramatic effect that the long struggle culminated in results that might be referred to as 'The Miracle of the Empty Beds.'

The volume is not a medical treatise on tuberculosis (those seeking medical information will find what they want in medical journals and textbooks). Here we are concerned with quite another approach to the conquest of what was once the most deadly of killers. When Sir William Osler persuaded a sufficient number of people that tuberculosis was a social disease with a medical aspect something new was born: a partnership between physicians and lay people, with a common cause of reducing and, if humanly possible, eradicating the disease. The story of their efforts provides the theme for the book.

Tuberculosis was the leading cause of illness and death during the first fifty years covered in the study. The astounding achievements realized through the combination of medical and social measures demonstrated among other things the benefits derived from public health departments, without which the needed services could not have been provided. Over the years the success of the tuberculosis program also convinced a wide range of people of the value of tax-supported services and provided a framework which was adopted by pioneers in socialized medicine. It is of some significance that Saskatchewan was the first province to provide a fully tax-supported plan for tuberculosis treatment in 1929 when, as a result of the stimulation triggered by the success of this program, medicare was introduced during the administration of Premier T.C. Douglas.

For over forty years it was my privilege as medical officer and executive secretary of the Canadian Tuberculosis Association and consultant to health departments, both provincial and federal, to have a 'ringside seat' from which to observe the campaign being waged in all the provinces of Canada. At the outset, I worked for four years in Saskatchewan as a medical officer dealing daily with clinical aspects of the disease as it affected people of all ages and walks of life in that part of Canada. The effects of the disease on the pioneers, the immigrants, and the Indian people were part of the daily concern of the Saskatchewan Anti-Tuberculosis League. Later, my task in New Brunswick, as a staff member of the Department of Health, was to develop the clinic services of that province. This led to an interest in the Canadian Tuberculosis Association and its program for stimulating antituberculosis work in all parts of Canada. Later still, as executive secretary of that organization, I represented Canada on the Executive Committee and Council of the International Union against Tuberculosis for twelve years and as a member of the Expert Committee on Tuberculosis of the World Health Organization from 1959 to 1972. This gave me an understanding of the world picture of the disease and the problems created by it. During these years it was my privilege to know personally nearly all of the leaders in the campaign. I also met many people engaged in this work in the United States and in the countries affiliated with the International Union.

As a young medical officer treating and advising tuberculosis patients and their families, I was often also emotionally involved in their troubles. I realized the hopelessness of the disease in so many cases, and the anguish and despair of families when their young people, and particularly their young women, became victims of the disease and so often succumbed to it. At the same time, I was impressed by, and admired, the courage with which so many of these afflicted people faced the problems presented by the disease and the months and years spent in isolation in sanatoria, often in exile from their homes and friends, and rejoiced with those who overcame their disease and returned to a normal way of life.

I have been greatly affected by the story of two young men, Angus and Edward, just out of their teens, whom I admitted to the sanatorium during my first month as medical officer at the Fort Qu'Appelle, Saskatchewan, institution, in 1924. Six years later, I was again serving the sanatorium. I was astonished to find both these young men still in the institution. For Angus, the disease had gradually run its course with the usual ups and downs. The lad remained in one of the ambulant pavilions, a favourite and a source of information for all the patients who came and went during that time. On the evening of his death, I had a curling game, and I called in to see him before I went. He said: 'Doctor, don't worry about me, go on to your game.' I called as soon as I finished and he said: 'Doctor, I think *you* would feel better if I went to the infirmary' (where more nursing care was available). He died during the night, his final thoughts being of others, that he should not be a burden to anyone.

Edward, during his six years in the sanatorium, had gradually got his disease under control, but still had a lot of pulmonary fibrosis, which left him too disabled to lead a normal life. The authorities decided that he could be cared for in a boarding house in Yorkton on welfare until 'light work' could be obtained. The prospect of obtaining work in 1931 was so bleak that this young man decided to finish the business, obtained a shot-gun and ended his life.

These are harrowing tales that, fortunately, could not occur fifty years later, after specific drugs had come into use and more adequate social care for the tuberculous had been developed.

In the position of executive secretary of the Canadian Tuberculosis Association, it was my duty to help all provinces in Canada to improve facilities by developing voluntary and official agencies to cope with the problem. I was particularly interested in the provinces and areas of the country where the disease was most prevalent. I was appalled by the amount of tuberculosis in the native races of Canada and was continually associated with the officials of the Indian and Medical Services of the Department of National Health and Welfare. After my retirement from the association I became a full-time consultant to the Medical Services of the department and was able to devote my attention to the problems of the Indians and particularly the Eskimos, and to see first hand the life of the Eskimo in the Arctic.

I became conscious of the fact that much of the history of the disease was going to be lost unless an effort was made to preserve the records of the hundred years of tuberculosis work, so the early records of the Canadian Tuberculosis Association were placed in the Public Archives of Canada, where they would be available for study. I then undertook to prepare the present volume by sifting through photocopies of this material and the wealth of other historical material in the records of other associations, such as the Canadian Medical Association and the Canadian Public Health Association, as well as in those of government departments, both federal and provincial.

The writing of the book had to proceed in several stages, because there was far more information available than could be accommodated in a reasonable number of pages. The structuring of the book also required consideration, and it was eventually decided to divide it into two parts, the first covering in various chapters matters of national concern and the second describing the development of the programs in the individual provinces. For ease in reference, the statistical tables and graphs showing variations in mortality rates over the years have been collected together as appendices. The references for individual chapters appear together under 'Notes' following the appendices, except for the chapter on BCG, which has appended to it a rather complete bibliography on the subject. An extensive bibliography on other aspects of tuberculosis in Canada is included as well, to assist anyone who is interested in further study.

In offering this social history of tuberculosis in Canada, it is my hope that it will be of interest to public health workers and lay people as well as to doctors, and that it may stimulate studies in other social problems.

G. J. W.

Acknowledgments

Many people and organizations have contributed to the preparation of this history. It is impossible to acknowledge adequately the part played by each, but it is also impossible to refrain from expressing gratitude for the help of some without whose encouragement and aid this volume would never have reached publication.

Among those friends in the voluntary and official organizations who suggested that while the experience of fifty years in various aspects of tuberculosis work was still fresh in my mind I should put it in a book, I must single out two for a special tribute, Dr Floris E. King and Mrs Eve Shulman, for without their encouragement and prodding the work would probably never have been started. Mrs Shulman provided a further push along the way when she helped prepare the first application for financial help from the Canada Council. She also directed the project during my absence at the University of British Columbia in 1971.

Research assistants included Mr Wayne Brighton, Mr A.J. Finlayson, Miss Lise La Barre, Mr Brian Norris, and Mr Pierre Verrette. Among them they collected more information than could be included, but it has all been catalogued and placed in the Public Archives where it is available for further study.

The chief burden has been borne by Miss Eileen Flanagan. Her long experience in all phases of the nursing profession and her ability to glean the last item of information of a historical nature from any source have been of inestimable value.

I would like to thank others who contributed to various chapters: Mr A.J. Finlayson, Miss Esther Paulson, Dr Owen Clark, Dr Stefan Grzybowski, Professor Armand Frappier, Mrs Nora Corley Murchison, and Miss Anne Grant. Mrs Murchison also ably assumed the task of coordinating the project, and Miss Jean Henderson, the clerk-stenographer throughout, did excellent work. During the later stages of revision of the manuscript, Miss Lorraine Ourom, Science Editor of the University of Toronto Press, gave valuable advice and assistance.

I am especially indebted to the Department of National Health and Welfare for providing the team with office space and facilities. I would like particularly to thank Dr J.H. Weibe, Dr Marion Webb, Dr Lyall Black, and Dr Wm Frost for advice and encouragement, and Mr Vaughan Russell, who prepared the graphs and tables.

At all times the section heads of Statistics Canada have given their full co-operation, specifically Mr Harry Page of the Vital Statistics Section and Mr Cecil Baldwin and Mr A. Bowden of the Public Health Section.

I am grateful for the help of my wife, Margaret, during the final revision of the manuscript and for the patience she displayed throughout. She also suggested the title for the book.

The research work on the volume was assisted financially by the Canada Council, the Physicians' Services Incorporated Foundation, the Sanatorium Board of Manitoba, the Saskatchewan Anti-Tuberculosis League, Merck Frosst Laboratories, and Dow Chemicals. Publication of the book has been made possible by grants from the Canadian Tuberculosis and Respiratory Disease Association and from the Hannah Foundation for the History of Medical and Related Sciences.

Finally, the Macmillan Company of Canada has graciously granted permission to quote from p. 194 of their publication *I Chose Canada* by J.R. Smallwood.

PART I

THE NATIONAL CRUSADE

1

Historical Background

A generation ago in Canada little attention was given to what is called public health. The individual was left to kill or cure himself by patent medicines and domestic remedies, varied by an occasional doctor's visit. To the prevention of disease little thought was given. No longer than twenty-five or thirty years ago epidemics of disease were popularly spoken of as visitations of Providence and punishment for sin. There has been a revolution since that time. Public Health is now the new gospel [Clifford Sifton, in Commission on Conservation, *Annual Report*, 1914]

Until the 1860s Canada was a vast, unconnected reserve of natural resources which housed a rural population of small towns and a few primary industries such as fishing, lumbering, and wheat-growing. Her large centres, Montreal and Toronto, could boast populations of but 90,000 and 45,000 respectively. Her placid existence was, however, threatened by her more mature and aggressive neighbour to the south, the war-torn United States. In response to this external threat as well as to internal malfunctioning, Confederation took place.

Confederation involved the drawing up of an entirely new set of rules and regulations for the functioning of government in Canada, guidelines which were to go relatively unchanged for the next 100 years despite the fact that conditions in Canada changed. Looking back with a twentieth-century bias, one notes a certain absurdity in the granting of administrative powers to the provinces for education, health, hospitals, and social welfare in the British North America Act without provision for financing. Yet Sir John A. Macdonald and his cohorts did not live in an environment of medicare or social welfare; theirs was an uneducated rural world in which social problems were looked after by the local community. Then, too, they were concerned with the building and protecting of a transcontinental nation, and minor problems could be overlooked. They also had analysed the American War among the states, which was seen to have been caused by the fact that individual states possessed too much power, and were determined not to make the same mistake in Canada: power would rest in the hands of the federal government.

Because Canada wanted to protect herself and thus of necessity had to become the equal of the United States, she embarked on a rapid expansion program, both externally and internally. 'Externally,' she quickly acquired the West and British Columbia, while 'internally' her gates were opened to receive any immigrant who was willing to come. In her desire to enlarge her population and market for economic growth, Canada sought to make it as easy as possible for immigrants to enter the country. Under the Immigration Act of 1869, each province was to set up its own rules regarding immigration, but the federal government was to provide and supervise quarantine stations in order to guard against those old enemies cholera and typhoid fever. To a large extent Canada hoped to attract European farmers who would settle her virgin lands and thus populate her vast geographical hinterland. However, Europe by this time had become highly industrialized and it was the poor urban worker who often made the journey. At the same time, Canada herself was undergoing a rapid transformation. From the 1860s onward, the steam engine, railways, and new manufactured goods were drawing more and more people from the land and into the city. In the 1870s alone the proportion of rural Canadians dropped from 80 per cent to 74 per cent of the total population.[1] This trend was to continue throughout the following decades at an even more accelerated pace, and Canada was placed in a dilemma: she wanted to increase her population as quickly as possible, yet her infant industries could not develop quickly enough to provide jobs for an ever increasing population. Added to this was the problem of disease. Immigrants who were sick or liable to become public charges were not allowed to enter Canada, but with poor knowledge of diseases, rapid urban growth, and lack of jobs, the country soon found itself with a slum problem.

As the numbers grew, so did the rates of crime and disease, a fact which did not go unnoticed by public-spirited individuals. As early as 1879, the press was attacking government policy of allowing in so many immigrants. The Department of Agriculture for that year reported:

As regards the suitability of the class of immigrants, it is necessary to remark that lately it was circulated in the press, and complained of by some agents, as well as private individuals, that paupers were coming into the country and were cast upon the community for support. Measures were therefore taken to stop such proceedings, which were apparently about to be extensively adopted through agencies unconnected with Government emigration service, and wholly unauthorized to make the statements put forth to induce the pauper class to emigrate to Canada as a refuge.[2]

By 1902 the Immigration Act had been considerably strengthened, but its main concerns were still the same, namely, the prohibition of those who might become public charges or who had contracted infectious diseases.

By this time medical knowledge had made great advances and tuberculosis was recognized as *the* great killer, and to be of an infectious nature. Yet persons with tuberculosis were still entering Canada. In 1903 Dr Peter Bryce, chief medical officer of the Department of the Interior, noted: 'It is evident that there are diseases such as epilepsy, insanity, incipient tuberculosis, all of the greatest importance, yet of which cases, in the necessarily rapid examination of the hundreds coming off a vessel, will not infrequently pass unrecognized.'[3] Because of this fact, Bryce came under repeated attack by a now concerned public, led by the press and community officials. In 1905 Dr Bruce Smith, inspector of hospitals and charities, protested: 'Too often of late years by the pernicious system of bonusing emigration agencies abroad, mental and physical degenerates have been landed on our shores and have finally drifted, either through mental, physical or moral deficiencies into one or other of our great public Charities.'[4] In 1907 Dr Bryce was again questioned because of the 'enormous proportion' of immigrants among tuberculosis patients in sanatoria in Ontario, and was even told that British officials were taking tubercular patients out of British sanatoria and sending them to Canada, where Canadians had to support them. Bryce replied that personal examinations were necessary to detect incipient tuberculosis, and that, because of the numbers involved, these were impossible.[5] Later, in investigating the number of immigrants in sanatoria, Bryce found that many of these persons had developed tuberculosis in Canada.[6]

Certainly the development of tuberculosis in Canada was as great a problem as, if not greater than, the problem of the immigrant. Owing to the rapid pace at which the country was moving, a fact which is perhaps the key to understanding the era, it is understandable that problems would arise and that the sheer lack of experience in these areas, not to mention the obstacles of social attitudes, would hinder any attempt to find an easy solution. As Sir Oliver Mowat remarked after passing the immensely important Public Health Act of Ontario in 1873: 'We have passed the legislation, but have little knowledge of just what there is to do.'[7]

Just what was the government to do? As has been mentioned, the legislation of 1867 was for the functioning of a rural society without provision for financing of hospitals, welfare, and education. Yet, within little more than a decade this became very much a problem and the financially strained provinces were crying out not only for money but for more power. Such a cry was anathema to Macdonald, the firm believer in a central authority, so there were repeated clashes between the federal government and the provincial leaders throughout the 1880s and 1890s on the question of jurisdiction and responsibility. When the new leader, Sir Wilfrid Laurier, took over, he found himself on a virtual keg of powder, and in his dream of consolidating Canadian unity he was led down the path of compromise, with major concessions being given to the provinces.

Not only was the matter of jurisdiction a problem. The basic question of determining the best solution weighed heavily on the government's mind. Also, afraid of acting lest someone be offended, the Laurier government needed to retain all the support it could get because of the racial tensions of the period, which threatened to break up the Canadian nation. It is understandable, therefore, that little initiative was shown before 1918. Even if the government had wanted to act, it could not until it had decided on the line of action to be taken, for there were two distinct schools of thought on the question of government aid and welfare. To the reformed, society was a social organism consisting of interrelated parts, and if one section became 'diseased' in some way, it must be helped before it infected the entire body:

The functions most proper to government no doubt are national defence, the maintenance of public order, the protection of the rights of property and repression of crime. But its actions cannot always be confined within these bounds; it must sometimes be paternal; it must, as in the case of children employed in factories, take care of those who cannot take care of themselves; it must enforce regulations which, through interferences with private habits, are essential to public health and comfort; it must sometimes interfere to save people even from the consequences of their own misconduct and prevent them from dying of hunger on the street, though their destination may be the consequence of their own faults and the penalty affixed to such faults by nature. Strictly to define duties of a government is impossible; they must vary with circumstances, with the character of the nation and the stage of civilization which it has reached. Government is the organ of the community for such purposes as it may be found, from time to time, expedient to effect by common action.[8]

Not all, however, agreed with this interpretation of government's role. In a century of revolt and attempts to escape from powerful, omnipotent governments, there were many who greatly feared a return to a 'tyrannical' system, even though it be accompanied by new bureaucratic paraphernalia. Such people treasured, above all, individual rights and saw in the rise of 'socialism' a great threat to liberty. One individual of this school of thought was Carroll Ryan of Ottawa, who asserted in 1879 that, unfortunate though it may be that people were unemployed, 'the very worst thing a government could do would be to teach them to look to the state for aid ... The Government should be dependent on the people, not the people on the government.'[9] Ryan feared that a paternal government would lead to the type of 'Frankenstein monster' which Bismarck had created in Germany. Similarly sixteen years later, in an era when class struggle was the theme of the day, Adam Shortt remarked in *The Queen's Quarterly* that 'the most demoralizing and illegitimate function of a government is either to step in and do the people's work for them ... or in forcing one portion of the people to contribute to the support of another.'[10]

It should also be remembered that these were the days when the urban immigrants were seen as the 'scum' or 'dregs' of Europe, and were believed to be such because of their inferiority or laziness. The system could not be blamed for personal faults; if these people were to rise, they must help themselves.

Given these opinions, is it any wonder that the government tended to tread softly in social matters? Government officials such as Lord and Lady Aberdeen, the governor general and his wife, who did take the lead in promoting better social conditions, were not looked upon favourably by the 'better' class of society. Lord Minto informs us that the Aberdeens absolutely upset society, to the extent that Queen Victoria herself advised Lady Minto not to get 'mixed up in any new venture which might be criticized.'[11] Lord Minto did, however, give every assistance in the organization of the Canadian Association for the Prevention of Consumption and Other Forms of Tuberculosis in 1900.

This lack of leadership from within society might appear unusual, but an analysis of society itself provides an almost endless list of obstacles. One such example was the opposition, or at least lack of co-operation, from the churches. Once the leaders of society, they clung desperately to their old charitable ways and did not adapt to the faster, more mundane world with new forms of recreation and problems. They still attracted the relatively unchanged portion of society – the upper classes – but lost touch with the populace. The churches should not emerge in a totally bad light, however. Like the leaders of the government and other leading citizens, many believed in the class structure of society and the need for people to raise themselves, and some did give assistance to the lower classes. The Salvation Army, for example, practised social work in the new industrial environment and was therefore a valuable ally of the social reform school.

The reform school itself was basically an environmentalist group of doctors, sociologists, and politicians who believed that social problems, be they material, structural, or ideological, were the product of living conditions. Seeing society as a unit, they believed that by relieving stress upon one of the component parts, possible friction on others was prevented and society thus improved. Taking a lead from the findings of the New York Medical Society, the *Sanitary Journal* of 1876 remarked that 'crime ... is often the direct and positive outgrowth of unsanitary conditions' and concluded that it was 'undoubtedly in the nature of man to be largely influenced by the physical conditions by which he is surrounded.'[12] Quoting from the Report of the Committee on Hygiene and on Relations of Unsanitary Conditions to Pauperism, Vice and Crime, the *Journal* noted that 'the filthiest parts of towns are inhabited by the most unhealthy and poorest people and that unhealthy surroundings are scarcely less potent in blunting the sensibilities and lowering the standards of morals than is diminishing the strength of the physical system.'[13] Basic to the thinking of the reform group was the belief that the well-being of the populace was the key to the growth of Canada because it was on the shoulders of the masses that the political and economic structures would rest. To the doctors, this involved a revolutionary change in attitude, one which stressed not the curing of disease but rather the prevention of it. Here was the link between doctors and reformers: public health.

As industrialism increased, the link between filth and disease became so apparent that epidemics of cholera soon moved governments to action. Canada, still a rural nation, had based its medical practice upon country practitioners who attended individual cases and attempted to prescribe a cure. With the growth of industrialism, however, doctors observed the examples of Britain and the United States and saw the need to prevent rather than simply cure a disease, and prevention became the first duty of a physician. This attitude was further acknowledged when the president of the Canadian Medical Association asserted, in 1877, that 'a knowledge of the laws of health should not be confined to the profession.'[14] The basis for this change was the increase in the number of patients attended by doctors, a fact which brought hospitals into existence, and the realization that the physician's efforts were often futile because of the ignorance of the family members attending the sick bed. Education of the public was therefore needed.

In 1877 the Canadian Medical Association was able to report, too, that 'the conviction is steadily gaining ground that a Board of Health should be established for the Dominion; Provincial Boards for each Province; and local boards for each municipality.'[15] Still, it was readily acknowledged that 'legislation is useless where people are totally uninformed on the most elementary health matters ... We must get those whom sanitary laws affect, to have some sort of intelligent appreciation of the principles they involve.'[16] The 'crusade' on behalf of public health was pushed ahead with great success during the 1880s and 1890s not only through the passing of public health acts and the establishing of boards across the country, but also by making attempts to educate the people themselves. At the same time, the medical advances of men such as Louis Pasteur and Robert Koch, to name only two, sent medical expertise racing ahead at speeds hitherto unknown.

It should never be assumed, however, that progress came easy, for as has already been mentioned, this same period was a time of provincial-federal squabbling over jurisdiction and responsibilities. Also, of course, there was the lack of experience of the groups themselves, not to mention the problem of educating the people in matters which we today would assume to be simply common sense. For example, doctors cried out for accurate records of vital statistics so that causes of death could be determined. Yet in 1879 it was noted that the registrars who attempted to get this information from the people were meeting great resistance. Such a response was not so unusual in view of the common tendency to equate sickness with punishment by God for leading a sinful life. By responding to the registrars, one would be placing a social stigma upon the family. Similarly, in 1885, when a smallpox epidemic was threatening Montreal and the authorities attempted to enforce compulsory vaccination, they were met with extremely strong resistance. This is once again understandable, remembering the lack of education of the people and the newness of the procedure. Not only would they have been sceptical of its curative worth, but the moral implications would no doubt be similar to those expressed by Jehovah's Witnesses to this day regarding blood transfusions.

Progress, however, was made and by 1901 the Provincial Board of Health of Ontario reported:

during the past twenty years there has been, on the whole, a very remarkable change in the habits of thought amongst the people of Ontario as regards disease prevention. Up to twenty years ago, smallpox was commonly treated by the family physician who, exciting more or less care, continued to attend at the same time his other patients. To-day, the public will practically boycott any physician who is willing to

attend smallpox. The reasons which have produced this situation are the direct result of sanitary education and on the whole are to be commended.[17]

It was not smallpox, however, that dominated the people's minds by this
time; it was consumption, the number one killer and the disease for which
there was no cure. This fact alone would give tuberculosis a starring role in
any discussion of the period, but its direct relationship to the social transformation which Canada was undergoing gives it an even greater prominence.

The campaign against bad living and working conditions was already
well under way. Even in 1879 people were surprised

that so many die during the latter part of winter, and in the early spring, with lung
diseases – consumption, inflammation and congestion of the lungs, bronchitis, etc.
But the weather is blamed for this increase in the death-rate from these diseases.
This is largely misplaced unjust censure. It is most difficult to get people to understand or comprehend how large a quantity of air around us, we, at every breath, render unfit to be drawn into our lungs. Herein lies the chief benefit of outdoor life: the
breath, as it escapes from the mouth in the open air, is usually at once dissipated
and carried away, so that no portion of it gets back into our lungs again: in close
rooms this is not the case.[18]

The seeming link between poor living conditions and consumption was also
brought out: 'A truly scrofulous disease is caused by breathing air vitiated
by respiration and ... it is not always necessary that there should be a prolonged stay in such an atmosphere. Often, a few hours each day is sufficient,
as sitting in a close schoolroom, or sleeping in a confined bedroom ... That
most frequent cause of death is without doubt, Pulmonary Consumption,
developed by respired air.'[19]

More and more people came to realize that destitution was not necessarily the product of laziness, but that there were just not enough jobs available. Canada, the land of vast resources and opportunity, was starting to be
seen in a more realistic light. As an example of this change in attitude, the
Commissioner Appointed to Enquire into the Prison and Reformatory System of Ontario wrote in 1891 that 'of the people who applied for assistance
during the winter season, from one-half to two-thirds would be willing to
work if they had the opportunity of getting it ... I question whether it is reasonable or right, that people who are simply in necessitous circumstances
should have to go to the police magistrate and be sent to gaol for periods of
three to six months.'[20]

Regarding the general living conditions of the poorer segments of the population several comments have been made. Close to the turn of the century, a visiting British MP, Henry Vivian, saw the slums of Montreal and remarked: 'Nothing in East London is worse than some of the conditions which I saw in Montreal yesterday; ... Montreal will become one of the greatest cesspools of human depravity in the world if action is not taken.'[21] Others described how workers lived in the midst of tall chimneys where the air hung heavy with smoke. Toronto was not much better, for it was noted: 'In our city at the present time there is scarcely a vacant house fit to live in that is not inhabited, and in many cases by numerous families; ... respectable people have had to live in stables, tents, old cars, sheds (others in damp cellars), where we would not place a valued animal, let alone a human being.'[22] Unsanitary conditions are vividly displayed in the reports of reformers working on the Commission on Conservation. For example, Dr C.A. Hodgetts reported on the lack of refuse collection and disposal in Toronto, a problem which led to the storing of solid wastes in barrels. Critical of civic authorities' interest in the problem, he wrote that the city's 'clean-up week' was really the health authorities' admission that there was no system for collection or disposal of refuse during most of the year and that the annual display of 'ridding' itself of the decomposing refuse showed their inefficiency.[23] Conditions in factories were no better. Most were overheated, dirty, smoky, and had no ventilation. Health and living conditions were becoming inseparably linked, with the result that government authorities were being attacked from all sides for ineptitude and even callous indifference.

The grave concern over the living conditions of the poor was compounded, of course, by the medical advances in the last quarter of the century which confirmed to the world that tuberculosis was indeed infectious. As early as 1877 the Canadian Medical Association was tossing around the concept of a 'germ theory' for the disease and in 1879 the *Sanitary Journal* reported that 'from numerous recent experiments, it appears that pulmonary consumption may be regarded as contagious; it is probable that a healthy person may contract this fatal disease directly by breathing the seeds of it – minute particles of tuberculosis, exhaled from the lungs of another suffering from it.'[24] Throughout the 1880s and 1890s the medical profession stressed the infectious nature of tuberculosis, and acclaimed experiments such as Dr Herman Brehmer's sanatorium and the policy of disposing of sputa, but did not offer a proven cure. The terror connected with consumption may be seen in the terms used to describe it. People were repeatedly told that they were in 'the jaws of death' or the 'clutch of consumption,' while consumption itself was termed the 'White Plague.'

Doctors feared for the survival of the race, and termed it a 'national disease' as public concern in health matters rose to a new level.

The problem became one of major concern, not only to those afflicted with the disease but to those who feared developing it. Anticonsumption leagues soared into existence, and the problem of cleaning up the slums received a great shot in the arm because of the new interest. Suddenly consumptives found themselves to be a type of 'leper' with whom none wanted contact. Shunned by their friends, their strength weakening every day and their chances for employment steadily diminishing, the sufferers were indeed a pitiable lot.

Wealthy consumptives could afford to enter a sanatorium where they would receive proper care and, if the disease was stopped early enough, perhaps could be cured. To the poor, however, there was no answer. Hospital wards closed their doors along with the rest of society. All had excuses for non-action: provincial authorities claimed to lack finances, charities said it was hopeless to attempt a task so big without government help, and municipal and federal governments claimed it was not their responsibility or under their jurisdiction.

It may be wondered why the pressure of public opinion itself did not force the governments to action, but the opinions presented concerning the nature of consumption and the remedies required were those of the educated, not those of the people. True, literature on sanitation had gone far, but the problem of tuberculosis was a distinct one, not like that of diseases such as cholera, which could be cured. Remembering the lack of education, the old pseudo-religious beliefs concerning disease and the wrath of God, and the general confusion of the time, it is understandable that the populace did not believe everything they heard about tuberculosis. Because of the constantly new discoveries, the medical world itself was in a constant state of flux, disproving one theory and advocating another. To the people, there still existed no proof that consumption was not hereditary. By the 1870s it was agreed that the marriage of persons with tendencies to consumption or insanity should be avoided or prevented as far as possible; it was a 'known fact' that babies were born with tuberculosis. In 1899 Dr John Hunter led an attack against this very problem in his attempt to obtain life insurance policies for people whose parents had had consumption.[25] To the uneducated layman who did not possess or comprehend the concept of 'germs,' it appeared perfectly obvious that families, not just individuals, were dying of tuberculosis, and that therefore it must be hereditary.

The press during these decades played a formative role in the development of all individuals, and in the realm of medicine it played a very important one. Policy in this period allowed advertisements naming cures and treatments for various diseases, which included the name, address, and office hours of a doctor. Quack doctors availed themselves of this opportunity to advertise and hence gained advantage over practitioners, who were unlikely to do so. This was a thorn in the medical profession's side from early times, and in 1877 the Canadian Medical Association was calling for the establishment of registration boards to set standards which should be met before medicine could be practised in a province. It was hoped that this would enable doctors to get rid of the quacks, but by 1899 the problem was still a major one. The quack could offer the one thing the doctor could not, particularly in the case of tuberculosis – hope. Dr Daniel Clark provides a good sketch of the prevalence and success of quackery in his article 'Medical Manias,' published in 1879. He noted that 'every city, town, and village is full of ignorant pretenders to medical lore and skill,' most publishing a highly sensational medical document of some sort, intended to frighten the reader into believing he was sick and should therefore run to him for help. Through the press, such a pretender gained a wide reputation before he even entered an area:

at this hour there is travelling in Ontario a licensed charlatan who puts placards on the fences, gates and barns of the back townships and villages, that he is the 'greatest physician of the age.' He puts in largest type, with ornamental headings, a list of diplomas and licenses, which strike with astonishment the unsophisticated rustic and his wife. He can intuitively tell what is the matter with a patient the moment he casts his eye on him ... His fame spreads far and near ... After a few visits ... the victims shamefully go back to the family physicians ... Experience shows that a lesson of this kind has no effect upon the public, for each brazen-faced successor of a similar type will gull the same neighbourhood and the same patients with equal facility to that of the first.[26]

For those who could not see the quack in person, there was the inevitable post-office box number accompanying the advertisement in the newspaper, telling where to send money.

This practice did not have only a fleeting popularity. Because of consumption's 'incurable' nature, it was the focal point of a great many products such as 'Burdock Blood Bitters,' 'Allen's Lung Balsam,' 'Extract of Cod Liver,' 'Piso's Cure for Consumption,' 'Campbell's Skrei,' 'Angier's Petroleum Emulsion,' 'Dr. Wood's Norway Pine Syrup,' and 'The Slocum Cure' throughout the 1890s. All were 'sure cures,' and usually contained testimonials as to their effectiveness to convince the willing public. In today's scientific age, it is perhaps too easy to pass over the gullible nature of the people of that era. They believed because they were desperate, and it was their only hope for finding a cure. Nor were the people who sought this relief all of the 'uneducated' calibre; even intelligent, well-educated, and highly thought of citizens patronized the quacks in a stealthy way. The greatest harm produced by the quacks was not through their medicines, which were usually harmless vegetable mixtures, but rather in the time wasted depending upon these worthless solutions when proper treatment could have been given by a qualified doctor. In the case of consumption, time was of the utmost importance.

As has been previously mentioned, the tuberculosis problem became one of public concern near the turn of the century. It was then that the various segments of the public health environmentalist school were able to co-ordinate their efforts and produce results. The members of the medical profession were at last united in their belief as to the nature of the disease, the sanitary movement had produced results, the seriousness of tuberculosis was finally being recognized because of the numbers involved, and anticonsumption leagues were joining charity and other volunteer groups. With more experience behind them, reformers and doctors at last began to move with common strides.

An additional stimulus to the crusade was provided by the example of the epidemic proportions consumption had reached among the Canadian Indians. This evidence at last placed consumption in the same category of seriousness as smallpox or cholera in the public mind, for there was a general fear that the Indians could infect the white settlements. Cries were made that the government should do something. The health problem among the Indians was not a new one for the government, their susceptibility to disease being well known, but it was only with the coming of the 1880s that tuberculosis was identified as the specific killer and the extent of the ravages realized. Adding to the problems were the Indians' own personal habits, which tended towards communal living, and their general lack of knowledge concerning sanitary habits. In their crowded, smoke-filled rooms in which tuberculous sputa often dried on the floor only to re-enter the air and hence the lungs of the inhabitants, the spread of consumption took place in much the same manner as it did among the poor urban classes.

Under new pressure and armed with a greater knowledge of medical science than ever before the political machinery began to function. Number one on its list of priorities, of course, was tuberculosis, 'the captain of all the men of death' in the words of John Bunyan.

Unfortunately, there are no over-all statistics on tuberculosis for these early years since there were no federal or provincial departments of health or of statistics. For some of the cities, however, particularly Montreal and Toronto, and for the province of Ontario, statistics covering mortality from tuberculosis are available from 1880 (see Appendices 1 and 2). These may well be indicative of an average since Montreal represents the province that had and still has the highest prevalence, while Ontario has always had the lowest prevalence in Canada. The mortality rate for Canada might therefore have been approximately 200 per 100,000 in 1880, and perhaps a little higher than this by 1900 (in any case it does not seem to have decreased during the twenty-year period, as it did in Great Britain). From 1900, however, when organized efforts to control the disease began to be made, the rate began to fall.[27] Reports from the Canadian Tuberculosis Association indicate that in 1901 the population of Canada was 5,371,315 and there were 9709 deaths from tuberculosis, a rate of 180 per 100,000, and that in 1908 the population was 6,500,000, the number of deaths 11,700, and the mortality rate 165 per 100,000.[28]

The toll in human lives in Canada and the United States to 1908 is vividly portrayed by Dr George D. Porter in reporting on his first visit to the offices of the National Tuberculosis Association in New York:

When I came to Broadway, I was stopped by a huge procession of one hundred thousand men who were marching up that great thoroughfare in honour of Mr. Taft who was then running for President. Every man carried a flag and each section was headed by a band of music of which there were over a hundred in the parade.

Then I thought, as I looked at them, of the hundred and fifty thousand men, women and children, every year in the United States, who marched, not with flags and banners, but in silence and alone, down to consumptives' graves.

As for Canada; in 1908 it was true that 'Every time the clock struck the hour in the daytime, one Canadian died from tuberculosis and every time it struck the hour during the night, two Canadians died of the same disease.'[29]

These were the sad realities that led to the formation of a national association to battle the disease. Fortunately, by this time many facts had become known about the disease, which made it possible to set up an effective program once the means were available.

Important discoveries had been made in France and Germany. In 1865 Jean Antoine Villemin showed that the disease was communicable, and was able to transfer it to animals. In 1882 Robert Koch of Berlin discovered the tubercle bacillus and established it as the cause of the disease, thus providing the basis for a scientific attack on the disease and laying to rest the theory that it was inherited. He explained how the disease was transmitted from a sick person to a healthy one and, in particular, to members of a family and close associates. Koch's discovery pointed the way for a program of prevention, aroused interest in treatment, and raised the hope that a 'cure' might eventually be found for the disease that had plagued the world since the time of Hippocrates.

Pathologists, including Robert Koch and Rudolf Virchow in Germany, studied the various forms of tuberculosis as it appeared in different parts of the body, such as the lungs, glands, bones, pleura, and peritoneum, as well as acute forms such as meningitis, and rapid types such as miliary disease. No matter what part of the body was affected, the various forms were shown to be due to one and the same germ, which in every case could be found in the lesions.

The germ gained entrance to the body either by inhalation or ingestion, or occasionally by inoculation, as in the case of butchers handling tuberculous meat from diseased cattle. Having gained entry, the germ might develop at the site of entry, set down somewhere in the lung, or be spread by the lymphatics or the blood stream to other parts of the body. The first lesion was in the form of a small nodule or tubercle; hence the name tuberculosis. These tubercles might be successfully attacked by the defences of the body (the white blood cells) and be destroyed; the tubercles might become healed; or several tubercles might coalesce and spread, enlarge, and eventually destroy the patient.

Following the spread of the original tubercles, the onset of active disease became manifest. Symptoms depended on the part of the body involved. In the commonest form – pulmonary tuberculosis – symptoms such as cough, expectoration, and/or spitting of blood usually developed. Fever, weakness, and wasting were later symptoms; hence the old name consumption. If the pleura was involved, pain on breathing was a symptom; if bones or joints were involved, pain in the joint was an early symptom; with tuberculosis meningitis, headache was the common symptom; and with tuberculosis of the lymph glands, their swelling was noted.

Tuberculosis meningitis and miliary tuberculosis, the latter spreading by way of the blood stream, were dreaded because they were invariably fatal. These facts were known to the medical profession around 1900, and methods of detecting and treating the disease were being introduced.

In 1890 Dr Koch prepared tuberculin, an extract of tubercle bacilli, and observed that if the substance was injected into the body of persons who had been infected there was a noticeable reaction in the form of oedema, or swollen tissues, at the site of injection (now known as a positive tuberculin test). He believed, erroneously as it turned out, that tuberculin could be used to treat the disease as well as to indicate its presence. Koch described the disease in man, cattle (bovine tuberculosis), and birds (avian tuberculosis), expressing the belief that these were the result of different germs, the latter two not being infectious to man. In 1907, however, it was firmly established that bovine tuberculosis often spread to man, particularly to children who drank milk from diseased cattle. This knowledge led to the development of a successful campaign against bovine tuberculosis by pasteurization of milk and the establishment of disease-free herds.

In 1907 Clemens von Pirquet introduced the tuberculin scratch test that bears his name, and the next year Charles Mantoux introduced the intracutaneous tuberculin test that likewise bears his name. In time, these tests formed a preliminary step in case-finding, indicating as they do whether a person, or animal, has been infected by the tubercle bacilli, and hence whether examination or other tests should be performed to determine whether the disease is active or not, and if treatment is required.

Other important milestones in the earlier control of the disease were the discovery of the stethoscope by Rene Laennec, the x-ray by Conrad Roentgen, and a method of staining the bacilli by Paul Ehrlich so that they could be recognized under the microscope. The value of open-air treatment, with rest and fresh air, was established by Herman Brehmer and Peter Detweiler in Germany in 1876, and by E.L. Trudeau in the United States. Trudeau established a sanatorium at Saranac Lake, New York, in 1882, thus beginning the sanatorium era which was to last for over fifty years until the discovery of modern drugs. The first sanatorium in Canada was the Muskoka Hospital, established in 1897.

Dispensary treatment – first advocated by Sir Robert Philip in Edinburgh in 1887 – was an important step as it recognized the social implications of tuberculosis. Patients were isolated at home and instruction in such matters as the proper disposal of infected sputum was given by public health nurses to prevent the spread of disease to other members of the family.

The above facts provided the basis for the early campaign against tuberculosis, and indeed, except for the introduction of the Bacillus-Calmette-Guerin, or BCG, vaccine in 1924, there were few new advances until the great discovery by Dr Selman Waksman and his associates in 1944 of streptomycin, a specific drug for the tubercle bacillus. Streptomycin was the first of some ten drugs which were to appear over the course of twenty years, which were effective in treating tuberculosis, and which, in fact, made it possible to think of eliminating the disease entirely.

2

The Development of the
Canadian Tuberculosis Association

At the time of Confederation in 1867 recurring epidemics were the main problems of public health and tuberculosis was the greatest cause of death. Boards of health, both provincial and local, were gradually established to cope with the many health conditions. In Ontario, in 1882 Dr Peter Bryce was appointed secretary of the Provincial Board of Health and was not only active in establishing local boards but also shared with others a deep concern for the enormous problem of tuberculosis and advocated that something be done about it.

The beginnings of an organized effort to deal with the disease were made in Ontario in 1896, when Sir William Gage founded the National Sanitarium Association for the purpose of building sanatoria for the treatment of tuberculosis. Its first sanatorium, the Muskoka Cottage Hospital, which opened the following year, was a step in the right direction for sufferers from the disease, who previously had to seek sanatorium treatment outside the country. Two other organizations were formed in the next few years – the Toronto Association for the Prevention of Consumption and Other Forms of Tuberculosis in 1898, and the Ontario Association for the Prevention of Consumption and Other Forms of Tuberculosis in 1900* – but it soon became apparent to concerned individuals that in order to achieve success the attack would have to be made on a national level. Dr Peter Bryce, Dr E.J. Barrick, and the Reverend E.S. Eby, along with others who were interested, then took steps to organize the Canadian Association for the Prevention of Consumption and Other Forms of Tuberculosis.

On 13 September 1900, at the annual meeting of the Canadian Medical

---

* For further details on these and other local or provincial organizations, see the appropriate chapter in Part II.

Association in Ottawa, a provisional national association was set up by Mr W.C. Edwards (later Senator Edwards), Mr J.M. Courtney, Dr H. Beaumont Small, Dr F. Montizambert, Dr Thomas Roddick (later Sir Thomas), Sir James Grant, Sir George Perley, Professor J.W. Robertson, and Dr R.W. Powell. The organizing secretary, the Reverend E.S. Eby, conferred with the governor general, the Earl of Minto, who agreed to undertake the formal organization of the association.

At the next meeting, held in February 1901, which is considered to have been the first regular meeting of the association, a full executive committee was named and approved by His Excellency, the Governor General, Earl of Minto. The first president was Sir James Grant; the Reverend E.S. Eby was appointed 'lecturer and assistant'; and Dr E.J. Barrick, Dr R.W. Powell, Dr F. Montizambert, Dr A. Lafferty, Dr C.J. Fagan, the Honourable R.R. Dobell, Professor J.W. Robertson, W.C. Edwards, E.B. Eddy, and J.M. Courtney were officers. The governor general was not present at this meeting but approved the minutes on 23 March 1901. A full-scale meeting of the executive committee, with the governor general and the president, Sir James A. Grant, in attendance, was held in the office of the governor general on 17 – 18 April 1902. At this meeting the Reverend E.S. Eby was appointed secretary, to act under the authority of an advisory committee. He proceeded with the organization of the association, with much support from interested individuals throughout Canada.

The second general meeting of the Canadian Association for the Prevention of Tuberculosis, which the association was then called, was held in Ottawa on 17 April 1902. The Earl of Minto gave the introductory address: 'Today, we are met for the first time as an organized association – The Canadian Association for the Prevention of Tuberculosis – and I hope on each succeeding anniversary of this occasion our President may be able to lay before you not only a greater knowledge of the mysteries of the fell disease we are combatting, but increasing proofs year to year that its ravages are at last giving way before that knowledge of treatment and precaution which we owe to scientific research and discovery.'[1] This was an important meeting because a full slate of officers was appointed for 1902–3. The meeting received reports of those committees which had been set up at the meeting in 1901.

At first the association faced many difficulties. The membership was small, composed mainly of a few altruistic men and women scattered throughout an enormous territory, with few incentives and opportunities for meetings and meagre funds. The inertia to be overcome in the separate communities was great, and the force that could be used too small for any noticeable momentum; nevertheless, planning and the establishing of goals and objectives were begun.

The Reverend Dr William Moore, who had retired from the ministry, succeeded Mr Eby in 1903 as secretary, organizer, and lecturer, on a full-time basis, with a salary of $1000 per year plus remuneration for travelling expenses. He worked with energy and enthusiasm, directing his efforts to anti-spitting campaigns, lecturing, holding meetings, writing pamphlets, and organizing local associations. In a letter on 3 October 1903 to C.B. Edwards, City Clerk of London, Ontario, he remarked on the start of these efforts: 'I rejoice to know that your City has passed the anti-spitting by-law and trust it may result in abating the nuisance.'[2] Dr Moore proved a good man at this early stage in the life of the association, for to him we owe its emphasis on education and the initial definition of responsibilities.

During his first year in office Dr Moore, after attending a Presbyterian assembly in Vancouver, visited every major town on the Canadian Pacific Railway line between Victoria and Sault Ste Marie, giving lectures where possible and interviewing leading citizens with a view to enlisting their interest in the association's work; he also visited several cities and towns in eastern Canada. He covered the Maritime Provinces the following year. Travel was not easy in those days, and often Dr Moore was obliged to shorten his stay in some places because he felt he was trespassing on the hospitality of friends who put him up on his visits, as shortage of funds prevented him from many long stays in hotels.

In the report of the Education Committee to the fourth annual meeting and convention in 1904[3] Dr Moore emphasized that the association's work had to be largely educational, and that the success of any practical efforts depended on the thoroughness of the education of the people. He recommended that an annual grant from the federal government be requested to augment the monies already received from membership fees and individual subscriptions. He also recommended that a library be set up to collect books and pamphlets on tuberculosis, as well as copies of pertinent laws, vital statistics, reports of boards of health, etc., and relevant current medical journals, and that efforts be made to collect information regarding the status of similar work being done locally throughout the dominion and the results of research on bovine and human tuberculosis done at scientific laboratories.

Educational work consisted primarily of the holding of lectures and the distribution of leaflets. The first prepared by the association, *How Persons Suffering from Tuberculosis Can Avoid Giving the Disease to Others* and *Rules for Consumptives and Their Attendants*, were issued in 1904. A third leaflet issued that year, *How to Prevent Tuberculosis*, was produced in both English and French.

Financing the organization presented great problems in the early years. Typical concerns were reflected in a personal letter of Dr Moore to C.A. McMullan, 17 May 1904: 'It has been my custom to ask the collection after the lecture and to "pass the hat" for it. The amount received, though small, has generally been sufficient to pay for enough leaflets to supply the municipality. The leaflets and envelopes together cost about $3.50 per thousand. I fancy that it would take about three thousand to put one in every household in Brockville.'[4] However, great effort was expended in those early years as illustrated in another letter from Dr Moore dated 6 October 1904:

Since its organization the Association has put into circulation 1,250,000 pages of literature relating to the causes and prevention of tuberculosis, and lectures have been given by the secretary in about 75 towns. Provincial associations, and associations in cities and towns located in provinces where there is no general organization, are affiliated with the Canadian Association. The affiliated organizations include the Montreal League, the St. Francis District League, Toronto Anti-Consumption Association and the British Columbia Association for the Prevention and Treatment of Consumption.[5]

It was soon recognized that the federal government had an important role to play in the health of the nation, despite the provisions of the British North America Act, and it was petitioned in 1905 to take at the earliest moment the measures deemed best to render aid to the tuberculous and 'to take some active steps to lessen the widespread suffering and the great mortality among the people of Canada caused by the various forms of tuberculosis.'[6] Because of this action, a resolution was immediately passed by the House of Commons on Monday, 20 February 1905: 'That in the opinion of this House the time has arrived when Parliament should take some active steps to lessen the widespread suffering and the great mortality among the people of Canada, caused by the various forms of tuberculosis.' On 6 April of the same year a similar resolution was passed by the Senate which stated that in their opinion 'the time has come when the State should take some active steps to lessen the widespread suffering and the great mortality among the people of Canada, caused by the various forms of tuberculosis and that a conference between the Dominion and Provincial Governments should be held at the earliest possible moment in order that the best mode of action in the premises be adopted.'*

---

* The only tangible result of the resolution was an annual grant to the Canadian Association

The association realized the importance of these developments and took immediate action. A deputation waited on Sir Wilfrid Laurier regarding the establishment of sanatoria throughout the country. Another deputation waited on the Honourable F.W.G. Haultain, premier of the Northwest Territories, requesting his co-operation in securing the erection of sanatoria in each province and territory. He assured the deputation of his readiness to assist them.

Requests for help in organizing local associations started coming in from all across the country. The secretary of the Prince Edward Island association sent an urgent appeal for assistance in working towards the establishment of a sanatorium there. It is of interest that Dr Moore's subsequent trip to the Island cost the association $35.00. A few meetings, where the hat was passed around, were also arranged to help defray costs.

In summary, the main function of the early years was to arouse public interest and a sense of responsibility in government members. This was accomplished through personal visits, lectures, pamphlets, deputations, petitions, and conferences. The association became well established and its few workers were devoted individuals.

Dr George D. Porter succeeded Dr Moore as organizer and lecturer of the association in 1908, while Dr Moore continued in the post of secretary until 1910, when Dr Porter assumed that post as well. Dr Porter worked without remuneration during the first year, on the understanding that his expenses would not exceed $600. After 1 June 1909 he received the magnificent sum of $2000 per year as salary, as well as 'free transportation over the lines of the railway throughout Canada.'[7]

Looking back on his career in 1940, Dr Porter wrote: 'for my work the remarks of President Theodore Roosevelt gave me the key when he said: "This modern crusade against consumption brings with it hopes and bright prospects of recovery to hundreds and thousands, who, under the old teaching, were abandoned to despair." So, with Hope for a slogan, I spent the next thirteen years as ... secretary, travelling from coast to coast and doing what I could to arouse public interest in the prevention of tuberculosis.'[8] His philosophy was aptly summed up in a comment in his memoirs: 'One needs to keep his own fire burning if he means to kindle one in others, and that takes a lot of doing.'[9]

---

for the Prevention of Tuberculosis. Initially the grant was $2000 but it increased each year until it reached $25,000 in 1925. In 1931 and 1932 it was reduced by 10 per cent and it has remained at $20,250 ever since.

Dr Porter's first efforts were directed towards organizing local associations. The arrangements in the early years were made by Dr Moore, with whom he shared a close, amiable relationship. Wherever he went, Dr Porter always found willing hands. For example, Dr Moore received the following letter on 21 September 1909 from J.B. Black of Windsor, Nova Scotia, in regard to Dr Porter's arrangements: 'I will do my best to arrange for Dr. Porter's meetings at Windsor, Wolfville, Annapolis, Digby and Yarmouth ... For Antigonish and Cape Breton I would be of little help as I know scarcely a physician or clergyman east of Truro.'[10]

Dr Porter was easy-going and had a cordial way with people, which was often helpful in working through difficult situations, such as one described in his memoirs: 'Next I decided to try a one-man invasion of Berlin, later named Kitchener, and was allowed the use of the town hall for a meeting, but the mayor refused to act as chairman. After lunch I went to a shoe shine place and, as I sat there, the mayor came in for a shine of his too. So we got talking together and, before we left, he said he would act as my chairman.'[11]

Besides lecturing Dr Porter was active in the establishment of sanatoria, the opening of dispensaries, and increasing the number of visiting nurses. Under his leadership thirty-five new leagues were organized, and much space was given by numerous newspapers to the topic of tuberculosis. It was during his term of office that interest in the international tuberculosis scene began. In 1919 Dr J.G. Adami, then president of the association, was appointed by the executive council to represent the Canadian association on the international committee which had been set up by the International Congress on Tuberculosis at its meeting in Washington two years before. A close working relationship was also arranged with the Canadian Medical Association and with nurses' groups, which led to the development of a sense of partnership between the medical and voluntary groups.

By 1914 the association had a growing relationship with the tuberculosis associations in the United States and England, and there was much keenness in working together. The outbreak of World War I, however, curtailed some of the association's activities, but not the enthusiasm.

During the fourteen years Dr Porter served as executive secretary of the association he addressed over 450 meetings, organized seventy-five local societies, and arranged twelve annual conferences throughout the country; he also prepared various reports and wrote pamphlets and papers. In 1921 he retired from the association to become the first director of the University of Toronto Health Service. His gift of oratory and his facility for organizing the public and getting support from health personnel in federal, provincial, and municipal areas have never been equalled. The groundwork had been well and truly laid.

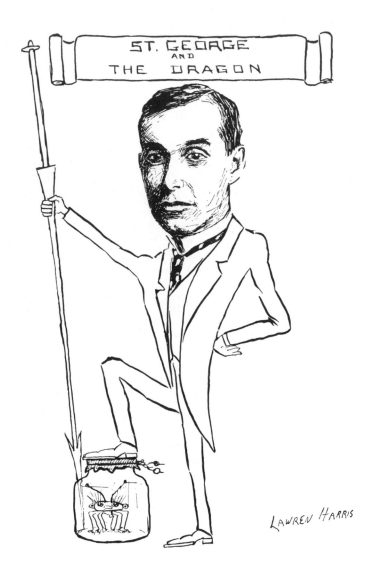

Dr Porter's crusade roused the enthusiasm of his friend, Lawren Harris, who made the above sketch in 1912. The young painter was later to become one of the famous Group of Seven which revolutionized Canadian art.

In July 1921 Dr Robert E. Wodehouse became the new executive secretary. The association was not new to him, however, for as early as 1913 he had begun co-operating with Dr Porter by organizing 'one grand tour across Ontario and bumper meetings in centres that would yield a good return,'[12] and engaging moving picture theatres where he hoped to attract more than the usual crowds.

Dr Wodehouse approached his new work with energy and enthusiasm. He immediately became acquainted with the international tuberculosis situation by attending the Third International Congress of the International Union against Tuberculosis in Brussels in 1922. One of his first projects was the publication of a periodical bulletin, aimed at professional workers and students in the hope that they might eventually take up the cause of eradicating tuberculosis. The *Bulletin* became a forum for literature on tuberculosis, as well as a source of reports on the numerous activities of the association.

Interest in professional education came to the fore at the annual meeting in Saint John in 1922, when the association recommended that the Canadian Association of Trained Nurses consider including three months' special tuberculosis training for student nurses before graduation. The Canadian Association of Trained Nurses passed a motion favouring this proposal the following June, which was then forwarded to all the training schools in Canada.[13]

A study was also made of medical training in tuberculosis. It was found that Dalhousie University gave lectures in the subject in the third, fourth, and fifth years; Laval University held clinics, gave lectures, and offered postgraduate work for both doctors and nurses; the University of Montreal had a chair of phthisiotherapy as well as clinics and lectures; students in the fifth year at Queen's University spent one afternoon a week at the Mowat Sanatorium; the University of Toronto, the University of Western Ontario and the University of Manitoba all gave clinics and lectures. In 1923 educational opportunities for residency in many sanatoria were arranged for medical undergraduates. By that year the association's educational program was costing $7500 a year, not including salaries and overhead, roughly one-quarter of the total budget.

Planning was beginning to be an important part of the development of the association's programs. In 1923 three committees were set up: one to prepare a conference in Ottawa for April of that year; another to investigate antituberculosis work among Canadian Indians; and the third to draw up recommendations for the administration of research work by the association. As a result of this planning, a serious look was taken at the local organizations and their effectiveness. It was true that many sanatoria owed their existence to the local organizations, but it was evident that few were still actively engaged in either sanatorium work or public education, and that some local associations existed in name only, were no longer an active force, and were in need of revival.

In May 1925 a subcommittee of the Canadian Tuberculosis Association (the name had been changed in 1923) drafted an outline for tuberculosis research in Canada. Seven points were listed: the tuberculosis problem, diagnosis, the vaccination question, chemotherapy and serotherapy, bacteriology and pathology, biochemistry of tuberculosis, and epidemiology. The association initiated two annual prizes of $250.00 each for work on a laboratory and a clinical subject. In October, at the first meeting of the National Research Council's Associate Committee on Tuberculosis Research,* Dr Wodehouse indicated that the twenty-eight sanatoria in Canada, representing an investment of $12,000,000, were extremely anxious to co-operate in any research work planned by the committee. Later the Council authorized an expenditure of $30,000 a year by the Associate Committee for tuberculosis research in the universities of Alberta, Toronto, Montreal, and Queen's, as well as at the London and Saskatchewan sanatoria. Five research projects were undertaken and three were submitted from the sanatoria for the two scholarships offered through the association.

Dr Wodehouse realized at the time of his appointment as executive secretary that the ordinary means of financing by memberships and donations were not sufficient for any sustained program. Though the grants solicited from various sources, such as the Canadian Red Cross and the provincial and federal governments, were helpful in the organization of demonstrations and *ad hoc* programs in all the provinces of Canada, support on a continuing basis was essential. He presented a convincing argument to the Life Insurance Officers' Association of the value of tuberculosis prevention and, with the strong support of such men as Mr E.E. Reid of the London Life, Mr V.R. Smith of the Confederation Life, and Mr T.B. MacAuley of the Sun Life of Canada, he was instrumental in having the Life Insurance Officers' Association set up a health committee with a special budget for health grants. This marked the entry of these companies into the health field in general. The tuberculosis problem was the first and the Canadian Tuberculosis Association the main beneficiary for some years. Over the years a total of nearly half a million dollars was contributed to tuberculosis work by

* For more information about this committee, see chapter 4.

the Canadian Life Insurance Officers' Association (see Table 1). These companies are still interested, but are now largely supporting other health programs.

The activities of the Canadian Tuberculosis Association during Dr Wodehouse's period of service were many: (a) x-ray surveys of school children in eight provinces were carried out with financial assistance from the Canadian Red Cross; (b) a committee was set up by the association and the Department of Indian Affairs for a study of Indian tuberculosis from which the Indian tuberculosis program developed, financed by the department; (c) a number of industrial surveys in Ontario were organized with the co-operation of the Provincial Bureau of Health and McGill University; (d) funds were provided for the first tuberculosis diagnosticians in the province of Quebec; (e) with funds from the Canadian Life Insurance Officers' Association the Maritime Tuberculosis Educational Committee with Dr G.J. Wherrett as director was set up, which instituted nursing and diagnostic services as well as an educational program; (f) the Prince Edward Island Department of Health was set up with financial assistance from the Life Insurance fund, the provincial branch of the Red Cross, and the provincial government; (g) a scholarship fund was organized with special funds from the Sun Life of Canada, which sent, for two months, thirty Canadian physicians active in tuberculosis work in Canada to the British Isles, France, Switzerland, and the International Union against Tuberculosis in Rome, which was followed by a return visit of thirty public health and tuberculosis physicians from the British Isles to all parts of Canada in 1930; (h) the Christmas Seal campaign was introduced into Canada in 1927 with the help of the National Tuberculosis Association of the United States, in the hope that it would eventually become the main financial source for the association.

Dr Wodehouse resigned in 1933 upon his appointment as federal deputy minister of pensions and health. His service to the tuberculosis cause during his period of twelve years as executive secretary was outstanding as it saw the beginning and development of an active program for diagnosis, treatment, and after-care in every province in Canada.

Dr George J. Wherrett was appointed to succeed Dr Wodehouse. His challenge at that time was to stimulate the tuberculosis control program in the provinces and to complete the organization of the Canadian Tuberculosis Association and its branches.

In the provinces the first task was to appoint full-time secretaries of the associations as well as other staff to carry out the program, which included case-finding, health education, and later rehabilitation, as well as to direct

TABLE 1

Special grants from the Canadian Life Insurance Officers' Association, the dominion government, the Red Cross, and the Sun Life Assurance Company, 1920–45*

Year	Revenue ($)	Expenditure ($)
1920	5,000 Red Cross 10,000 Dominion government	
1921	10,000 Dominion government	
1922	10,000 Dominion government 10,000 Red Cross	1,000 to each province for school survey
1923	15,000 Dominion government 10,000 Red Cross	3,000 grants to provincial surveys
1924	20,000 Dominion government 5,000 Red Cross 2,500 Sun Life Ass. Co.	5,000 Three Rivers Demonstration 2,500 Three Rivers Demonstration
1925	500 Red Cross 2,500 Sun Life Ass. Co.	2,500 Three Rivers Demonstration
1926	5,000 Dominion government 5,000 Red Cross 5,000 Sun Life Ass. Co.	9,500 Three Rivers Demonstration
1927	15,000 Can. Life Ins. Off. Ass. 5,000 Dominion government 10,000 Red Cross 5,000 Sun Life Ass. Co.	20,000 Three Rivers Demonstration
1928	1,000 Sun Life Ass. Co. 15,000 Can. Life Ins. Off. Ass.	1,000 Sun Life Scholarship 15,000 Maritime Tuberculosis Educational Committee
1929	5,000 Red Cross 15,000 Can. Life Ins. Off. Ass.	5,000 Three Rivers Demonstration 15,000 Maritime Tuberculosis Educational Committee
1930	18,000 Can. Life Ins. Off. Ass. 4,500 Sun Life Ins. Co.	18,000 Maritime Tuberculosis Educational Committee 2,500 Quebec diagnosticians 2,000 CTA printing
1931	2,500 Sun Life Ass. Co. 18,500 Can. Life Ins. Off. Ass.	2,500 Quebec diagnosticians 15,000 Maritime Tuberculosis Educational Committee 500 CTA general expenses
1932	18,000 Can. Life Ins. Off. Ass. 2,500 Sun Life Ass. Co.	18,000 Maritime Tuberculosis Educational Committee 2,500 CTA general expenses
1933	12,000 Can. Life Ins. Off. Ass.	12,000 PEI
1934	9,000 Can. Life Ins. Off. Ass.	9,000 PEI
1935	15,000 Can. Life Ins. Off. Ass.	15,000 PEI

TABLE 1 (continued)

Year	Revenue ($)	Expenditure ($)
1936	12,000 Can. Life Ins. Off. Ass.	12,000 PEI
1937	12,000 Can. Life Ins. Off. Ass.	12,000 PEI
1938	10,000 Can. Life Ins. Off. Ass.	5,000 PEI
		5,000 Quebec
1939	10,000 Can. Life Ins. Off. Ass.	10,000 Quebec
1940	10,000 Can. Life Ins. Off. Ass.	10,000 Quebec
1941	5,000 Can. Life Ins. Off. Ass.	5,000 Quebec
1942	5,000 Can. Life Ins. Off. Ass.	5,000 Quebec
1943	5,000 Can. Life Ins. Off. Ass.	5,000 Quebec
1944	7,500 Can. Life Ins. Off. Ass.	933.88 Alberta
		600.00 British Columbia
		2,000.00 Quebec
		321.37 Saskatchewan
		2,311.20 Pamphlets
		930.70 Film
		402.85 Staff education
1945	10,500 Can. Life Ins. Off. Ass.	2,466.12 Alberta
		1,200.00 British Columbia
		2,000.00 Ontario
		500.00 PEI
		2,000.00 Quebec
		300.00 Saskatchewan
		1,300.00 Pamphlets
		733.88 Staff education

* G.J. Wherrett, personal file, 1945

the very important Christmas Seal campaign throughout each province, the proceeds of which made all the other projects possible.

The reorganization of the Canadian Tuberculosis Association was a major activity. Miss Margaret Grier had been assistant executive secretary during the term of Dr Wodehouse and at the time she resigned in 1935 to accept a similar position with the St John's Ambulance Association, the demands and duties of the new programs were such that it was necessary to have a Seal sale director and an office manager. The association was fortunate in securing Miss Hazel A. Hart to fill the former position. She made an outstanding success of this operation in Canada, and won the complete cooperation of the Seal sale forces in the United States. She became well informed on all the newer methods of conducting the campaign. Miss Elizabeth Sutherland, who had been on the staff since 1927, was appointed office manager and held that position until she retired in 1972. Because of her ability and charisma she had the goodwill and confidence of all tuberculosis workers throughout Canada.

Miss Ann Grant was employed in 1943–5 as Seal sale director in the absence of Miss Hart, and became director of education on Miss Hart's return. She had an excellent background of teaching and newspaper experience and a degree of Master of Public Health from Ann Arbor. She wrote the booklet *Grist for the Teacher's Mill*, a complete report on the tuberculosis campaign in both national and international fields. This booklet is an outstanding contribution to health education, and was in its fifth edition and tenth reprinting by 1969. Following her service with the Canadian Tuberculosis Association Miss Grant served for three years with External Aid, Department of Public Health, at the University of the West Indies in Jamaica.

Meanwhile, the numbers of doctors and nurses engaged in tuberculosis work had increased tremendously. This was due to the staff required for the growing numbers of institutions and services. The association had grown in membership and a management committee, composed of doctors and laymen from the provincial associations, directed its affairs. This committee met twice a year and reported to the council at the annual meeting of the membership.

Because of the enlarged attendance at the annual meeting it became necessary to change the format to provide for meetings of special groups which formed sections within the association. The medical section, which was the first to be formed (in 1946), proved to be very useful and eventually became the Canadian Thoracic Society in 1958. The nursing section, formed in 1948, had become the largest section of all by 1954 and was of much interest to the nursing profession. The non-medical full-time staff of the various associations, and the board members, both national and provincial, also formed a section which became designated as 'the tuberculosis workers' section.' In 1960 a research committee was formed to stimulate research in respiratory diseases. This is now an important part of the program of the Canadian Tuberculosis and Respiratory Disease Association. All these activities of the association had become possible with the ever-increasing Christmas Seal sale (Table 2).

As the association and its work expanded, the function of the executive secretary became that of a consultant to the many institutions for case-finding and treatment and to the provincial health departments. Consultation services were also made available to federal departments, such as Health and Welfare, National Defence, and Veterans Affairs. Considerable

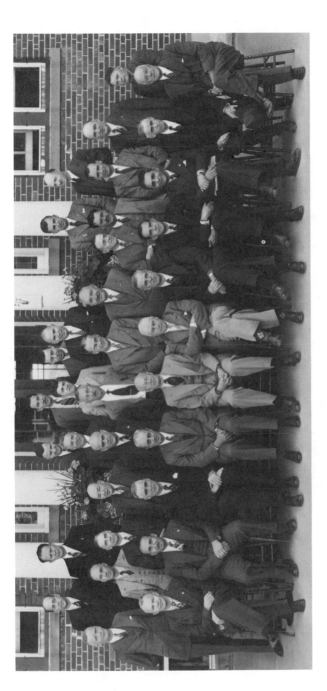

First meeting after World War II to reorganize the Medical Section of the Canadian Tuberculosis Association (later to be renamed the Canadian Thoracic Society), Calgary, 1946. *Front row:* Dr H.A. Doyle, Dr H. Meltzer, Dr R.G. Ferguson, Dr G.C. Brink, Dr A.H. Baker, Dr R.M. Bow, Dr G.J. Wherrett, Dr W.H. Hatfield, Dr M. Matas, Dr R.F. Stewart, Dr G.R. Johnson. *Second row:* Dr H.E. Burke, Dr L.M. Mullen, Dr H.C. Boughton, Dr J. Orr, Dr A.B. Simes, Dr W. Barr Murray, Dr G.F. Kincade, Dr W.S. Barclay, Dr A.M. Clark, Dr R.G. Huckell, Dr D.L. Scott, Dr C.C. Simpson, Dr J. Strauchler. *Third row:* Dr G.H. Hames, Dr A.C. Sinclair, Dr E.L. Ross, Dr P.E. Kozak, Dr J.D. Galbraith, Dr G.E. Miller, Dr H.H. Stephens. *Back row:* Dr J.W. Wright, Mr C.R. Dickey, Dr P. Schragge

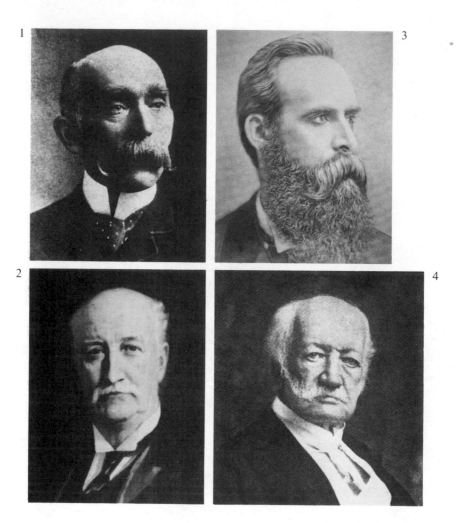

1 Dr Peter H. Bryce, secretary of the Ontario Board of Health 1882–1902, chief health officer for the Department of the Interior and Indian Affairs 1902–12, and promoter of the formation of a national association to combat tuberculosis

2 Sir William Gage, builder of the first sanatorium in Canada at Gravenhurst (1896), the Toronto Hospital at Weston (1904), and the Gage Institute in Toronto (1914)

3 The Reverend E.S. Eby, secretary and organizer of the Canadian Association for the Prevention of Tuberculosis, 1900–3

4 Sir James A. Grant, first president of the Canadian Association for the Prevention of Tuberculosis, 1901

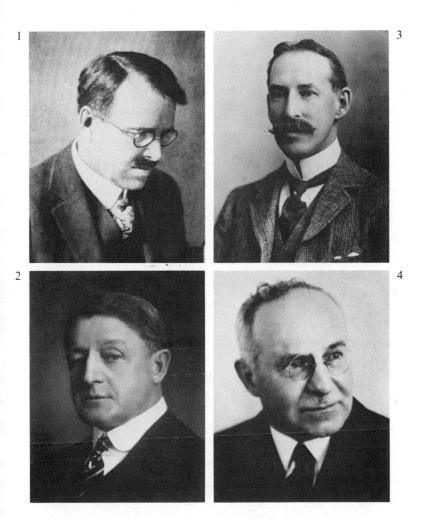

1 Dr David A. Stewart, medical superintendent of the Manitoba Sanatorium Board, 1910–37

2 Sir Adam Beck, organizer of the London Health Association and financer of the building of the Queen Alexandra Sanatorium in 1910

3 Colonel Jeffrey Burland, moving spirit in the Montreal League for the Prevention of Tuberculosis in 1902 and the Royal Edward Institute

4 Dr J. Arthur Jarry, medical superintendent of the Bruchesi Institute, Montreal, in 1912, and president of the Quebec Provincial Committee for the Prevention of Tuberculosis in 1937

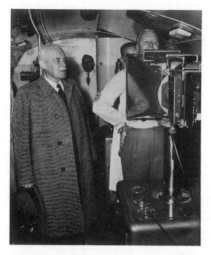

The Right Honourable Louis St Laurent, the prime minister of Canada, watches as the Honourable George Drew, leader of the Opposition, has his chest x-rayed during a survey in the early 1950s (Photo courtesy of Andrews-Newton Photographers, Ltd., Ottawa)

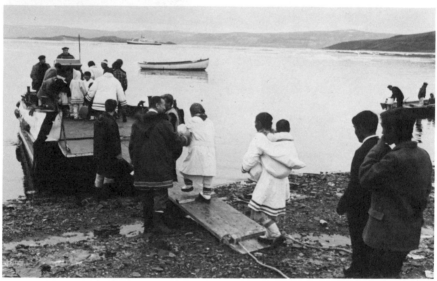

When the CGS *C.D. Howe* sailed north on the Eastern Arctic Patrol, doctors were aboard to bring medical services to the people of the settlements, including tests and x-rays for tuberculosis (Department of National Health and Welfare photograph)

TABLE 2
Canadian Christmas Seal Campaign returns, 1927–72*

Year	Returns ($)	Year	Returns ($)	Year	Returns ($)
1927	141,312.75	1943	577,252.00	1959	2,533,379.00
1928	196,914.05	1944	729,753.39	1960	2,519,132.00
1929	223,344.60	1945	912,293.00	1961	2,536.242.00
1930	232,222.86	1946	1,218,224.00	1962	2,601,278.00
1931	179,223.01	1947	1,397,396.00	1963	2,755,303.00
1932	146,250.20	1948	1,488,515.00	1964	2,784,036.00
1933	135,535.41	1949	1,427,374.00	1965	2,924,276.00
1934	152,721.01	1950	1,355,954.00	1966	2,878,296.00
1935	156,251.00	1951	1,646,253.00	1967	3,059,777.00
1936	171,391.20	1952	1,823,496.00	1968	3,198,423.00
1937	191,495.17	1953	1,945,884.00	1969	3,112,325.00
1938	197,122.35	1954	1,961,533.00	1970	3,251,872.00
1939	219,677.47	1955	2,110,940.00	1971	3,385,027.00
1940	273,940.23	1956	2,255,970.00	1972	3,702,551.00
1941	327,265.13	1957	2,437,249.00		
1942	431,179.28	1958	2,508,415.00		

* In CTA Records, PAC

time was given to problems of the Indian and Eskimo medical services and the Canadian Pension Commission. The Canadian Legion also requested advice on pension problems. The service given to these departments was appreciated, and their respect and confidence in the association were gratifying.

An important duty of the executive secretary was liaison with many other medical bodies, such as the Canadian Medical Association, the Canadian Public Health Association, and the Royal College of Physicians and Surgeons of Canada. This meant attendance at many meetings, but provided an opportunity to keep abreast of the ideas of modern medical thought in the field of tuberculosis control.

The international program also took a more prominent place in the executive secretary's activities, since he represented Canada on the International Union against Tuberculosis from 1948 to 1963. In addition, close association with the National Tuberculosis Association of the United States was maintained.

The Christmas Seal sale was of utmost importance (for the annual returns from the campaign, see Table 2). It financed the programs of the national, provincial, and local associations, particularly after 1945 when grants from the Canadian Life Insurance Officers' Association came to an end. These programs were mainly educational, using the term in its broadest sense. It also financed some tuberculosis clinic services and many of the mass survey campaigns which were carried out in Canada, until such programs were taken over by the provincial governments.

The coming of the new drugs in the treatment of tuberculosis drastically changed the whole medical approach to the disease. No longer were new facilities for treatment necessary, and case-finding methods were subjected to critical appraisal, particularly the mass survey program.

When Dr C.W.L. Jeanes succeeded Dr Wherrett as executive secretary in 1962, the program of the Canadian Tuberculosis Association had two outstanding problems. The first was the need to include all non-tuberculosis respiratory diseases, recognition of which led to the change in name from the Canadian Tuberculosis Association to the Canadian Tuberculosis and Respiratory Disease Association in 1969. The second was the need for greater involvement on the international level, as had become clear during the meeting of the International Union against Tuberculosis in Toronto in 1961. This, too, has received subsequent attention. Both Dr Jeanes and Mr E.J. O'Brien, executive director of the Ontario Tuberculosis Association, who had been prominent in organizing the Toronto meeting, have gone on to promote Canadian participation in projects in Africa and the Far East, and the association designated Mr O'Brien as consultant on the Far East program of the International Union against Tuberculosis in 1965.

With these changes in the program of the association have come further changes in the administrative structure. In 1962 an additional staff member, the executive director, was added to look after routine activities so that the former executive secretary, now known as the medical director, would be free to focus attention on the over-all direction of the association and the Canadian Thoracic Society, as well as on the research program. Increasing attention to the program of the International Union against Tuberculosis has also led to the involvement of the medical director as a consultant and advisor to the Director of External Aid of the Department of External Affairs.

In 1972 Dr Jeanes resigned as medical director to become full-time consultant with External Aid. He was succeeded by Dr J.J. Laurier, who resigned in 1974. Dr E.S. Hershfield was appointed medical director in 1975. Dr Hershfield is well qualified to direct the program of the association into the wider field of chest diseases. Trained in internal medicine, he has had wide experience in Manitoba in respiratory diseases, both as medical director of the tuberculosis program for the Sanatorium Board of Manitoba and later as director of the Respiratory Centre, Health Sciences Centre, Winnipeg. From 1967 he also served as a member of the management committee of the association and of the Canadian Thoracic Society.

3

Medical Care of the Tuberculous

DIAGNOSIS AND CASE-FINDING

Early diagnosis is of prime importance in the control of tuberculosis, but there are few symptoms in the early stages of the disease which would lead an infected person to seek medical help. For those people who paid regular visits to their physician, there was hope of detecting the problem soon enough to effect some control, but for people in the lower economic strata, many of whom did not have a regular physician, the situation was bleaker – and the disease was particularly prevalent in this group.

At the outset, the care of the tuberculous was in the hands of the general practitioner, who lacked the laboratory facilities and x-ray machines necessary for the diagnosis of the disease. To meet the situation, the tuberculosis dispensary came into being. First organized by Dr R.W. Philip (later Sir Robert) in Edinburgh in 1887, dispensaries soon occupied an important place in the tuberculosis program. Following the example of Edinburgh, dispensaries were set up in Canada, the first being the Royal Edward Institute in Montreal in 1909 and the Gage Institute in Toronto in 1914. Prior to this, as early as 1903, out-patient clinics had been set up in Toronto hospitals, which performed a similar service. Later, other cities also established regular tuberculosis clinics, usually in the out-patient departments of general hospitals.

In the beginning the clinics were supported as a rule by the voluntary tuberculosis association in the district and had the backing of the local health officer. Later, as local health departments grew in importance, many clinics were taken over by the official agency, although some continued to be supported by voluntary effort. Indeed, there was a regrettable tendency for voluntary associations to maintain the programs long after they should have been handed over to the official department in the best interest of good administration.

As individual clinics became fully equipped and able to carry out the functions required, case registers were set up, laboratory services added, and nursing and welfare services developed. All of these still form the background for a complete program for tuberculosis control, including diagnosis, treatment, and follow-up of ex-patients and contacts.

The next stage was the development of some form of travelling clinic to serve areas that were distant from established clinics. The first such clinic was organized in Ontario in 1923, and it was not long before they became general in all the provinces. Promotion of the travelling clinic became an important project of the Canadian Tuberculosis Association, which provided assistance in the form of grants, equipment, and demonstrations. At first, attendance at the clinics was confined for the most part to suspects, contacts, and patients referred by doctors and did not include the presumably healthy population. The service provided valuable assistance to the general practitioner in diagnosis.

Gradually, the concept was developed that if an examination of apparently well people or those apparently not so healthy was carried out the disease could often be recognized in earlier stages, particularly by the use of x-rays. With this as a guiding principle x-ray surveys of various groups of the population were organized and developed. Among the first to be surveyed in Canada were nurses, teachers and students in schools and universities, military recruits, teachers in training, and persons subject to occupational hazards, such as hard rock miners. Community surveys later became general in all provinces, with certain groups, such as the Indians and Eskimos, receiving particular attention. The surveys were mainly on a voluntary basis in Canada, but the movement received such acceptance that in some countries, such as Australia, periodic x-rays became compulsory. The surveys in Canada became an important function of local and provincial tuberculosis associations, who bought equipment and employed personnel to organize community participation using funds derived from the Christmas Seal sale. In some instances they were most successful, achieving a community participation of close to 95 per cent, but the participation could be as low as 40 per cent.

In order of historical development, the surveys of apparently well people which have been carried out are as follows:

1 / *School children* In 1922 the Canadian Tuberculosis Association, using funds from the Canadian Red Cross Society, instituted surveys of representative school children in each province, which were conducted over the course of the next few years.

2 / *Industrial groups* The routine survey of hard rock miners was introduced in Ontario in 1922 by Dr J.G. Cunningham, director of the Division of Industrial Hygiene. This formed the basis of the program for prevention of tuberculosis and silicosis among miners in Canada.

3 / *University students* Beginning with Mount Allison University in New Brunswick in 1925, the surveying of students became a general practice in most universities in Canada. Examination included the tuberculin test and x-ray, the latter usually taken by a portable machine using a full-sized film.

4 / *Indians and Eskimos* Indian groups were examined in British Columbia in 1925, and travelling clinics were used to examine Indian bands in Manitoba, Saskatchewan, and Alberta from the late 1920s. After World War II the surveys were intensified in major case-finding programs among Indians and Eskimos; these included the periodic x-ray of the Eskimo population at clinics transported by sea and air, beginning in 1946. These periodic examinations have been invaluable in the diagnosis and treatment of the disease in this highly infected group.

5 / *Nurses in training, medical students, normal school students, and teachers* These groups were gradually added to the diagnostic services and became a valuable part of the early preventive program.

6 / *Community surveys* The next major project was a full community survey undertaken in Saskatchewan in the town of Melville in 1941, when the entire population was covered. Similar programs followed in other provinces.

7 / *World War II recruits* Perhaps the greatest single case-finding project was the x-ray examination of recruits for World War II introduced in 1939 by the Department of National Defence at the suggestion of the Canadian Tuberculosis Association. Later, x-ray examinations were extended to cover those discharged from the armed forces as well. In all, some three million x-rays were taken for the three services. Of the recruits, about 1 per cent were rejected because of evidence of tuberculosis, and in approximately one-third of these the disease was active.

8 / *Hospital admissions* A routine chest x-ray on admission to general hospitals was instituted in 1950. This proved to be a valuable procedure, as previously undiagnosed cases of tuberculosis were found among people who were being admitted for other reasons. In 1965, the total x-rayed reached 825,000.

9 / *Other institutions* Other groups, such as patients in mental and convalescent hospitals, and inmates of gaols and correctional institutions, have been included in the program.

10 / *Immigrants* Examination of immigrants before admission to Canada became an established procedure by 1947.

All the above extensive case-finding programs proved to be very valuable, particularly since they were being carried out most effectively at the particular time when drugs for the successful treatment of tuberculosis came into general use. It proved possible to treat and render non-infectious many more open infectious cases than could otherwise have been done. The community surveys also had a beneficial educational side-effect in making the population at large 'tuberculosis conscious.' With such comprehensive case-finding services (see Table 3 for the extent of their coverage) there was no reason why tuberculosis should escape detection.

The value of such extensive surveys, except among certain groups, is much reduced today because the number of newly discovered cases is so low that the expense is not justified. For the same amount of money one can maintain permanent clinics for the supervision and treatment of all known cases and contacts, and provide prompt examination of everyone suspected of having the disease.

TREATMENT SERVICES

Early efforts at treatment were little more than an attempt to relieve symptoms such as cough, expectoration, and haemorrhage, and pain when pleurisy was present, and to improve the appetite with dietary adjuvants such as cod liver oil and tonics. Those sufferers who were financially able to do so were advised to seek a warmer and drier climate. The classical picture of the consumptive is portrayed by Keats in his 'Ode to a Nightingale.' In superb poetry he describes the feelings of the far advanced patient and his wanderings in search of a southern climate. Frustration and despair are evident, too, in the poignant epitaph on his tomb in the Protestant cemetery in Rome: 'Here lies one whose name is writ in water.' The wanderings of Robert Louis Stevenson in his search for health is another example.

In Canada, many were advised to go to the dry belt of British Columbia or to Alberta. It was the accumulation of consumptives in these areas that accounted for the development of the Tranquille Sanatorium near Kamloops in 1908. It is now considered questionable whether any actual benefit derived from the choice of a dry climate. Indeed, it is felt that patients would have been better off at home in congenial surroundings rather than living, and in many cases dying, in exile. In a paper given in 1925, Dr A.D. Lapp[1] analysed the conditions of those treated in the dry belt in British Columbia and summed up his opinion thus: 'It is the tale of blasted hopes, told by these disappointed people, that is largely responsible for adding numbers to the ranks of those who maintain that climate is not even a minor factor in the treatment of tuberculosis.'

TABLE 3
Tuberculosis examinations in Canada, 1944–65

	Examination by clinics and dispensaries*			Examination by x-ray surveys†				x-ray of general hospital admissions		
Year	Canada	Cases detected†	Rate per 1,000 examinations	Canada	Rate per 1,000 population	Cases discovered	Rate per 1,000 examinations	Canada	Cases discovered	Rate per 1,000 examinations
1944	314,618			439,610	36.8					
1945	432,767			526,413	43.6					
1946	444,739			1,027,221	83.6					
1947	538,033			1,465,666	116.8					
1948	522,882			1,613,496	125.8					
1949	545,904			1,745,546	129.8					
1950	514,579			1,888,145	137.7			306,347		
1951	542,112			2,039,064	145.6			439,192		
1952	582,371			1,932,700	133.7			489,824		
1953	611,685			1,928,403	129.9			559,606		
1954	590,551	59,700	101.1	1,992,519	130.3	13,694	6.9	632,864	4,865	7.7
1955	628,947	75,275	119.7	1,752,298	111.7	12,345	7.0	686,324	4,598	6.7
1956	505,243	77,370	153.1	1,817,318	113.0	15,005	8.3	710,586	4,716	6.6
1957	658,352	73,764	112.0	1,785,282	107.5	16,616	9.3	749,707	4,676	6.2
1958	563,079	64,084	113.8	1,494,333	87.5	14,854	9.9	637,838	4,219	6.1
1959	548,976	57,138	104.1	1,483,164	84.8	14,206	9.6	586,251	4,548	7.8
1960	543,275	59,720	109.9	1,594,532	89.3	15,223	9.5	524,062	3,994	7.6
1961	558,966	65,119	116.5	1,770,208	97.1	12,042	6.8	562,397	5,159	9.2
1962	507,394	63,681	125.5	1,670,011	92.2	12,026	7.2	571,901	4,825	8.6
1963	377,360	60,033	159.1	1,060,580	79.0	18,986	17.9	559,770	6,516	11.6
1964	727,264	74,970	103.1	1,550,237	80.6	20,632	13.3	559,804	6,808	12.3
1965	663,403	82,613	124.5	1,484,562	75.9	14,584	9.8	825,109	8,591	17.3

* Includes Newfoundland general hospital x-rays on admission

† Includes old cases, regardless of activity

SOURCE: *Tuberculosis Statistics* (Ottawa: Institutional Branch, Statistics Canada, 1965)

In most instances the patient remained at home, nursed by relatives during the final stages of illness and, in too many instances, infecting other members of the family or nursing attendants. The introduction of home nursing services and dispensaries, following the pioneer ones of Sir Robert Philip in Edinburgh and Dr Joseph Pratt in Boston, brought some order to the situation of untreated tuberculosis in the homes and slums of the cities. Too frequently in our own country the dying tuberculosis patient was left in the home. This was particularly so among the Indian population between 1870 and 1890, when it appeared that the race would be decimated by two diseases, smallpox and tuberculosis.

In this situation of despair, the advent of the sanatorium offered some hope. The sanatorium organized by Dr E.L. Trudeau at Saranac Lake, New York, in 1884, and the one in Canada at Muskoka, organized by the National Sanitarium Association in 1896, were beacons in the darkness. They demonstrated the value of rest, fresh air, and good nutrition in arresting the disease in some instances, and stimulated interest in creating similar conditions for the thousands who were unable to find such havens.

The sanatorium occupied a unique place in the tuberculosis program in North America and Western Europe, and nowhere was it as well developed as in Canada and the Netherlands – countries that were eminently successful in the control of the disease. At one stage in the program it was thought that enough sanatoria could be developed in Canada to treat every case of tuberculosis. This actually happened in Saskatchewan, Manitoba, and Alberta, but in the other provinces it was not until the drug era that there was a sufficient number of treatment beds.

There are many reasons why the sanatorium became the focal point in the campaign. The development of the sanatorium concept by Trudeau at Saranac Lake was well publicized. This had a profound effect on the early pioneers in Canada, many of whom had been treated there and had become imbued with the crusading spirit of Trudeau and his disciples Lawarson Brown, Fred Heise, and Hugh Kinghorn. Such men as Charles Parfitt, D.A. Stewart, Fred Miller, H.A. Farris, R.J. Collins, Roderick Byers, and A.H. Baker, together with outstanding surgeons such as Edward Archibald and later Norman Bethune, returned to Canada as keen disciples; most of them developed sanatoria of their own, and were outspoken in their opinion that the sanatorium was the ideal situation in which to treat tuberculosis. The institutions were directed and developed by this group of physicians, who gathered around them a number of important laymen who constituted the boards of directors for the sanatoria. They also greatly influenced health departments and politicians, who supplied ever-increasing budgets to pay for the operation of these services.

The members of the medical staff in those days were often former tuberculosis patients who had recovered after sanatorium treatment and had learned the value of the sanatorium routine. These men were an example to their patients and encouraged many to persist until the disease was arrested.

One of the great success stories of sanatorium treatment and rehabilitation is that of Dr D. MacDougall King. The tale of his recovery from far-advanced tuberculosis is told vividly by his brother, the Rt. Hon. W.L. Mackenzie King, in the introduction to Dr King's second book, *Nerves and Personal Power*.[2] Dr King's first book, *The Battle with Tuberculosis and How to Win It*,[3] written during his convalescence, was one of the best publications presented from the standpoint of the patient and was widely read by patients everywhere. It was ironic that after successfully overcoming his fight against tuberculosis and returning to medical practice, Dr King developed muscular dystrophy, which proved fatal. His second book was written for the encouragement of those who can rise above a hopeless prognosis and still make a contribution to assist others similarly afflicted.

During the long, trying period which many spent in sanatoria without signs of improvement, feelings of discouragement and despair were not uncommon. It was no easy task for the medical and nursing staff to keep alive the spirit and the will to persist in a sanatorium routine that could, and usually did, become tedious and hard to bear. Fortunate, indeed, were those institutions that provided moral support and made good use of all their facilities for entertainment, as well as diversionary and educational means of passing the time, in order to help make sanatorium life bearable if not even pleasant. Some patients were loathe to leave these places of refuge for they had neither the same facilities in the outside world nor the resources to sustain themselves. It is hard now to realize the months and years that patients spent in these institutions. The marvel is that so many of them stayed the course until success was achieved. The depressing thing was that for many the treatment facilities were not available, or they actually refused to accept the routine and left against advice, to die in their own homes.

Over the years new techniques were added to sanatorium treatment. The first was 'pneumothorax' or collapsing of the lung. If the lung movement could be controlled the lesion healed more readily, just as does a broken bone when splinted. This control could be brought about by injecting air into the pleural space, thus collapsing the lung and putting it at rest; air refills had to be given at certain intervals. The use of this procedure became general, although it was not suitable for all patients. For instance if adhesions had developed between the lung and the chest wall or if the disease was advanced in both lungs it was not desirable to carry it out.

Other surgical procedures also became available for reduction of the pleural space. A resection of portions of the ribs could be done so as to reduce the size of the chest cavity and thus collapse the lung. The diaphragm could be paralysed by cutting or injecting the phrenic nerve supplying it, thus enabling it to rise and thereby reduce the pleural space. Although these devices were helpful in some patients, they were not adaptable to even the majority of them.

The movement to secure sanatorium accommodation for all tuberculosis patients was a tremendous task, and the degree to which the objective was attained is remarkable. Looking back on the results achieved in curing or arresting the disease during the pre-drug treatment era, one can marvel at how many recovered, though, in the final analysis, failures outweighed successes. An analysis of the 2519 tuberculosis patients treated in Saskatchewan between 1917 and 1929 showed that although 488, or 19.37 per cent, died in the sanatorium upon first admission, of the remaining 2031 patients discharged alive, one-half could be listed as 'well and working' and the other half as 'apparently cured,' 'apparently arrested,' or 'arrested,' and only slightly more than 10 per cent of the latter had relapsed one to thirteen years after their discharge.[4]

Apart from the recovery of many after sanatorium treatment, a great benefit was derived from the isolation of the infectious from their families who might otherwise have spread the disease had they remained at home.

The extent to which sanatorium treatment became available in Canada is well set out in the reports of the Dominion Bureau of Statistics from 1937 to 1971. Comparative tables show how the total number in sanatoria reached the figure of 17,364 in 1953, the peak year, which was just before the effect of the new drugs began to be felt.

As the number of sanatoria and sanatorium beds increased most patients were treated in sanatoria. The length of treatment was prolonged, varying from six months to two years, the highest being among the Eskimos from the Arctic, who were kept in institutions for their entire period of treatment until, of course, domiciliary drug treatment became practical in the Arctic.

In the development of sanatoria in Canada several phases were evident. The first institutions were built on the pattern of Dr Trudeau's sanatorium at Saranac Lake in the Adirondack Mountains of New York state. They were generally far removed from urban centres, since it was argued that the advantages of isolation included purer air and better rest for patients, who were undisturbed by the attractions of the cities, and that patients would learn to accommodate themselves to the lack of visitors resulting from their remoteness. These institutions usually developed a social life of their own, and many patients found it easier to take treatment in company of other patients. However, the disadvantages, such as lack of contact with loved ones, often outweighed the benefits.

The first such institutions included the Muskoka Sanatorium in Ontario, opened in 1897; the Kentville Sanatorium in Nova Scotia (1904); the Mountain Sanatorium in Hamilton (1910); the Tranquille Sanatorium in British Columbia (1908); the Ninette Sanatorium in Manitoba (1910); the Beck Sanatorium in London (1910); the Lake Edward Sanatorium near Quebec City (1911); the Jordan Memorial Sanatorium in New Brunswick (1913); the short-lived Dalton Sanatorium in Charlottetown, PEI (1916); the Fort Qu'Appelle Sanatorium in Saskatchewan (1917); the Three Rivers Sanatorium (1923); the Laurentian Sanatorium at Ste Agathe, Quebec (1925); the St John's Sanatorium at Top Sail Road, in Newfoundland, when Newfoundland was still an independent dominion in 1917. Rather late in the development of sanatoria others were built in remote areas (1938–50), such as those at Noranda, Mont Joli, Gaspé, Roberval, and Dorchester in the province of Quebec, and at Ste Basile and Bathurst in New Brunswick.

With regard to the location of sanatoria, the philosophy gradually developed that, by establishing these institutions nearer to the centres of population, they would be more convenient for the patients and their families, and it would be easier to obtain staff and consultation services from near-by general hospitals. The importance of obtaining necessary supplies easily was another incentive. Examples of conveniently located institutions in Ontario would be the Royal Ottawa Sanatorium, the St Catharines Sanatorium, the Freeport Sanatorium, the Brant Sanatorium, the Essex County Sanatorium at Windsor, the Cornwall Sanatorium, the Sudbury Sanatorium, and the Fort William Sanatorium. In other provices there were the St Boniface Sanatorium in Manitoba, the Prince Albert and Saskatoon sanatoria in Saskatchewan, the Pearson Sanatorium in Vancouver, and the tuberculosis units in Victoria.

The modern concept of treatment of tuberculosis is that it should be in the environment of a general hospital. The tuberculosis institutions in Saint John, Montreal, Quebec City, Sherbrooke, and Hull, the Willow Chest Centre in Vancouver, the D.A. Stewart Chest Centre in Winnipeg, and the Aberhart Hospital in Edmonton fall into this category.

In addition to the above institutions there were a number of others which were acquired or built by the Indian and Eskimo services of the Department of National Health and Welfare. The Indian hospitals at Fort Qu'Appelle, Moose Factory, and Frobisher Bay were built by the department. Some were buildings converted from other purposes, such as schools at Sardis, BC, and Selkirk, Man. Others were acquired from the Department of National Defence at the end of World War II. These included hospitals at Nanaimo and Prince Rupert in British Columbia, North Battleford in Saskatchewan, Brandon and Clearwater in Manitoba, and the Charles Camsell in Edmonton. Other hospitals were acquired by the provincial services in St Hyacinthe, Quebec; Sussex and Moncton in New Brunswick; and Shelburne and Point Gray in Nova Scotia. In Newfoundland, the Naval Hospital in St John's was acquired by the near-by St John's Sanatorium, and was a useful addition.

The story of the rise and fall in the number of beds available in Canada for the treatment of tuberculosis is told in the annual reports, *Tuberculosis Statistics*, compiled by the Institutional Branch of the Bureau of Statistics. Until 1965 the reports published the clinical records of patients admitted and discharged, the drugs used year by year, and the surgical treatments carried out. They were of great value to the people who played such an important part in the program for tuberculosis control: provincial directors of tuberculosis control, sanatorium superintendents, and clinicians interested in the effectiveness of the services provided by the institutions.

With the advent of drug therapy after 1950, there was a drastic reduction in the need for and the use of surgical procedures such as pneumothorax, phrenic nerve interruption, lung collapse by thoracoplasty, and lung resection. After 1965 domiciliary drug therapy became the order of the day, and patients were discharged for home treatment as soon as they lost their infectivity. In consequence, during the past twenty years, there has been a quiet revolution, characterized by curtailment of the use of sanatoria and tuberculosis hospitals, which can be truly described as the 'miracle of the empty beds.' For proof one need only compare the figures for 1953 and 1971 given in Table 4.

The construction of sanatoria depended on what financial help was available. It was first undertaken by laymen on the suggestion of physicians and health officers, and some outstanding institutions were built. Often grants came from the cities in which sanatoria were located, and later from the provinces. During the two world wars assistance was provided by the federal government in the way of hospitals for veterans, many of which were later converted to use as sanatoria, mainly for Indians. Institutions for Eskimos were almost totally built from federal funds. The Federal Health Grants of 1948 included funds to assist in the building of sanatoria.

Cost was perhaps the greatest problem in the treatment of the disease. In the early days paying the cost of sanatorium care was the responsibility of the patient, and there was no over-all scheme to assist those who were un-

TABLE 4

Number of patients in institutions, 1953 and 1971

	1953	1971
Canada	17,364	1,894
Newfoundland	766	66
Prince Edward Island	132	5
Nova Scotia	922	117
New Brunswick	844	58
Quebec	5,506	670
Ontario	4,361	417
Manitoba	1,125	98
Saskatchewan	814	85
Alberta	1,044	214
British Columbia	1,467	125
Northwest Territories	384	37

able to pay. Support did come, however, from charitable organizations such as the IODE or the Every Woman's Fund of Saskatchewan. Later urban and rural municipal pools were set up for the purpose, until complete free treatment of tuberculosis was instituted on a provincial basis. Saskatchewan was the first to do so in 1929, followed by Alberta in 1936. Manitoba and Ontario partially followed suit at the same time, and British Columbia and Quebec liberalized their municipal and provincial assistance programs during the 1930s. Immediately after World War II, New Brunswick and Nova Scotia adopted free treatment. In 1948, under the program of Federal Health Grants, four million dollars were made available to the provinces for tuberculosis work. One of the conditions was that free treatment be progressively adopted by each province that received the grant, which also made available the newer drugs for all patients. All provinces have free treatment now.

In the early days, financial assistance for the poor and indigent and for everyone who found the cost of treatment beyond their means was a perpetual problem, not only for the patient but also for his or her family. The local authorities were responsible for the treatment of indigents but, often lacking sufficient funds, they would question the exact meaning of the term. Would a person need to dispose of all assets before he could be considered worthy of assistance? An important judgment was made by Judge Lamont in the Saskatchewan Supreme Court, which stated that a person was indigent when unable to provide that for which he was in need.

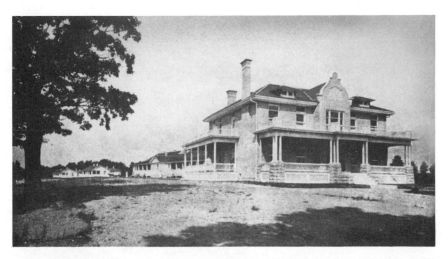

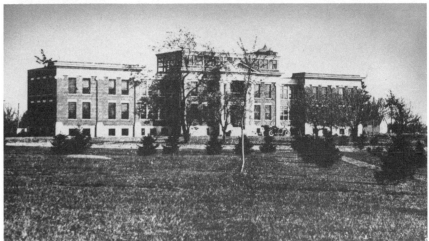

TOP Queen Alexandra Sanatorium, London, Ontario

BOTTOM The Queen Mary Hospital for Tuberculous Children, Weston, Ontario, erected by the National Sanitarium Association, 1913

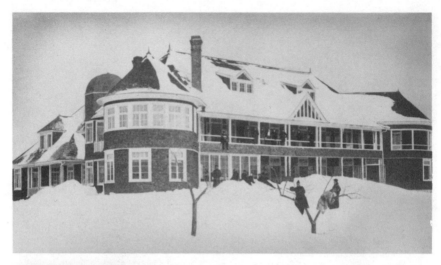

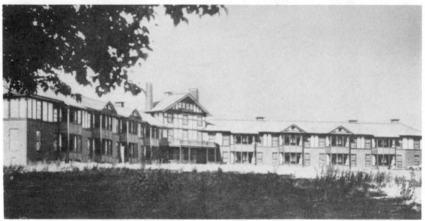

TOP Kentville Sanatorium, Nova Scotia
BOTTOM King Edward Sanatorium, Tranquille, British Columbia

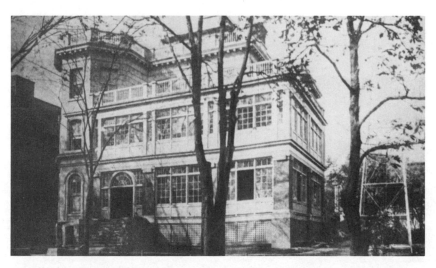

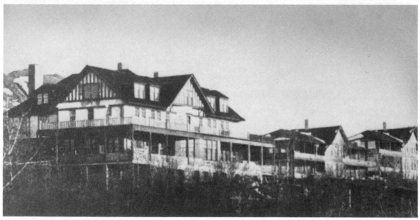

TOP Royal Edward Institute, Montreal
BOTTOM Ninette Sanatorium, Manitoba

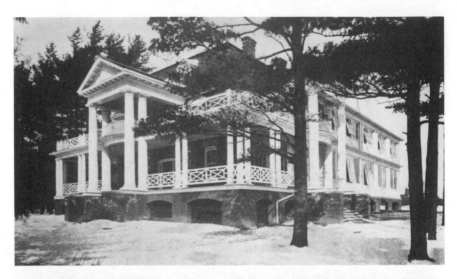

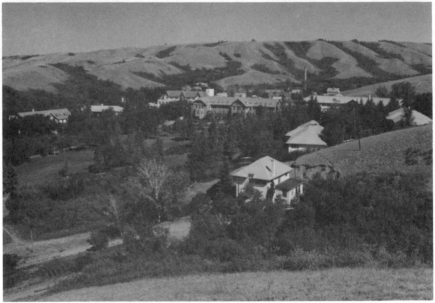

TOP Imperial Order of the Daughters of the Empire Preventorium, Toronto

BOTTOM Fort Qu'Appelle Sanatorium, Saskatchewan (Saskatchewan Government Photograph)

Institutions were operated at extremely low per capita cost in comparison with general hospitals. Although it might seem that prolonged institutional treatment was an expensive way of attacking the problem, the costs in the earlier years were not beyond the reach of western countries.

The coming of free hospitalization and medicare has profoundly affected the cost of institutional treatment of tuberculosis. Today the disease is mainly treated in special wards of general hospitals where costs are comparable to other wards, staff are on union rates of pay, and medical services are paid under the prevailing standard fee schedules and not often provided by full-time physicians on a lower salary schedule as was true in earlier years. All this has been of benefit to staff, but has increased the cost to the taxpayer, who must bear the ever-increasing burden of medical costs.

Perhaps there is a lesson to be learned by hospital administrators in their search for means to stem the ever-rising tide of hospital and medical costs. Sanatorium boards and medical directors early recognized the value of auxiliary nursing services. The routine treatment of tuberculosis – even in patients requiring surgery – could be carried on with a minimal number of graduate nurses and trained nurses' assistants. In such departments as radiology, the main burden was carried by the regular medical staff who were proficient in the reading of chest films and were usually as proficient as the trained radiologist. The training of a doctor in radiology was required for films of other conditions. In 1965, the year when the case-finding agencies x-rayed the greatest number of persons – nearly three million – most of the interpretation was done by regular tuberculosis medical staff. It can be estimated that the same service would have cost at least $15,000,000 if a radiologist had been employed at standard fees.

For the complete story of sanatorium financing one can consult the annual reports of the Bureau of Statistics (Statistics Canada), *Tuberculosis Statistics*. They show all phases of treatment from 1937 to 1965, when the institutions began to decrease in size rapidly and the information became irrelevant. The reports also show that at pre-inflation prices the cost of sanatorium treatment reached a peak of $33,000,000 for Canada as a whole before the newer drugs became effective and domiciliary care became a practical possibility. One shudders to think what would have been the situation if the new drugs had not suddenly come upon the scene.

THE COMING OF THE NEW DRUGS – A MODERN MIRACLE

One theme that appears continuously throughout the history of medicine is the search for methods of treatment that would cure without risk of further damage to the patient. If the cause of the illness was unknown such measures had to be directed to relief of symptoms, perhaps the removal of diseased organs, and general support and strengthening of the patient in his combat for survival. No disease demonstrated the desperation of this battle better than tuberculosis, which attacked young adults in the prime of life and destroyed them.

It is difficult to realize now that the cause of tuberculosis was unknown until 1882, when Robert Koch discovered the tubercle bacillus and proved that it was present in patients with tuberculosis could be transmitted to others, and could then cause disease anew in an unfortunate contact. Up until then consumption was considered a consequence of a variety of causes – heredity, evil spirits, odours from foul sewage or swamp lands, vapours and corruption within the body – including possibly germ infection. Treatment included hypnosis, in addition to the purging, blood-letting, and other desperate measures still used in the nineteenth century.

Once Koch's great discovery was believed, the search began for a drug that would destroy the germ without harming the patient. Of the many substances tried, from umkalabo, the bark of an African tree, to gold itself, none proved to have the ability to kill, inhibit, or even delay the growth of the bacillus. Indeed, even when the era of chemical therapy dawned with the use of arsenicals, prontosil, the sulpha drugs, and penicillin, the wax-coated bacillus remained invulnerable.

In 1944 Professor Selman A. Waksman made the discovery for which so many thousands of patients and doctors had been waiting: from a soil fungus, *Streptomyces griseus*, he isolated a substance, which he called streptomycin, that was bacteriocidal for the tubercle bacillus. The impact made by this discovery, its effect upon the whole management of tuberculosis control, and its encouragement to tuberculosis workers throughout the world were fantastic, especially in Canada where streptomycin soon became available for clinical trials. This was the first drug with a definite curative effect on tuberculosis; for the first time physicians were able to watch the clearing of x-ray shadows of advanced disease, and even the arrest of meningeal tuberculosis, which until then had been 100 per cent fatal.

Thus the era of chemotherapy for tuberculosis began; within a decade a dozen different drugs had been developed and recommended for treatment. All the previous advances made in early diagnosis and treatment services, including sanatoria and surgical facilities, were insignificant compared with the rapid advance now made. Credit must be given to the medical research centres and pharmaceutical firms throughout the world for immediately turning their energies to developing this new possibility.

The development of suitable programs of chemotherapy was not without difficulties, for in the early stages there was no way to estimate correct dosage. One of the most serious toxic effects of streptomycin is damage to the VIIIth cranial nerve, causing dizziness, loss of balance, and deafness. At first, most patients who showed improvement were severely disabled by these effects, which were particularly prevalent in children treated for miliary or meningeal tuberculosis. Initially, a daily adult dose of 3 grams of streptomycin was used, but this was subsequently reduced to 1 gram with almost complete elimination of the toxic symptoms.

Development of bacterial resistance to the drug was a more serious complication, one that had also been noted with other antibiotics, such as penicillin, and which is due to the survival and multiplication of some strains of bacillus. In such patients, not only would treatment become ineffective before the disease was cured, but there was also the risk of infecting other people with a resistant organism against which the drug would again be ineffective. Fortunately, the remedy for this was soon found. If two or more drugs were used in combination for an adequate period of time, resistance did not develop and in due course the disease was arrested. Two such effective supplementary drugs were rapidly discovered: first para-amino-salicylic acid (PAS) in 1946 and then isonicotinic hydrazide (INH) in 1952. These two drugs, along with streptomycin, soon formed the basic regime of chemotherapy, as they continued to do for twenty years. Indeed, they are still widely and successfully used in Canada, and more particularly in developing countries where economy, as well as effectiveness, is a vital factor.

The three drugs act in different ways: streptomycin and INH are bacteriocidal (that is, they destroy the germ) whereas PAS is only bacteriostatic (that is, it inhibits the growth of the germ but does not necessarily destroy it).

During the 1950s and 1960s at least a dozen other drugs were tested and found to have some beneficial effect; among these pyrazinamide, ethambutol, ethionamide, and kanamycin probably found the most supporters. In some European countries, notably Holland, blockbuster regimes using six or seven drugs at a time were in favour, especially for chronic advanced disease. On the whole, the original three drugs, used in regimes lasting for eighteen to twenty-four months, were preferred in Canada; the results of such treatment certainly bore comparison with results anywhere else in the world.

The important procedure in treating tuberculosis was to test the organism in order to ascertain the drugs to which it was sensitive, and then to use the correct drugs, in proper dosage, for the correct period of time. Unfortunately, despite the repeated and urgent warnings of all those who had experience, this procedure was often ignored, with the result that the number of patients with 'resistant organisms' increased and the problem of control became more complicated.

Another drug, or a new combination of drugs, which would be comparable to INH was required. Success was achieved in 1968 when Lepetit Laboratories in Milan produced the group of drugs known as the rifampicins. These proved to be as effective and almost as non-toxic as INH or streptomycin, though much more expensive. After development and initial testing in Europe, rifampicin was licensed by the Canadian Food and Drug Directorate for use in Canada in 1973, following trials done in 1970.

At the present time, opinion in Canada remains divided on the most suitable initial drug regimen. There are those who claim that since streptomycin, INH, and PAS have proved their worth and can be expected to give 100 per cent sputum conversion in suitable cases, there is no need to change to other drugs. These drugs are cheap and relatively non-toxic as well. However, the necessity for extramuscular injections of streptomycin, and the cumbersome, rather nauseating bulk of PAS are disadvantages, though these have to some extent been overcome by the development of combined products of INH and PAS that are more palatable while also ensuring that both drugs are taken. Streptomycin is usually discontinued after three months, provided culture sensitivities are satisfactory.

The other 'first-line' attack is to use rifampicin, INH, and ethambutol. This has the probable advantage of more rapid sputum conversion, easier medication, and equal efficacy, but is, unfortunately, more costly.

As yet, there is no clear preference in Canada, or indeed in Europe, where cost is not a dominant factor; in the poorer countries the first alternative is preferred. Both these regimes demand daily medication and must be continued for a minimum of twelve months after sputum conversion. In Canada a total period of eighteen to twenty-four months is the official policy, which implies relying on patient co-operation in taking the drugs conscientiously at home.

The so-called 'Madras Trials,' which were conducted by the British Research Council in the early 1960s in Madras, India, demonstrated that little benefit was derived from treating patients in hospital rather than at home, even in the very poor social conditions of Madras, provided there was adequate supervision to ensure that patients treated at home took the drugs regularly. In other words, it was the effect of the drugs that was all important, not the benefit of hospital care, extra nourishment, rest in bed, or other apparent advantages of hospitalization. This lesson was most difficult to learn. Indeed, ten years later it had not really been accepted and acted upon either in prosperous or poorer countries, and even today hospitalization is still considered an integral part of treatment of pulmonary tuberculosis.

It may be asked whether chemotherapy has eliminated the need for hospital care. The answer to this question is quite clear and simple, and can be summarized in three sentences: (1) A sick person may need hospital care because he is a sick person. (2) Hospitalization may be the simplest method for isolation until the patient is non-infectious. (3) Problems of drug management may require close supervision because of toxicity, drug resistance, or non-co-operation by the patient, and hospital care is then indicated. These principles have particular relevance in Canada because of the great variations in development and medical facilities across the country, and should be borne in mind when planning for the future. What the Madras trials have done is to prove the supremacy of chemotherapy if properly applied, and to show that treatment at home can be as effective as in the hospital. The ideal of treatment is 100 per cent cure, and this should be pursued wherever possible, though a compromise is frequently necessary to meet individual circumstances.

The most difficult problem in chemotherapy is to ensure that drugs are regularly taken as prescribed and over a period as long as 18 to 24 months, even after the patient has returned to all the distractions of living at home and resuming work. In developing countries, where medical facilities may be widely scattered and individual instruction and supervision are difficult, the problem becomes compounded. In view of such circumstances research has gone into developing regimes whereby drugs could be taken once or twice a week, which would make supervision less of a problem. Such techniques have received much study, especially by the Medical Research Council in East Africa and Southern India, as well as in most developed countries.

No intermittent regimen has proved as consistently 100 per cent effective as the recognized standard daily regimes. Nevertheless there are many situations where it is better to ensure supervision and co-operation for an intermittent program than to hope for an ideal that will not be achieved; even under the relatively ideal conditions of this country a decision to use intermittent regimes will often be wise. Nearly all the main drugs have been tried in such programs in various dosages and combinations, but the success rate has not exceeded 85 to 95 per cent. In any event, it is strongly urged that treatment should start with at least three months of daily therapy.

Any discussion of chemotherapy would be incomplete if it did not admit that failures occur and attempt to explain them. It would be easy to attribute failure to drug resistance, but this explanation would not be valid in many instances. Bad drug administration is in fact a much more important cause of failure, as has been shown by trials in many countries and most classically in Hong Kong, where the incidence rate of tuberculosis is one of the highest in the world. Indeed, drug resistance is usually the result of an incorrect choice of drugs or failure to supervise and ensure that they are taken correctly. It is rare for treatment to fail because of initial complete drug resistance, although admittedly there were in Canada in 1974 a hard core of about 300 known patients with active tuberculosis in whom the organism was resistant to all available drugs.

With the discovery of streptomycin and the battery of other antituberculous drugs the outlook for a patient changed in a manner that was dramatic beyond the wildest hopes of older physicians: a disease that once carried a mortality rate of between 50 and 100 per cent, according to circumstances, suddenly became curable. Indeed, the treatment of tuberculosis in any country today is not a question of knowledge but of organization and funding.

There have been some disappointments in the use of modern drug treatment. Although it is successful for individual patients, it has not eliminated all the sources of infection and the disease has not disappeared in any country in the world, even though drug treatment has been in use for over twenty-five years.

However, control of the disease has always been directed as much towards prevention as cure. Early detection, isolation of active cases, vaccination or regular supervision of those at risk – these have always been the bases of control, because it has been realized that only a small proportion of infected persons develop active disease immediately. In the great majority of cases the primary infection is overcome and controlled, but viable bacilli remain almost indefinitely in the body, ready to cause disease in the future. The tuberculin test and the chest x-ray are still valuable tools.

Could drug treatment prevent the disease from developing? The philosophy of preventive drug therapy – chemoprophylaxis – has been widely applied to specific groups of people known to be at special risk and the immediate results have shown statistically confirmed benefits. The principle is simple and easy to apply: isoniazid is used alone in an adult dose of 300 milligrams once daily for a year. This is acceptable to patients who can understand the reason for taking preventive measures, and they usually co-operate well; it is also essentially free of complications and in no way limits normal activity.

The groups to whom chemoprophylaxis is offered are essentially those with evidence of recent infection, i.e, those showing recent tuberculin test

TABLE 5
Growth of prophylactic drug treatment, 1966–71

	1966	1971
Canada	1,939	11,504
Newfoundland	5	82
Prince Edward Island	20	37
Nova Scotia	75	270
New Brunswick	46	187
Quebec	432	2,098
Ontario	860	5,212
Manitoba	65	1,019
Saskatchewan	91	121
Alberta	17	370
British Columbia	321	687
Northwest Territories	7	1,421

conversion, or those who have evidence of old disease that has not been adequately treated in the past but who show no evidence of current activity. In addition, chemoprophylaxis is sometimes advised in certain situations such as during steroid therapy, and during treatment for diabetes, after gastrectomy (resection of the stomach), and during the course of the disease pneumoconiosis which occurs in hard rock miners, according to the clinical situation at the time.

This is a new and active approach to preventive medicine which still needs to be prudently and impassionately assessed: large-scale trials, especially in the United States, have undoubtedly proved its value in specific cases, and in Canada the principle is being widely adopted in all provinces. It is probably the most valuable preventive measure in force, though certainly not the only one needed. It would be folly to encourage indiscriminate and inexperienced chemoprophylaxis either in Canada or, more particularly, in countries where tuberculosis control is still in a very undeveloped state. The number of patients on prophylactic drugs rose from 1939 in 1966 to 11,504 in 1971, as shown in Table 5.

The principles of chemotherapy for lung disease apply equally well to non-pulmonary tuberculosis, such as that involving the kidneys, bones, or joints. In patients suffering from these types of tuberculosis the isolation of the bacillus, its culture, and assessment of drug sensitivities are always more difficult and are often not done. It is therefore difficult to estimate progress, to anticipate relapse, or to determine the development of drug resistance. For these reasons, many specialists may not appreciate the need for prolonged treatment; indeed it is very difficult to assess how essential it is. However, since tuberculosis is a widespread disease, it is strongly recommended that the same regimes should be used as for pulmonary disease, with special emphasis on combined drug therapy and at least one year of medication after apparent cure of the active process. As a result of successful chemotherapy, surgery for non-pulmonary tuberculosis is less frequently required now even though it can be done with greater safety when accompanied by drugs.

It is little more than twenty-five years since the first effective antituberculosis drug became available, and its effect upon the whole pattern of tuberculosis control, and especially upon the individual patient, has been revolutionary. It is difficult to think of any other discovery in medicine that has had such a world-wide and dramatic impact and led to so many changes. Hospitals have been closed, surgical intervention has almost been discontinued, and the social and economic disaster of consumption has been removed, at least in Canada and most of the opulent and well-developed countries of the world.

The responsibility for Canadians in the future is to ensure that this weapon is not wasted by misuse in our own country, and to continue to give maximum support to the control of tuberculosis in those countries where it is still epidemic, and where, through a combination of good organization, available funds, and professional expertise, the new drugs could be put to wider and more effective use to reach the same goals that we have achieved in Canada.

REHABILITATION

Anyone who has had anything to do with the care and treatment of tuberculosis patients in the past is, of necessity, very much aware of the great problem of rehabilitation which the disease presented. One was particularly conscious of a number of factors connected with the disease which contributed to the problem. The advancement of disease when it was discovered, the uncertain prognosis, the tendency to relapse, and the severe disability that followed, all made the lot of the patient a difficult one. The long period of treatment caused the depletion of the patient's and the family's resources, and after such a length of time, it was likely that, if the patient was the breadwinner of the family, someone else had been given his job. It was no wonder that the patient often lost confidence and was afraid to attempt to make the necessary adjustment, particularly if it was necessary for him to change his occupation or he felt shunned by his fellow workers.

Sanatorium staff would have had to be less than human not to have been distressed by such a bleak prospect facing a patient. Many of them gave thought, time, and energy to plans designed to assist patients; they suggested suitable avenues of employment and some tried to lend a hand in opening them up. Occasionally, through a combination of industry, persistence, and luck, they were successful.

Notwithstanding the success stories, too often the physician and other members of the staff, though aware of the problem, were unable to find a solution. The patient and the patient's family were left to struggle alone with their dilemma, without the support of enlightened community interest. Sometimes these courageous though handicapped fighters were rewarded with marvellous success, but often they met with defeat, evidenced by relapse, frustration, depletion of individual and family resources, and a costly increase in the relief rolls.

The picture has now changed. The factors contributing to the altered situation each carry such weight that it is difficult to grade them in first, second, or third place. The difference made by early diagnosis is important; that made by drugs is most important. The realization gradually came that every patient was potentially a rehabilitation subject and that all patients could benefit, either psychologically or materially, from a rehabilitation service, and that rehabilitation is as inseparable from the rest of the program as are diagnosis and medical treatment, the treatment effect shown in the rehabilitation conference being as important as that shown in the medical conference.

There are some basic facts which should be noted briefly before proceeding to a fuller discussion of the topic. First, let us remind ourselves of that well-known but cogent proverb: 'An ounce of prevention is worth a pound of cure.' It may seem superfluous to point out that the person who never develops tuberculosis never becomes a tuberculosis rehabilitation problem, but we need to remind ourselves of this fact periodically. We were more conscious of it in the old days, when we had only a fraction of the facilities needed for all phases of a control program. Lack of funds was indeed one of the reasons why a rehabilitation program lagged behind other phases. Our position then was rather like that of a general who knew that he had not the troops to attack all the weak places, but had to determine the disposition that might make the greatest impact. Quite rightly, we massed our strength on prevention and treatment, and for many years gave rehabilitation comparatively little attention.

Eventually it was possible to close in on all sides. The resources of the campaign expanded so that we could launch frontal, rear, and flank attacks; but the basic attack had lost none of its importance. Early diagnosis, prompt treatment, painstaking follow-up of contacts, these were not neglected, no matter what new aspect of tuberculosis control aroused our enthusiasm. On the contrary, common sense decreed that even more earnest attention be given to these facets of control at the same time as we were putting more vigour into rehabilitation.

The basic problem had been helped in other ways. In the field of rehabilitation, the first blessing for which thanks can be given is the fact that, due to earlier diagnosis and the revolutionary changes made by drugs, tuberculosis is not the disabling disease it once was. The results of modern treatment are presented in terms of the dramatic way in which the death rate has fallen. Perhaps we should be equally thankful that, not only were lives saved, but also the kind of life to which the patient was accustomed was salvaged.

Many of us remember when only about 15 per cent of patients were diagnosed in the minimal or early stage. Most patients never appeared in a doctor's office until the disease was moderately or far advanced. Inevitably there was a great deal of damage which could not be undone and, though the patient's life was saved, it was all too often a shadow of what it had once been: circumscribed and restricted. This was the group from which came the 'maximum benefit case,' the 'old chronic,' or the 'disabled chronic,' according to which term was in use at the time.

That gloomy picture gradually became strikingly altered. Within the doctor's reach more and more facilities for early diagnosis became available. The net of case-finding spread by mass surveys, hospital admission radiographs, examination of contacts, and pre-employment examinations tipped the scales in favour of finding cases early. Formerly, at least 50 per cent of patients admitted to sanatoria were in a far advanced stage and many were hopeless; now no one with the disease is hopeless.

A concrete example will perhaps illustrate the difference in the patients' prospects, even by a relatively early date. In 1940 Weston Hospital in Toronto made a study of the post-sanatorium occupation of a group of its patients. It was discovered that all but 3 per cent had either returned to their former job or gone to another in the same field. This would have been quite unbelievable a few years previously.

It would be unrealistic to ascribe this change entirely to improvement in detecting the disease early, or even in subsequent years to early detection and the new drug therapy. It was to some extent due to the remarkable way in which the whole work picture has altered. One does not walk many blocks these days without being confronted with some machine doing work that once was done by men with shovels, picks, or axes. Every day tons of dirt, gravel, and rock are lifted mechanically that formerly would have been moved by men. Cement is mixed, piles driven, weights lifted – all by machines. We are now in a machine age. On the other hand, one has only to stand on any city street from eight to nine-thirty in the morning or from five to six-thirty at night to be almost overwhelmed by the number of office workers needed to keep the modern world going. The demand for workers who put brain rather than brawn into their jobs would stagger our grandfathers. This has expanded the job opportunities for the ex-patient enormously.

There are other non-medical factors which have an important bearing on the rehabilitation pattern, and for which we should be thankful. Social legislation has made valuable contributions. Tuberculosis still imposes financial hardship, but there is a great difference between hardship or strain and financial ruin – and financial ruin is not too strong a term for what once happened to many a family hit by tuberculosis. We have realized the wisdom of giving enough tax-supported help to enable a family to weather the storm. There is, first of all, relief from the burden of treatment costs. There is no longer need for a patient to curtail treatment for lack of funds. Veterans' allowances, after-care allowances, mothers' allowances, and family allowances have helped patients to continue treatment in a way that was impossible some years ago. There is no denying the fact that at one time some patients did leave the sanatorium prematurely, provoked by the knowledge of want and even poverty at home. While all the holes in the dikes have not been plugged, there has been great improvement. Legislation in 1949, such as the post-sanatorium care program in Ontario, was a great advance and such care programs in other provinces are much superior to previous ones. It is now possible to take treatment and continue one's occupation without a break.

But nothing perhaps is fundamentally more important than a change in outlook concerning the potential for rehabilitation of the average person. Not so long ago our faith in what the average adult would or could do in the way of learning was pretty meagre and summed up in the tag: 'You can't teach an old dog new tricks.' Maybe we did not give enough thought to the fact that we were teaching neither dogs nor tricks. We were helping human beings to do something of importance to them, either economically or emotionally. We now realize that rehabilitation is one department of adult education, and that adults can learn and are the better for it. This realization has come slowly, but surely and convincingly. With it has come the conviction that every patient needs rehabilitation advice, not only the minority who must face decreased activity or change their occupations, but the many men and women who will return, with no appreciable physical impairment, to the same workaday world.

It was sound therapy and sound economics to have the patient use his time in hospital to better himself. Of course, this is another area where advances in treatment have revolutionized the possibilities. The antibiotics have done a great deal toward making a patient feel well enough to use his time advantageously. Twenty years ago patients in sanatoria were generally too ill to employ their time as many do at present, even had educational and rehabilitation courses been available. Now we have to think of such rehabilitation programs as being outside the institution.

But rehabilitation did more than equip the patient to cope better with life than he could otherwise. Discussion of future activities served as a constant reminder that recovery was certain, and that the patient would leave the sanatorium within a short time. This psychological approach formed part of treatment.

It is some satisfaction to know that the Canadian Tuberculosis Association, through its provincial branches, was able to pioneer the rehabilitation program over a period of years. The educational program necessitated by the large number of children and young adults under treatment has been in operation since 1930.

The first rehabilitation officer was appointed in Manitoba in 1941 by the Sanatorium Board and in British Columbia and Alberta in 1947. The rehabilitation program of the Department of Veterans Affairs, started in 1946 under the direction of Major Edward Dunlop, was a great stimulus to the program generally. A number of rehabilitation officers first employed by the department were later available for the provincial tuberculosis programs.

All the provinces had rehabilitation programs. Some were under the direction of the department of health, labour, or welfare, and some were directed or operated by tuberculosis associations. All were assisted greatly after 1948 by the Federal Health Grants, and further strengthened in 1954 by the appointment of provincial coordinators on a nation-wide scale. This established a bond of unity between all rehabilitation agencies. The program benefited from the stress laid on vocational training by this co-ordinating plan.

Programs varied in different provinces but all followed a similar pattern. First, there was the in-sanatorium program, now rarely needed. Stress had moved from occupational and diversionary activities to educational and vocational courses. There was still opportunity for studying design, and doing leather and copper tooling and similar crafts, but much more attention was given to academic work and pre-vocational and vocational courses. How extensive these courses were can be judged from the fact that some students completed their high school education, and even a few years of university as well, while in sanatoria. Such was the interest in rehabilitation during the lengthy periods of inactivity in the pre-drug era.

The post-sanatorium program now utilizes other community resources and agencies. Where training or retraining of ex-patients is required, assistance is forthcoming under the Vocational Training Act. The special placement officers of the National Employment Service have shown a willingness to co-operate in finding suitable employment for former tuberculosis patients. Their usefulness is greatly extended where there is close liaison with other rehabilitation officers, counsellors, and supervisors who have a more intimate knowledge of the ex-patient and his capabilities.

There are few rehabilitation failures and unmet needs, but there is still the older disabled patient whose lack of education has fitted him only for a manual job which he is no longer able to do. This is just a part of the whole problem of an aging population, but the lessening of the tuberculosis problem in the younger age groups, and particularly in women, sets out in bold relief this problem of the older male.

Only when such problems are added to recurring regional unemployment problems is there still difficulty. For example, in the Maritime Provinces and Newfoundland there are fishermen who are prevented from following the strenuous life at sea they once led, and for whom the village or the outport holds little in the way of useful employment. Loggers in British Columbia and miners in other provinces have similar problems. Equally serious is the problem confronting the Indian and Eskimo, untrained for jobs in the white man's world and yet not equal to the rigours of their former life. It is encouraging that the federal government is tackling this one.

There is still a great need for a continuous educational program to allay the fears of the public, based on conditions of former years. We need to instil a feeling of confidence in the stability of the ex-patient. The truth is that he is one of the safest of employees on the score of contagion. He or she is in effect certified to be free of contagious disease, and when ex-patients are referred to an employer he can be sure that, from the medical standpoint, they are fully capable of doing the particular job for which they are applying. We need also to approach the problem from the point of view that the trained ex-patient is an asset to any employer, and that he has something to sell in full competition with the so-called unimpaired.

4

The BCG Vaccine in Canada*

No history of tuberculosis in Canada would be complete without a discussion of BCG vaccine, for its production after years of patient research represents the origins of organized medical research in this country. The series of events in Canada which followed the publication, in 1924,[5] of the first results obtained by Dr Albert Calmette and his group in newborn babies immunized with BCG (Bacillus-Calmette-Guérin) vaccine in France is yet another example of the eagerness of Canadians and their research organizations to take an early interest in the most daring public health innovations and, furthermore, to take advantage of them as soon as they have proved useful.

I am deeply indebted to Dr Armand Frappier, CC, OBE, for providing me with the complete history of the development and use of BCG vaccine in Canada which has been summarized in this chapter. Until his retirement in 1975, Dr Frappier was professor of Bacteriology at the University of Montreal and also in charge of the Institute of Microbiology and Hygiene, renamed on his retirement 'The Armand Frappier Institute' in recognition of his outstanding work during his professional career. From 1933, Dr Frappier was responsible for the production of BCG vaccine and its distribution to all parts of Canada.† The careful research necessary to maintain the vaccine as a safe biological product required constant vigilance on the part of Dr Frappier and his staff. It is regretted that space does not permit mention of the many dedicated workers who assisted him over the years. Dr Frap-

---

* Superscript numbers in the text of this chapter refer to the corresponding item in the appended bibliography.

† After the freeze-dried type of vaccine was developed (see below) the Connaught Laboratories in Toronto and other commercial firms also produced and distributed BCG in liquid and freeze-dried form.

pier has also prepared a complete bibliography, appended to this chapter, which provides an excellent source of material for those who wish to study the subject.

In 1924 Dr Albert Calmette and Camille Guérin of the Lille branch of the Pasteur Institute, Paris, announced the development of a vaccine which prevented active tuberculosis. This vaccine was a strain of a virulent bovine tubercle bacillus which had become attenuated by 230 successive transplantations on an ox bile potato medium over fifteen years. The vaccine, although mild, produced increased resistance to a virulent infection without producing active disease. In other words, BCG is an attenuated live vaccine, the attenuation having become fixed. It loses its viability within a few days so must be used soon after its preparation.

In 1925 the National Research Council of Canada began to organize, coordinate, and subsidize what was then one of the largest programs of research on BCG. Cattle breeders' associations throughout the country were worried about the prevalence of bovine tuberculosis and had pressured the Department of Agriculture to organize a study of the new vaccine. The initiative taken was daring because it meant testing, first in animals and then in man, the innocuousness and effectiveness of a vaccine made with live, albeit attenuated, tubercle bacilli. BCG was the first live bacterial vaccine to be seriously considered for human use, to say nothing of use on the weakest, the newborn. It would have been easier for politicians or official bodies to wait, without risking anything, while scientists in other countries carried out the necessary research, but they did not and Canada played a leading role in the eyes of the world.

The involvement of the National Research Council came about on the advice of an *ad hoc* committee to the minister responsible for the council, the Honourable Thomas A. Low, who authorized the council to form an associate committee on tuberculosis, under the chairmanship of Dr H.M. Tory, president of the council and formerly president of the University of Alberta. Shortly after the committee first convened in May 1925 a tuberculosis research program was drawn up, the fifth article of which dealt with vaccination and suggested that Canada repeat the original tests made by Calmette and Guérin on cattle.

Before the associate committee was formed, two Canadian researchers had already begun to study BCG in cattle: Dr A. Watson, VS, chief pathologist, Department of Agriculture, Ottawa, and Dr A.C. Rankin, CMG, professor of Bacteriology and Hygiene, director of the Provincial Laboratory, and dean of the Faculty of Medicine, University of Alberta, Edmonton. Dr Watson had been trying to develop an antituberculosis vaccine on his own, and had also obtained the BCG strain from Calmette and Guérin in 1924 for research purposes. He was extremely cautious with the vaccine. Dr Rankin had also obtained BCG vaccine in 1924 and, under the auspices of a research committee on tuberculosis of the province of Alberta, had begun inoculating a herd of cattle as early as March 1925. In October of the same year, he reported to the National Research Council committee that he had already inoculated ninety-eight calves without any harmful effects.

At the second meeting of the executive of the Associate Committee on Tuberculosis in 1925 Dr J.A. Baudouin, professor of Hygiene in the Medical Faculty, University of Montreal, offered to direct the project. He proposed the repetition of the vaccination tests of Calmette and his group, but using newborn babies from tuberculous families in Montreal. His proposal was accepted; thus, using vaccine prepared under the direction of Dr A. Pettit in the Department of Bacteriology at the University of Montreal based on the strain brought from the Pasteur Institute, Dr Baudouin began a series of clinical trials before the end of the year. The success of the project led to its renewal year after year until 1947 under Baudouin's supervision. Miss A. Séguin assisted him, and he also had the co-operation of the Bruchesi Institute (an antituberculosis dispensary), the Royal Edward Hospital, the Assistance maternelle (a volunteer organization giving home care to women in confinement), and several hospitals including the Ste Justine Hospital for Children, Notre Dame, St Luc, and Verdun.

Dr Baudouin, a former Rockefeller Foundation Fellow at Johns Hopkins University, was a pioneer worker and a promoter in the field of public health and social hygiene in Quebec. His BCG research work was concentrated on the epidemiological and statistical aspects and in 1948 he made detailed reports on the progress of his trials to the National Research Council, the Pasteur Institute, and the International Conference on BCG. During the twenty years of his research, he published several papers on his work,[2,3] but because of a decision of the associate committee, some of the early statistical data which he accumulated were published under the name of J.W. Hopkins, statistician of the National Research Council, in the *American Review of Tuberculosis*,[26] to ensure that the report would be independent and objective.

In 1933 Dr R.G. Ferguson, medical director of the Saskatchewan Anti-Tuberculosis League, proposed to the committee that vaccination trials be carried out among Indian babies of the Fort Qu'Appelle Indian Health Unit in Saskatchewan. At that time in Canada, the death rate from tuberculosis in the Indian population was ten times higher than in the non-Indian population. The death rate for newborn Indian babies, as calculated by the health unit, was 1018.3 per 100,000. The project was approved and turned out to be one of the better-controlled BCG trials conducted to that time. As in Quebec, the vaccine was first given by mouth, but soon the intradermal method was used because the results were likely to be more uniform. Families were divided into two groups: infants in one group were vaccinated one year while the other group served as controls, the groups being switched the following year. Later, the vaccinations were extended to include nurses and hospital attendants in Saskatchewan hospitals who had previously had a high incidence of tuberculosis.

Dr Ferguson, as well as being a tuberculosis specialist, had a keen interest in epidemiology and extensive knowledge of the clinical and epidemiological aspects of tuberculosis. In co-operation with Dr A.B. Simes, medical director of Fort Qu'Appelle Indian Health Unit, he published his work in the *American Review of Tuberculosis*,[11] *Tubercle*,[13] and the *Canadian Journal of Public Health*.[12]

While vaccinations of humans were under way in the two provinces, Dr Watson and Dr Rankin continued their experiments with BCG in cattle. Dr Rankin reported to the Alberta committee and the Associate Committee on Tuberculosis that he had found BCG to be innocuous and that it conferred a high degree of immunity. In 1928 Dr Watson expressed concern that BCG might regain its virulence,[60] though his experiment had not been based on a sufficient number of cattle to prove whether this was indeed true. In 1934 the associate committee declared that BCG was innocuous but that the vaccine was not of practical value in eliminating bovine tuberculosis. (The policy adopted in eliminating bovine tuberculosis is described in the chapter on 'Bovine Tuberculosis.')

Dr Pettit spent only a few months in Montreal when he brought the BCG strain from Paris in 1925. Dr A. Breton, professor of Bacteriology at the University of Montreal, then took over the supervision of the preparation of BCG. On his death in 1932 he was succeeded by Dr P.P. Gauthier, professor of Bacteriology, who remained in the position until 1933, when Dr Armand Frappier took over the responsibility. Dr Frappier had just completed studies in the United States and with Calmette at the Pasteur Institute in Paris as a Rockefeller Foundation Fellow.

When Dr Frappier assumed responsibility for the production of the vaccine, his first objective was to confirm the innocuousness of the strain that had been used in Quebec since 1925, and also of the new strain which he had brought from the Pasteur Institute earlier in 1933. The strains were checked meticulously to ensure that they had not become virulent or lost their effectiveness. The recent Lubeck tragedy in Germany, when a number of children who had been vaccinated with BCG died as a result of the contamination of the vaccine by a virulent strain of tubercle bacilli, was one that could not bear repeating. Though this disaster was caused by unforgivable negligence by the people responsible for the production of the vaccine (indeed, some were given gaol sentences) it did shake the confidence in BCG for a time, until the effectiveness of careful techniques such as those of men like Dr Frappier was demonstrated.

The tuberculosis situation was serious. In 1926 the death rate of the non-Indian population in Canada was 82.5 per 100,000 and in Quebec it was 118.6 per 100,000. In the Indian population it was ten times greater. In 1930 there were 3350 deaths from tuberculosis in Quebec alone. There were few sanatoria, and the campaign against tuberculosis was as yet undeveloped. The number of new cases per year was not known, as medical practitioners did not always report the disease and avoided disclosing it on death certificates. Fifty per cent of tuberculosis patients died within five years of the diagnosis of the disease. In this discouraging situation Dr Baudouin and Dr Frappier could see no other solution than to recommend mass BCG vaccination, as is now being recommended in underdeveloped countries. However, before recommending a policy of general vaccination, the safety and efficacy of BCG in animals and man had to be thoroughly assessed as well as the various methods of administration. This was done.

The next move was the establishment of a BCG clinic in Montreal, in 1935, by Miss H. Hamilton, head of the Assistance maternelle, for the express purpose of vaccinating the newborn of tuberculous families. The babies were isolated for two or three months and then returned to their families when the post-vaccination reaction had reached its peak. The clinic was administered by Mrs Simonne David-Raymond, and the first medical director was Dr A. Guilbeault, professor of pediatrics at the University of Montreal. This clinic was an important development because it demonstrated how successful BCG vaccination was if infants were vaccinated at birth and isolated until the tuberculin test had become positive, indicating that the vaccination had taken. Dr Baudouin and Dr Ferguson had demonstrated that BCG vaccination in infants was about 70-80 per cent successful even when they were not isolated. Similar results were obtained in studies carried out by Dr N. Vézina in Montreal,[58] Dr G. Grégoire of the Quebec Anti-Tuberculosis Dispensary,[23] and Dr G. Lapierre of the Ste Justine Hospital.[33]

BCG was also being administered to other groups in Canada. It was given by Dr G.F. Kincade[30] of British Columbia to medical students and nurses, and by Dr C.B. Stewart and Dr C.J.W. Beckwith of Halifax to the same groups. It was also being given by health services and dispensaries in Quebec: the Bruchesi Institute and the Royal Edward Hospital as well as the BCG clinic in Montreal, and the Quebec Anti-Tuberculosis League Dispensary. A program of vaccination of children entering and leaving school was undertaken by the health units of Quebec in 1953 and vaccination was offered to newborn infants: about 35 per cent were vaccinated each year.

In 1949, to expedite the BCG vaccination of school children, the Quebec health minister called upon the Institute of Microbiology and Hygiene of Montreal (which had been founded in 1938) to place mobile school vaccination teams of four to six people at the disposal of the health units and municipal health services. The institute was also put in charge of the technical management of operations, of the doctors and nurses of the health services who were involved, and of the administrative organization and the rotation of teams.

In the meantime Dr Frappier and his group were engaged in studies of the experimental and epidemiological aspects of BCG vaccine and of the methods for immunization. In particular, they investigated the stability of BCG in animals[14] and tested transcutaneous methods of immunization[16] and the development of post-vaccinal allergy in both man and other animals.[18,20] They pioneered the use of radioisotopes in their experimental work.[53] The Montreal Laboratory (at the University of Montreal from 1926 to 1938 and thereafter at the Institute of Microbiology and Hygiene of Montreal) became prominent among the few research centres specialized in experimental tuberculosis and BCG.

In 1957 Dr E.H. Lossing, epidemiologist in the Department of National Health, presented an over-all view of the vaccination program in the Canadian provinces to the annual meeting of the Canadian Tuberculosis Association.[38] Dr J.W. Davies, epidemiologist of the same department, on the basis of a survey, published in 1965, of about twenty epidemics of tuberculosis in Canada, representing 6 per cent of all new active annual cases, advised a rational use of BCG to prevent such outbreaks.[7]

The use of BCG vaccine varied in the different provinces, depending primarily on the views of the program directors. For some time, in both Canada and the United States, the influence of critics of BCG, such as Dr S.A. Petroff of New York and Dr J.A. Myers of Minnesota, prevented not only the use of BCG but also the development of experimental studies of the vaccine. Dr Petroff considered the vaccine potentially dangerous because he had found a strain of virulent bacilli in his original culture, but this was not subsequently found by him again or by anyone else.

In 1948, after the First International Congress on BCG in Paris, the situation began to change. The health ministers of Quebec and Newfoundland, on the advice of their deputy ministers Dr J. Grégoire and Dr J.M. McGrath, both of whom relied on the Canadian experience and the technical advice of Dr Frappier and his colleagues, came out in favour of systematic BCG vaccination and integrated it into their programs of preventive medicine. Other provinces opted for selective programs of vaccination for tuberculosis contacts and others exposed to the disease, such as nurses-in-training and medical students.

At about that time, the federal department responsible for the health of Indians and Eskimos in Canada, in collaboration with Dr Frappier, undertook a survey of the possibility of using BCG systematically in this particularly vulnerable population. This service was supported by Dr P.E. Moore, director of Medical Indian Health Services, and was subsequently instituted and maintained in many Indian reservations, including those in the province of Quebec. In later years this policy has not been systematically enforced because of waning interest in tuberculosis control as well as a substantial decline in mortality and morbidity rates. It is, however, the conviction of many people that the time is not yet ripe for the abandonment of any procedures likely to assist in the complete control of tuberculosis in native races.

From 1926 to 1949 many studies were made on BCG vaccination in Canada in addition to those mentioned above. Dr Baudouin and Dr Guilbeault reported their findings when they attended the BCG International Conference in Paris in 1948. Dr Baudouin's report confirmed his earlier findings (the observation period was now more than twenty years) for matched groups of vaccinated and unvaccinated controls living under conditions as nearly identical as possible (for example, 75 per cent were brother and sister living in the same family). The vaccinated had 70 per cent less mortality and morbidity from tuberculosis than the unvaccinated. These results were confirmed by an independent statistical study made from Dr Baudouin's data by a five-member panel appointed by the National Research Council of Canada and reported by Dr J.W. Hopkins. Dr Guilbeault reported that there were no recorded deaths among 477 babies vaccinated and isolated at birth. The group was compared with 751 unvaccinated controls from the same families who were not isolated. The controls had a death rate of 93.8 per 100,000 for the whole group and 160.6 for those where there was an open case of tuberculosis in the family.

In 1947 the Institute of Microbiology and Hygiene of Montreal developed a freeze-dried vaccine to facilitate the preservation of BCG when transported outside the province, though it continues to use the fresh or liquid vaccine on the spot. Thus the institute has been able to keep ampoules of freeze-dried vaccine in which BCG is still living after twenty-five years.

Also in 1947 Dr Frappier and Dr R. Guy introduced the Cuti-BCG allergy test, which they believed to be a more rapid and sensitive test than the tuberculin tests which were and still are commonly employed. The test consists of making one scarification across a drop of bacilliary suspension at a concentration of 50 mg/ml. Cuti-BCG has the advantage of requiring no syringe, no sterilization of instruments, no dilution, and no special care over preservation of the antigen. No palpatation of the skin is necessary in observing the reaction to the test, and quantitative results are observed after twenty-four hours. The test has been used in Quebec and Newfoundland since 1949, but so far has not been adopted in other provinces.

The total annual number of BCG vaccinations, including revaccinations, was about 135,000 in 1974, of which 115,000 were in Quebec. Obviously the use of BCG is limited in other provinces at present. A total of 4,000,000 individuals have been vaccinated, or revaccinated, in Canada since 1926, about 3,200,000 of them in Quebec.

It should be mentioned here that Dr Paudouin set up a file for each vaccinated and unvaccinated control subject, and that the Institute of Microbiology and Hygiene later set up a BCG index on perforated cards using the file. The index includes every person vaccinated in the province of Quebec since 1926 and is most useful for epidemiological surveys. For a few years the institute maintained a similar index for Newfoundland and for the federal department responsible for the health of Indians and Eskimos.

Over the years Dr Frappier has become increasingly involved in international studies on BCG. In 1958 the International Union against Tuberculosis and the International Childhood Centre in Paris made the Institute of Microbiology and Hygiene of Montreal responsible for organizing the first interlaboratory experiment on 'Experimental Methods for the Study of BCG.' One of Frappier's colleagues at the institute, Professor M. Panisset, MV, was co-ordinator of this international experiment in which some fifteen specialized laboratories participated. The results of the joint experiment were reported at a meeting in Montreal in 1961 at which all participants were present as well as other tuberculosis researchers from several countries, thanks to a generous grant from the Medical Research Council of Canada. The proceedings were published jointly by the Montreal Institute and the Pasteur Institute of Lille.[28]

At this meeting, the Montreal group was given the responsibility of organizing another interlaboratory experiment in which the activity of certain BCG strains in animals and in laboratories would be compared, including the strain at the Montreal Institute. The results, together with a report of Dr S. Grzybowski's comparative study of the use of BCG in developing versus developed countries, were presented in 1971 at a conference organized by the Fogarty Health Centre of the United States National Institutes of Health and later published under their auspices.[46]

It is noteworthy that in 1957 Dr Frappier and Dr Panisset published, in the form of a brochure, an exhaustive study on BCG.[22]

A number of experiments have been carried out in foreign countries using the Canadian BCG strain, particularly the freeze-dried vaccine produced by the institute in Montreal. One was done by Dr M. Dworski of the Will Roger's Hospital at Saranac Lake,[10] and Dr H.N. Vandivière made a human field trial in Haiti[57] which showed an 80 per cent reduction in the incidence of tuberculosis in BCG-vaccinated individuals.

Dr H. Brown of the Connaught Laboratories in Toronto obtained a strain of BCG from Dr Frappier for the purpose of producing a freeze-dried vaccine to carry out experiments on the administration of the vaccine. The results were published by Dr S. Landi, Dr F.H. Fraser, and Dr F.O. Wishart,[32] and by Dr S. Grzybowski and Dr M.J. Ashley.[24] Dr C.O. Sieberman also conducted experiments on the vaccine.[52]

Freeze-dried BCG vaccine prepared by the Connaught Laboratories is at present undergoing tests with BCG vaccines from other laboratories in a clinical trial under the aegis of the World Health Organization. Tests of the capacity to elicit immune responses have also been done on the dry vaccines made at both the institute in Montreal and the Connaught Laboratories, along with others, by Dr G.B. Mackaness of the Trudeau Institute in Saranac Lake.[39] The two BCG vaccines, which originated from the same strain, behaved consistently well in this comparative experiment.

Of considerable interest are a number of reports describing the effects of BCG vaccination on certain forms of tuberculosis and other diseases. In 1962 Drs Frappier, L. Frappier-Davignon, M. Canton, and F. St Pierre[17] published an evaluation of the effects of the BCG vaccination program on mortality from tubercular meningitis among children up to ten years of age, between 1949 and 1953, in the province of Quebec. The mortality was reduced to almost nil in the group of vaccinated subjects. In 1971 the same authors, with Dr P. Robillard and T. Gauthier, RN, published 'BCG Vaccination and Pulmonary Tuberculosis in Quebec.'[15] This study, which covers the period from 1956 to 1961 and deals with the population under thirty years of age, showed that the protection given by BCG was 50 to 85 per cent effective in that age group.

Studies on the prevention of leukaemia have also been undertaken. In

1962 and the following years, Dr P. Lemonde and his collaborators showed that, for spontaneous leukaemia in mice induced by the polyoma virus, early vaccination with BCG prevented up to 50 per cent of the mortality and prolonged the survival of dying animals.[35-37] Other authors have made similar observations using transplanted tumours.

Using the 1960-63 figures for populations of children vaccinated with BCG and those unvaccinated, in the 0–4 and 0–14 age groups, Frappier and co-workers found a 50 per cent reduction in mortality from leukaemia among those who were vaccinated. This observation was published in 1970 in the *Lancet*[8,9] and aroused much interest. Other researchers[4,6,31] did not confirm the figures, but Drs H. Th. Waaler, G. Hems, A. Stuart, S.R. Rosenthal, and the British Medical Research Council group[25,50,51,59,62] reported that they, too, had found the same percentage reduction in leukaemia. As a result of these reports, further studies are going on in France[40] and the United States.[41] In 1971 the Montreal Institute of Microbiology and Hygiene took the initiative and convened a meeting of the interested group in the province of Quebec to draw up general protocol for conducting clinical immunotherapy trials for certain types of cancer using BCG. Representatives of the Medical Research Council of Canada and the National Cancer Institute attended the meeting as observers. As a result, in 1972 the Medical Research Council of Canada created a special committee, the Advisory Committee on Cancer Immunotherapy, with Dr J.W. Thomas of the University of British Columbia as chairman and Dr H.E. Taylor of the Medical Research Council as secretary and moderator. Interested workers in Toronto are collaborating in the study. In all studies the manufacturers of BCG in Canada have adhered to the requirements of the World Health Organization.

In looking back on the history of BCG vaccine in Canada, one is impressed with the interest which has been aroused in and centred around the work of Dr Frappier. It is doubtful whether the value of BCG in the preventive tuberculosis program would have been proved without his work. His group was the first to note the possible use of BCG as a preventive immunotherapeutic agent in cancer and the first to observe that vaccination of the newborn provides protection against leukaemia. It is gratifying that Dr Frappier's contribution was recognized in Paris on the occasion marking the fiftieth anniversary of the announcement by Calmette and his collaborators of the beneficial effects of BCG, at which he was invited to speak.

The work on BCG opens up avenues for future solutions of medical mysteries.

BIBLIOGRAPHY

1 Baudouin, J.A., 'Vaccination contre la tuberculose par le BCG à Montréal,' in
   Vaccination préventive de la tuberculose de l'homme et des animaux par le BCG, 6th
   ed. Rapports et documents, Institut Pasteur (Paris: Masson et Cie, 1932): 103–13
2 – 'Vaccination against tuberculosis with the BCG vaccine,' *Canad. J. Pub. Hlth.* 27
   (1936): 20–6; 31 (1974): 362–6
3 – 'Vaccination antituberculeuse au BCG,' *Union Méd. Canada,* 70 (1941): 750–1;
   71 (1942): 375–8; 73 (1943): 826–30
4 Berkely, J.S., 'BCG vaccination and leukaemia mortality,' *Hlth. Bull.* 29/3 (July
   1971): 167–9
5 Calmette, A., C. Guérin, B. Weill-Hallé, A. Boquet, L. Nègre, Wilbert M. Léger,
   and R. Turpin, 'Attempts at immunization against tuberculosis,' *Bull. Acad. Nat.
   Med. (Paris),* 91 (24 June 1924): 787–96
6 Comstock, G.W., V.T. Livesay, and R.G. Webster, 'Leukaemia and BCG – A controlled trial,' *Lancet II,* Nov. 1971: 1062–3
7 Davies, J.W., 'B.C.G. vaccination – Its place in Canada,' *Canad. J. Pub. Hlth.* 56
   (June 1965): 244–52
8 Davignon, L., P. Lemonde, P. Robillard, and A. Frappier, 'BCG vaccination and
   leukaemia mortality,' *Lancet II,* Sept. 1970: 638
9 Davignon, L., P. Lemonde, J. St Pierre, and A. Frappier, 'BCG vaccination and
   leukaemia mortality,' *Lancet I,* Jan. 1971: 80–1
10 Dworski, M., 'Efficacy of Bacillus Calmette-Guérin and isoniazid-resistant Bacillus Calmette-Guérin with and without isoniazid chemoprophylaxis from day of
   vaccination,' *Amer. Rev. Resp. Dis.* 108 (1973): 294–300
11 Ferguson, R.G., 'BCG vaccination in hospitals and sanatoria of Saskatchewan,'
   Amer. Rev. Tuberc. 54/ 4–5 (Oct.-Nov. 1946): 325–39
12 – 'BCG vaccination in hospitals and sanatoria of Saskatchewan,' *Canad. J. Pub.
   Hlth.* 37/11 (Nov. 1946): 435–51
13 Ferguson, R.G., and A.B. Simes, 'BCG vaccination of Indian infants in
   Saskatchewan,' *Tubercle,* 30 (Jan. 1949): 5–11
14 Frappier, A., 'Some experimental and clinical observations on the stability of BCG
   vaccine,' *Proceedings of the Fourth International Congresses on Tropical Medicine
   and Malaria,* Washington, DC, May 10–18, 1948 (Bethesda, Md.: National Institutes of Health): 187–201
15 Frappier, A., M. Cantin, L. Davignon, J. St Pierre, P. Robillard, and T. Gauthier,
   'BCG vaccination and pulmonary tuberculosis in Quebec,' *Canad. Med. Assoc. J.*
   105 (Oct. 1971): 707–10
16 Frappier, A., and J. Denis, 'La résistance antituberculeuse du cobaye vacciné au
   moyen du BCG par des piqûres superficielles et multiples de la peau,' *Rev. Canad.
   Biol.* 4/3 (1945): 334–45.

17 Frappier, A., L. Frappier-Davignon, M. Cantin, and J St Pierre, 'Influence de la vaccination par le BCG sur la mortalité par méningite tuberculeuse des enfants de 0 à 10 ans dans la Province de Québec,' *Canad. Med. Assoc. J.* 86 (May 1962): 934–41

18 Frappier, A., and V. Fredette, 'Influence de la voie d'inoculation et de la virulence des bacilles tuberculeux sur le développement et l'évolution de la sensibilité dermique à la tuberculine chez le cobaye,' *Compt. Rend. Soc. Biol.* 131 (10 juin 1939): 760–3

19 Frappier, A., and R. Guy, 'A new and practical BCG skin test (the BCG scarification test) for the detection of the total tuberculous allergy,' *Canad. J. Pub. Hlth.* 4 (Feb. 1950): 72–83

20 Frappier, A., R. Guy, and R. Desjardins, 'Variations du degré d'allergie par rapport aux méthodes de vaccination et aux doses de BCG,' *Rev. Tuberc.* 16/9 (1952): 749–62

21 Frappier, A., R. Guy, R. Desjardins, O. Roy, and C. Painchaud, 'L'emploi courant de la Cuti-BCG pour la sélection des sujets aptes à la vaccination contre la tuberculose,' *Rev. Hyg. Méd. Soc., France,* 3/2 (1955): 95-110

22 Frappier, A., and M. Panisset, *La souche du BCG* (Montreal: Institut de Microbiologie et d'Hygiène de l'Université de Montréal, 1957)

23 Grégoire, G., 'Le BCG: expérience faite dans un dispensaire,' *Notes sur la tuberculose,* publication du Comité provincial contre la tuberculose 6 (1 sept. 1943), PQ

24 Grzybowski, S., and M.J. Ashley, 'Report of a crash tuberculosis program in a high incidence area,' *Canad. J. Pub. Hlth.* 56 (1965): 527–30

25 Hems, G., and A. Stuart, 'BCG and leukaemia,' *Lancet I,* Jan. 1971, 183

26 Hopkins, J.W., 'BCG vaccination in Montreal,' *Amer. Rev. Tuberc.* 43/5 (May 1941): 581–99

27 Institut Pasteur, Paris, *First International Congress of BCG,* June 18–23, 1948: 108, 213, 244, 255

28 Institut Pasteur, Lille, and Institut de Microbiologie et d'Hygiène de l'Université de Montréal, *Méthodes expérimentales d'études du vaccin BCG,* Résultats d'une expérience interlaboratoires et discussion de Table Ronde, 1963

29 International Seminar of BCG Research Techniques, 'Methods for the study of BCG vaccination,' Paris, 1958, discussed by the International Union against Tuberculosis and the International Center of Childhood, *Bull. Intern. Union against Tuberc.* Feb. 1960: 10–12, 14–20, 23–8, 164, 278–88, 298–9

30 Kincade, G.F., 'Vaccination program for student nurses in Berkeley, California,' *Canad. Nurse,* 49/2 (Feb. 1953): 110-12

31 Kinlen, L.J., and M.C. Pike, 'BCG vaccination and leukaemia – Evidence of vital statistics,' *Lancet II,* Aug. 1971: 398 – 402

32 Landi, S., F.H. Fraser, and F.O. Wishart, 'Vaccination with freeze-dried BCG' *Canad. Med. Assoc. J.* 91/8 (1964): 372–3
33 Lapierre, G., 'Quinze années de BCG à l'Hôpital Ste-Justine,' *Union Méd. Canada,* 76 (mars 1947): 328–31
34 League of Nations Health Organization, Report of the Technical Conference for the Study of Vaccination against Tuberculosis by Means of BCG, *Publ. League of Nations Hlth.* 111/17 (1928): 50
35 Lemonde, P., 'Inhibition of experimental leukaemia by a combination of various factors,' *Lancet II,* Oct. 1966: 946–7
36 Lemonde, P., and M. Clode, 'Effect of BCG infection on leukaemia and polyoma in mice and hamsters,' *Proc. Soc. Exptl. Biol. Med.* 111 (1962): 739–42
37 – 'Influence of Bacille Calmette-Guérin infection on polyoma in hamsters and mice,' *Canc. Res.* 26 (1966): 585–9
38 Lossing, E.H., 'Summary of Canadian B.C.G. vaccination program,' read at meeting of Canadian Tuberculosis Association, Vancouver, BC, June 1957
39 Mackaness, G.B., D.J. Auclair, and P.H. Lagrange, 'Immunopotentiation with BCG–I. Immune response to different strains and preparations,' *J. Nat. Canc. Inst.* 51 (1973): 1655–67
40 Mathé, G., J. Amiel, L. Schwartzenbert, M. Schneider, A. Catton, I. Schlumberger, M. Hayat, and F. de Vassal, 'Active immunotherapy for acute lymphoblastic leukaemia,' *Lancet I,* April 1969: 697–9
41 Morton, D., F. Eilver, R. Malmgren, and W. Wood, 'Immunological factors which influence response to immunotherapy in malignant melanoma,' *Surgery,* 68/1 (July 1970): 158–64
42 Myers, J.A., 'The latent or smouldering stages in tuberculosis,' *Amer. Rev. Tuberc.* 36 (1937): 355–75
43 – 'Primary infection in adults,' *Amer. Rev. Tuberc.* 39 (1939): 232–5
44 – 'Tuberculosis in students,' *Amer. Rev. Tuberc.* 44 (1941): 479–86
45 – 'A summary of the views opposing BCG,' *Adv. in Tuberc. Res.* 8 (1957): 272
46 National Institutes of Health, Bethesda, Md., Fogarty International Center Proceedings no. 14, 'A status of immunization in tuberculosis in 1971,' *Report of a Conference on Progress to Date, Future Trends and Research Needs:* 127–37, 157–78
47 National Research Council of Canada, Associate Committee on Tuberculosis Research, Reports from 1925 up to 1936
48 – Proceedings of the Seventh Meeting of the Associate Committee, June 1936: 5
49 Rankin, A.C., 'Vaccination des bovidés par le BCG,' *Vaccination préventive de la tuberculose de l'homme et des animaux par le BCG,* 6th ed., Rapports et documents, Institut Pasteur (Paris: Masson et Cie, 1932): 114–20
50 Rosenthal, S.R., 'BCG in cancer and leukaemia,' *Bull. Inst. Pasteur,* 70/1 (1972): 29–50

51 Rosenthal, S.R., R.G. Crispen, M.G. Thorne, N. Piekaski, N. Raisys, and P.G. Rettig, 'BCG vaccination and leukaemia mortality,' *J. Amer. Med. Assoc.* 222/12 (Dec. 1972): 1543–4

52 Sieberman, C.O., 'Experiments with killed antituberculous vaccines derived from BCG and Vole bacillus,' *Acta Tuberc. Pneumol. Scand.* Supp. 58 (1964): 35–46

53 Sternberg, J., and A. Frappier, *Proceedings of the 1st Isotope Technique Conference, Oxford 1951* (London: HMSO, 1: 317–37

54 Stewart, C.B., and C.J.W. Beckwith, 'Lack of association between hypersensitivity and immunity following BCG vaccination,' *Canad. Med. Assoc. J.* 83/1 (July 1960): 1–5

55 Thistle, Mel, *The Inner Ring* (Toronto: University of Toronto Press, 1966): 167

56 Turcotte, R., and M. Quevillon, 'Effects of BCG and two of its phenotypes on Erlich tumor,' *J. Nat. Canc. Inst.* 52/1 (Jan. 1974): 215–17

57 Vandivière, H.M., M. Dworski, I.G. Melvin, K.A. Watson, and J. Begley, 'Efficacy of Bacillus Calmette-Guérin and isoniazid-resistant Bacillus Calmette-Guérin with and without Isoniazid chemoprophylaxis from day of vaccination,' *Amer. Rev. Resp. Dis.* 108 (1973): 301–13

58 Vézina, N., 'Vaccination anti-tuberculeuse: le BCG,' *Union Méd. Canada*, 73/11 (féb. 1944): 1330–5

59 Waaler, H. Th., 'BCG and leukaemia mortality,' *Lancet II*, Dec. 1970: 1314

60 Watson, E.A., 'Research on Bacillus Calmette-Guérin and experimental vaccination against bovine tuberculosis,' *J. Amer. Veter. Med. Assoc.* 73 (Nov. 1928): 799–816; *Bull. Inst. Pasteur*, 27 (Jan. 1929): 302–3

61 – 'Studies on Bacillus Calmette-Guérin (BCG) and vaccination against tuberculosis,' *Canad. J. Res.* 9 (1933), 128–36; *Bull. Inst. Pasteur,* 32 (1934): 47

62 WHO, Health Report, 'BCG and Vole bacillus vaccines in the prevention of tuberculosis in adolescence and early adult life,' *Bull. Wld. Hlth. Org.* 46 (1972): 371–85

5

Medical Education in Tuberculosis

The development of the sanatorium movement resulted in the separation of the treatment of tuberculosis from the main stream of medicine. The sanatoria were generally built in isolated places away from general hospitals and schools of medicine, which created problems in the teaching of medical students and nurses.

Although isolation probably did not affect the teaching of basic subjects such as anatomy and pathology, since these were taught in the regular medical course, difficulties arose in the day-to-day teaching of clinical medicine in relation to tuberculosis. General hospitals tended to discourage the admission of tuberculosis patients and, whenever possible, discharged them to the sanatorium at the first opportunity; hence the medical student was deprived of the opportunity of observing tuberculosis on a regular basis with other diseases, and students could only indirectly observe the changes taking place in the diagnosis and treatment of the disease. Many medical men felt that they had graduated with only a smattering of knowledge in the diagnosis and care of the disease, having had only a few lectures and clinics during their course work. Unless they had served as medical officers in sanatoria, for example, they would not have participated in or observed the wide use of pneumothorax, as practised over some twenty-five years in the treatment of tuberculosis. Years later they were likewise often ignorant of the procedures for use of the new drugs in treatment, particularly for the first years after their introduction.

The problem was considered by a symposium held during the annual meeting of the Canadian Tuberculosis Association in April 1924. Representatives of the schools of medicine of the University of Toronto, University of Montreal, and McGill University – Professor Duncan Graham, Dean T. de Lotbinière Harwood, and Dean C.F. Martin, respectively – and three sanatorium superintendents – Dr D.A. Stewart from Manitoba, Dr A.F. Miller from Nova Scotia, and Dr W.B. Kendall from the sanatorium at Gravenhurst in Muskoka – took part in the discussion. In addition, Dr J.H. Elliott from the Chest Clinic, Toronto, discussed the subject of the use of the sanatorium in the teaching of medical students. Although all agreed on the value of a short term of residence for students, they recognized the difficulties, mainly the distance from the medical schools and the limited clinical material presented at the sanatoria for diseases other than tuberculosis.

Dr Martin made a number of observations at the meeting. He felt that too early specialization was dangerous for a medical student, who should be given as broad an outlook as possible on the numerous aspects of medicine. He also felt that adequate contact with patients was essential, as opposed to extended classroom and laboratory study. In other words, the student should be encouraged to cultivate the utmost utilization of his eyes, ears, hands, and fingers in the practice of his profession, while retaining the heart and interest to give his patients the best treatment possible. Dr Martin was of the opinion that the numerous subjects of the medical curriculum should not be divided into 'water-tight compartments' so that allied conditions of individual diseases might not be neglected. For example, regarding tuberculosis, since its protean manifestations were found throughout the tissues and organs of the body, and not confined to the lungs, he felt it was necessary for students to work in medical, surgical, and gynaecological wards of hospitals as well as in dispensaries, clinics, and public health departments. This view being clear, Dr Martin also felt that it was incumbent upon the medical schools to teach the elements of diagnosis in chest diseases and to give students an opportunity to examine patients in the hospitals so that they might learn to distinguish early changes in lungs and appreciate their significance as well as to recognize the early signs of tuberculosis.

It is true that there were a few 'tuberculosis wards' which were near, if not part of, teaching hospitals, but the great majority of patients were treated in isolated institutions which were only indirectly connected with a teaching complex. This affected medical teaching of the disease. Patients with tuberculosis of the bones and joints and of the genito-urinary tract were retained in the departments of orthopaedics and urology in the hospitals, so teaching of these manifestations presented no problem. Pediatrics suffered, however, because tuberculous children were withdrawn from hospitals or other institutions that had pediatric or separate childrens' wards. To offset this, great use was made of diagnostic chest clinics in teaching hospitals such as the ones associated with Toronto hospitals. The sanatoria encouraged the use of their facilities for the teaching of medical students, and Manitoba pioneered in the sending of medical students for short periods to sanatoria for special instruction in tuberculosis.

Chest surgery for tuberculosis was first done in the general hospitals with the patient being admitted on a short-term basis. Later, many sanatoria developed their own surgical facilities, but these were manned by a specialist staff and not always available for the routine teaching of students and junior housemen. Gradually, however, the situation was remedied, and in many university centres tuberculosis units or even sanatoria were set up which established teaching services for this and other pulmonary diseases. A sketch of developments in various provinces (from east to west) follows in the next few pages.

In the 1930s the Halifax Tuberculosis Hospital served as an adjunct to Dalhousie University for the teaching of medicine, under such directors as Dr T.M. Sieniewicz and Dr C.J.W. Beckwith.

In the province of Quebec excellent university affiliations were established in Quebec City at the Laval Hospital and the Quebec Anti-Tuberculosis League dispensary which was organized in 1912. Dr Roland Desmoules and Dr Georges Grégoire were among the pioneers in this work. Later Dr Alphonse L'Esperance made Laval Hospital one of the most complete teaching units in Canada by adding facilities for thoracic and cardiac diseases and setting up an institute of clinical research. He was appointed medical superintendent in 1948.

In Montreal both the French and English groups had facilities for instruction in tuberculosis from an early date. From its founding in 1912, the Bruchesi Institute, first under Dr J.A. Jarry and later under his son Gaetan, was an important teaching centre for the French-speaking physicians affiliated with the University of Montreal. The Royal Edward Institute, from its inception in 1910, was a centre for teaching, and after its affiliation with McGill University in 1925, it became a research centre as well, first under the direction of Dr E.S. Harding and later under Dr Hugh E. Burke.

The first in Canada to take advantage of Koch's discovery of the tubercle bacillus in 1882 were the professors on the medical faculties of the universities. Immediately Dr William Osler (later Sir William) had students identifying the bacilli in his classes at McGill University, and Dr Emmanuel Persillier-Lachapelle was soon giving the same instruction at Laval. Other professors also joined the ranks of the evangelists. There were Dr Thomas Roddick (later Sir Thomas) of McGill and Dr Odilon Leclerc, who not only preached the gospel to medical students but organized the first antituberculosis league in Quebec City. Dr John George Adami, the brilliant head of

McGill's pathology department, was another of the enthusiasts who did not limit his educational efforts to the classroom but stirred up Montrealers to undertake the setting up of facilities for treatment, which resulted in the opening of Canada's first tuberculosis clinic there in 1909. Dr Adami, like many others whose names appear in the next few pages, served a term as president of the Canadian Tuberculosis Association.

The talents of the men who were in the vanguard ranged over a wide field. They were not only excellent physicians but writers, lecturers, and often scholars in fields other than medicine. They could turn their hand to administration and, as was proved a few years later, to practise their profession in the very different situation of battlefield care of the wounded.

We must not forget the outstanding thoracic surgeon Dr Edward William Archibald (1872–1945), who pioneered tuberculosis work in Montreal and in fact in North America. He was the first surgeon to perform a thoracoplasty in America, and became known as the 'father of thoracic surgery.' But he had other capabilities beyond surgery. He was a gifted lecturer and had considerable skill as a linguist, being able to speak with equal ease in English and French. Dr Archibald was typical of the men who came into tuberculosis work in the late nineteenth and early twentieth centuries in that he had himself contracted the disease and had been successfully treated at the Saranac Lake Sanatorium.

An important contribution made by Dr Archibald was his training of Canada's first chest surgeons. A number of these men achieved renown: Dr Alexander (Sandy) Mackintosh, Archibald's successor as the leading chest surgeon in tuberculosis; Dr John Allingham of Saint John, NB; Dr F.L. Schaffner of Wolfville, NS; Dr G.M. Brownrigg, the first thoracic surgeon in St John's, Nfld; and the world-famous Dr Norman Bethune, who was associated with the Royal Edward Institute and the Royal Victoria Hospital before becoming chief thoracic surgeon at the Sacred Heart Hospital at Cartierville, where his associate was Dr Georges Deshaies. Dr Bethune had become seriously ill with tuberculosis in 1926 and was a patient at Saranac Lake for two years, where he was given pneumothorax which he credited with saving his life. He returned to Montreal to work with Dr Archibald and later took up his duties as chest surgeon at the Sacred Heart Hospital. Although a difficult and controversial man, Dr Bethune was years ahead of his time in his attitude and approach to tuberculosis; he was also an advocate of socialized medicine. He resigned from his post at the Sacred Heart Hospital in 1937 to serve as a volunteer in the Spanish Civil War, where he developed the blood transfusion service which played such an important role in that bitter struggle. Dr Bethune returned to Canada in 1937 an avowed communist, and in 1938 went to China to serve with Mao's Red Army, tending the wounded soldiers, enduring hardships, and eventually losing his life from septicaemia after performing an operation without gloves. His work in China, which received recognition from Mao Tse-tung, made him a hero of the Chinese Communist Revolution and caused him to be hailed in China as the most famous Canadian of his time.

Mention should also be made of Dr Armand Frappier, Professor of Bacteriology at the University of Montreal, for his contribution to the development of the BCG vaccine (see chapter 4). His long service and many publications rate him as an outstanding scientist and teacher, and have led to acclaim not only in Canada but internationally.

Ontario, with its excellent tuberculosis centres, developed one of the most complete services in Canada for the treatment and control of the disease under the leadership of Dr G.C. Brink, who was appointed director of the Division of Tuberculosis Control in 1935. The prominence of the clinicians and public health and social services in that province was not excelled anywhere. Such services could not help but impress and give leadership to tuberculosis work everywhere, but, unfortunately, the services were usually too far removed from major teaching centres to make a lasting impression on undergraduates. It was only after 1960 that chest services were established in teaching hospitals and undergraduate teaching became greatly improved.

A number of clinics did, however, develop in Ontario in the early years, and these assisted in the medical education of undergraduates. In Toronto two chest clinics were organized by Dr H.D. Parsons, one at the Toronto General Hospital in 1906 (which was run later by Dr W. P. Warner until he left for war service in 1940), and one in the Sick Children's Hospital (which was later under the direction of Dr Gladys Boyd and then Dr Peter Turner). One was organized also at St Michael's Hospital, by Dr Jabez H. Elliott, and Dr John Paterson set up another clinic at Western Hospital and later at Sunnybrook. In 1910 a chest clinic was organized as well in the Victoria Hospital in London.

To Manitoba goes the credit for first establishing and promoting the teaching of undergraduate medical students and also the public. In 1921 the Ninette Sanatorium, which was some distance from an urban centre, introduced the practice of having medical students pay short-term visits during their undergraduate years. Soon every medical student of the University of Manitoba was participating in the program either at Ninette or at Fort Qu'Appelle in Saskatchewan. So impressive was the teaching that a study of medical personnel in tuberculosis work in the 1950s indicated that more doctors came from the University of Manitoba than from any other school, and that their interest had probably been aroused during their undergraduate training.

Manitoba, having established the first sanatorium in the Prairie Provinces, trained many of the personnel who served in all three. Dr David A. Stewart was a leader without parallel in the crusade. True to its traditions, Manitoba is still proving to be a leader, for today it is one of the outstanding centres on this continent for the study of, research into, and treatment of pulmonary diseases generally.

In Saskatchewan, the teaching of tuberculosis to undergraduates at the university in Saskatoon has been carried on by the staff of the sanatorium in that city since 1925. A new university professorship has now been established, however, with the financial assistance of the Saskatchewan Anti-Tuberculosis League: the George Ferguson associate professorship with particular interest in the teaching of chest diseases.

In Alberta, the staff of the Aberhart Sanatorium has assisted in the teaching of tuberculosis to undergraduates at the University of Alberta. Today the medical services at the sanatorium are directed by Dr B.J. Sproule, an authority on respiratory diseases, who is also in charge of undergraduate medical education in chest diseases. A similar set-up is planned at the university hospital in Calgary.

In British Columbia, the staff of the Vancouver unit of the Division of Tuberculosis Control has assisted in undergraduate medical education. In 1969, an associate professorship, with special interest in chest diseases, was established by the University of British Columbia and attached to the tuberculosis unit to encourage the teaching of tuberculosis and other respiratory diseases to both undergraduates and postgraduates. The first incumbent is Dr Stefan Grzybowski.

With the decline of the sanatorium, attention in postgraduate teaching is now being focused on the smaller tuberculosis unit attached to a general hospital. It is here that younger staff members should find an opportunity and a challenge. The task of the tuberculosis clinic is becoming one of establishing a liaison with doctors in other fields to ensure that tuberculosis and related respiratory diseases receive adequate attention. This is not a new concept. The British service now recognizes that these diseases should be treated in general hospitals instead of through public health departments. With the change has come a greater appreciation of the significance of other lung diseases such as chronic bronchitis, emphysema, and lung cancer. It has also brought awareness of the importance of pulmonary function and the effect of environment on the aetiology of pulmonary disease.

More thought is now being given to the problem of medical education and research in the field of tuberculosis and respiratory diseases in general. This was first prompted by the situation in regard to tuberculosis and the difficulties in obtaining adequate staff, and later by the necessity for a broader view of the treatment and prevention of respiratory diseases generally. It is obvious that the role of teaching in the fields of diagnosis and treatment of these diseases, including tuberculosis, will in the future be taken more and more by the internist trained in the field of respiratory disease. For this reason, more opportunities for training and co-ordination of effort need to be made available. Now that the rate of mortality and to a lesser extent the rate of morbidity for tuberculosis have been greatly reduced, younger physicians are not being enticed into the service. Some of us remember when applications for positions far exceeded the vacancies and tuberculosis services were staffed with keen, dedicated workers.

The importance of specialized training in tuberculosis was such that the Royal College of Physicians and Surgeons of Canada in 1953 granted recognition to those physicians who were acknowledged as outstanding authorities on the disease by giving them certification in Internal Medicine (Tuberculosis). After that date certification or fellowship could be obtained by meeting the usual requirements in internal medicine.

The author is one of those who believe that the field of respiratory diseases should be an integral part of internal medicine. Without the active support of a group who will devote a good deal of attention to the problems of these diseases, however, they will not receive the attention they deserve. The present situation in regard to tuberculosis and other respiratory diseases has required a drastic revision of our thinking. We need to recognize clearly the fields where full-time tuberculosis services are still applicable and where an integrated service should be encouraged. In general, it seems to me that the full-time services required for tuberculosis work should consist of a director of provincial services and sufficient clinic service staff to continue the diagnostic and follow-up service so necessary for many years to come. Some of the clinic service could be on a part-time basis, and the treatment services should be largely on a part-time basis and integrated into the medical services of the community. More and more the work of sanatoria, except for certain institutions, will be done by tuberculosis units attached to general hospitals.

With the integration of the treatment of tuberculosis into community medical services, the younger internists and general practitioners should find an opportunity and a challenge. Previously neither had been given the responsibility or, in many instances, the training to accept fully this assignment, so there will be need for the tuberculosis clinic director to provide assistance. It has been noted that this is the recognized practice in Britain, where clinics and treatment services form part of the chest service, which includes under its purview other respiratory diseases as well. Whereas formerly a tuberculosis officer could have simply a diploma in public health, and be attached to a health department, those who are now responsible in Great Britain are clinicians with higher qualifications in internal medicine. This has become the recognized practice of the Veterans Administration of the United States as well, and, in our own country, such a service is in operation in Quebec, Alberta, and British Columbia and will soon be instituted in other provinces.

Even a casual study of the subject of respiratory diseases indicates the increasing magnitude of the problem. While we are continually reminded of the increasing incidence of lung cancer, the present interest in chronic diseases and geriatrics underlines the extent to which chronic respiratory disease exists. The closer we look at such problems as upper respiratory disease, bronchitis, and emphysema, the more it appears that too often these are the result of a gradual evolution and would have been preventable at some earlier stage of development. Deaths in the older age group may be preceded by months and years of symptoms, many of which could have been attenuated or prevented if detected earlier. We are now taking a definite stand on the problem of smoking, both as a cause of lung cancer and because of its effect on other respiratory diseases, notably bronchitis and emphysema. More and more the problem of air pollution comes to the fore, with the growth of industry and larger and larger urban centres. It increases daily with the increase in numbers of motor cars and buses.

There is no lack of interest or stimulation in the field of diagnosis, treatment, and research in respiratory diseases. This is evident from those few centres where a training program is undertaken. How much more interesting and valuable it would be if it included also the field of tuberculosis. I believe that we should be combining these services in a fellowship training program in order to produce the physician of the future trained fully for the wider field.

THE CANADIAN THORACIC SOCIETY

The events leading up to the establishment of the Canadian Thoracic Society are of sufficient interest to merit recording. Medical thought played an important role in the development of the tuberculosis campaign in Canada, on the part not only of public health officers but also of practising physicians who were active members of the Canadian Medical Association. They, in turn, interested the lay people who were so influential in developing early facilities for the diagnosis and treatment of the disease.

The need for a medical section of the Canadian Tuberculosis Association became evident as the attendance of both medical and lay members at the annual meetings increased. Medical interest in tuberculosis and related problems was growing, so in 1946 a program committee arranged for a medical section where items of purely medical interest could be discussed. The desirability of formalizing this section as a separate medical group was discussed at subsequent meetings, and as a consequence a study of medical personnel was undertaken in 1953. In the United States two organizations were already active – The American Trudeau Society (now the American Thoracic Society) and the American College of Chest Physicians – and the medical members of the association deplored the lack of a similar Canadian organization.

At the meeting of the association in 1954, a plan drawn up by the executive secretary, with a suggested constitution, was submitted to a list of interested physicians throughout the country, as well as to those from the tuberculosis services and the public health group and also to those in private practice who were working mainly in internal medicine. A committee, with Dr C.A. Wicks as chairman, reviewed this material and drew up a report for the meeting in 1955, which was adopted. A constitution and by-laws were then drafted later that year, but it was not until the meeting in 1958 that the final constitution was approved and the first official meeting of the Canadian Thoracic Society took place.

There had been several early efforts to organize local and provincial societies for those interested in the clinical and scientific study of tuberculosis and related diseases. Groups met in Manitoba, Quebec, and Nova Scotia, and an important one, the Laennec Society, had been organized in Ontario in 1916 following the meeting of the Ontario Medical Association. This society was started by Dr Frank Neal of Peterborough, who had had personal experience with tuberculosis. It has been said that its founding should be recognized as the beginning of the Ontario Thoracic Society and be so recorded.

Much of the thought that lay behind the organization of the Canadian Thoracic Society evolved because there existed a great need to solve the problems of medical education and research in the field of tuberculosis and other respiratory diseases. Increasing difficulty was being experienced in obtaining experienced staff because of the decline in the incidence of tuberculosis, and there was an obvious need for a broader viewpoint on the treatment and prevention of respiratory diseases in general.

The Canadian Thoracic Society is now growing rapidly and attracting the attention of the younger university men interested in the clinical and research phases of respiratory diseases. These men will eventually be responsible for these diseases in general, including, of course, tuberculosis.

6

Tuberculosis Nursing

Nurses and the nursing profession have held an important place in the history of tuberculosis in Canada, and have been an integral part of the long struggle waged against the disease. Right from the beginning, at the turn of the century, members of the medical profession were keenly aware that all their efforts would fail without direct contact with individuals, families, and the public. As a result nurses soon became involved, both in the area of patient-care and in education and conducting surveys. They cared for patients at home and in hospitals, sanatoria, schools, clinics, and dispensaries, and worked with the Indians and Eskimos. Their role has ever been an essential one, and it is even more vital today, now that treatment of the tuberculous consists largely of administration of drugs in the home situation.

VICTORIAN ORDER OF NURSES

The Victorian Order of Nurses, founded in 1897, became involved in the campaign for the prevention of tuberculosis from the very start. The executive council of the Canadian Association for the Prevention of Tuberculosis reported in 1902–3 that a pamphlet on the social and medical aspects of tuberculosis by Dr A.J. Richer of Montreal, as well as a large number of tracts issued by the Pennsylvania Association for the Prevention of Tuberculosis, were issued to the public by members of the order, who gave them to all their patients. It was not only necessary to educate the public, noted Dr T.G. Roddick, MP, speaking for the Montreal League for the Prevention of Tuberculosis in 1903, but also to consider thoroughly the humane side of the question. The league planned to give relief to indigent patients by co-operating with the established charitable organizations, such as the Victorian Order of Nurses. This was accomplished gradually, but only to a limited extent.

In 1906 the Ottawa Association for the Prevention of Tuberculosis, founded the previous year, reported that it had no financial resources for building and maintaining a sanatorium and therefore recommended that graduate nurses be employed to work in the homes of the stricken.[1] Miss Edith C. Rayside, a graduate of St Luke's Hospital, Ottawa, was engaged, and she made her headquarters at the Victorian Order offices on Somerset Street. Miss Rayside's distinguished nursing career included being an instructor at the Montreal General Hospital and later matron-in-chief of the Canadian Army Nursing Services, which earned her the order of Commander of the British Empire. However, while working for the Ottawa association she drew a salary of $337.50 for nine months, plus an allowance of $225.00 for board and $25.00 for carfare, a total of $587.50!

Dr George Porter, executive secretary of the Canadian Association for the Prevention of Tuberculosis, paid tribute to the order in his 1919 report 'Crusade for Good Health,' pointing out that 'to the Victorian Order of Nurses many a consumptive owes much for their care and attention, and scattered here and there in outlying districts their nurses have been the only "sheet-anchor" for some of these neglected cases.'[2] Earlier, in his report to the association in 1914, Dr Porter wrote: 'We are pleased to note the growing interest in our housing problem, and to congratulate the Conservation Commission upon its educational efforts along this line, and also those organizations undertaking a practical interest in this great social problem. The extension of the domiciliary visits by district nurses is a noteworthy improvement in this campaign. Some of these nurses are under the auspices of the Local Anti-Tuberculosis Societies, others under the local Boards of Health, others again belong to the Victorian Order of Nurses, who are doing such splendid work over the whole Dominion.'[3] These references to the work of the Victorian Order in the campaign served to emphasize the importance of nursing services, and the great contribution of public health nursing to the cause. The order continued its distinguished work in the tuberculosis field for many years.

EARLY VISITING NURSE SERVICES

Early nurses in the field of public health were greatly occupied with the serious problem of tuberculosis, though today it is only one of the many diseases to be coped with by the public health nurse. The new emphasis on providing health education to the public was based on what was known about tuberculosis. The causative agent, the tubercle bacillus, had been discovered, and certain, if not specific, treatment had been applied with effect.

Yet, in spite of this knowledge, the disease and its often fatal consequences were familiar in every community.

It was one of the numerous duties of the public health administrator in the person of the medical officer of health to recognize the situation. He was responsible for the health of his community. He knew that in order to attack the problem of controlling the incidence of tuberculosis, and indeed of other diseases, by provision of treatment for those who had the disease and by preventing its development in those who had been exposed to it, it was necessary to teach both the individual concerned and the community in general the nature of the disease, the methods of control, and the necessity for their application. Realizing that the public health nurse was the most efficient instrument available to him for such a purpose, he enlisted her services and commissioned her to go into the community to instruct the public concerning these matters. The public health nurse was therefore active in the field of tuberculosis prevention and cure in all stages.

In March 1905 the Ottawa Association for the Prevention of Tuberculosis was established, which led to the systematic visiting of patients in their homes (see above). In the following May it was decided to begin work along the lines laid down by Dr Philip of Edinburgh, Scotland, in 1887, namely, to pay personal house-to-house visits to the sick and provide sufferers individually with instructions regarding the means by which their condition might be improved and their families protected from infection.[4]

Tuberculosis nursing was, however, specialized work, and, at the turn of century, it was a new idea to have individual nurses visiting patients in their homes. The advantages were readily seen, however. First, regarding the matter of cost, it was found that the money spent to keep one patient in a hospital bed for a whole year was equal to the annual salary of a nurse who could visit some four to five hundred patients over the same period. Secondly, the number of available hospital beds was limited, and by no means large enough to accommodate all patients, so for many help had to be given at home. It was realized that the majority of tuberculosis patients could be treated at home, but the condition of the home, the attitudes of both the patient and the members of the family, and the proper form of treatment and the best manner of implementing it were of prime concern. The benefits derived from fresh air, nourishing food, rest, and care of sputum had to be taught, and constant watchfulness kept to ensure that these conditions were maintained. The needs of home patients varied, and each one had to be handled individually, and to do this it was necessary to have trained personnel who would give their full time, thoughts, and energies to their work, in other words dedicated people who understood the meaning of, and were imbued with, the spirit of the new crusade against the universal disease.

As Dr Osler, who is credited with originating the idea of having nurses visiting patients in their homes, so succinctly put it:

In its most important aspects the problem of tuberculosis is the home problem. In an immense proportion of all cases the scene of the drama is the home; on its stage the acts are played ... The battlefield of tuberculosis is not in the hospitals or the sanatoria, but in the home where practically the disease is born and bred ... probably not two per cent of such cases can take advantage of sanatorium or climatic treatment. What has our knowledge to say to the remaining ninety-eight per cent?[5]

In 1898 Dr Osler had had two young women medical students in Philadelphia follow up tuberculosis patients in their homes to see that the physicians' instructions were being carried out and that other members of the family were being protected.[6] Aware of this, Mrs Osler raised a fund in 1902 to help finance the program. The first specially trained tuberculosis nurse then went on duty under the Instructive Visiting Nurses Association in Philadelphia, replacing the medical students who had been doing the job until then. It was not long before the value of such nursing became apparent and the number of nurses gradually increased everywhere.

The need for trained nurses on the Indian reservations was recognized in the first decade of the twentieth century, when Miss Johnston (who seems to have no recorded first name) was sent to the Saulteaux Waywayseecappo Reserve in Manitoba to establish a tent hospital.[7] A log cottage, protected by the forest, was acquired near a lake, and two double-walled tents erected. Since this small establishment was so far from the nearest source of medical help and supplies, some twenty miles away, it called for someone with great courage and resourcefulness to run it. Luckily, Miss Johnston was equal to the challenge. At first she did not have a single patient to care for, which was as she had expected since she had been told that the Indians would not come to her tent hospital. But soon a chronic case arrived, probably out of curiosity. Later a boy with a tubercular knee turned up, and the moccasin telegraph took little time to spread the news that the reserve had a wonderful and kind nurse. By 1908 the reserve's 'sanatorium' had fourteen patients and room for another six was made by erecting another tent.

Fully appreciating her responsibility, Miss Johnston visited patients on foot throughout the reserve, eventually being supplied with a pony so that her ever increasing duties could be carried out more efficiently. The medical officer performed operations with great success, and, with fresh air and good nursing, it was not only possible, but relatively easy, to manage the tent sanatorium – even in temperatures of 40 and 50 degrees below zero – to the advantage of the patients, without inconvenience to the nurse, and at reasonable cost to the provincial health department.

The contribution of the visiting nurse in her various roles could not be too highly esteemed. Her work grew in scope and usefulness, and with her co-operation so did institutional care, dispensaries, educational propaganda, and knowledge of hygiene and sanitation. High qualifications were ideal for the work: a love and sympathy for suffering humanity, a desire to better conditions and bring peace and happiness where turmoil and misery existed, and, along with these, ability, character, tact, energy, and education. Professional qualities were necessary, too, the efficiency and skills acquired from good hospital training being invaluable. Added to all these accomplishments the tuberculosis nurse also needed the training or work experience which gave her familiarity with the problems of her service, as well as a knowledge of the lives, character, and habits of the poor, of their general housing conditions, and of other elements which predisposed them to the disease. To be most successful, she also had to be familiar with all agencies at her disposal to prevent or correct poor living conditions, and to be aware of local laws and the benefits which could be derived from schools, churches, charitable societies, as well as dispensaries, hospitals, and sanatoria. Obviously the ideal tuberculosis nursing specialist was a paragon!

By 1928 nursing agencies were gradually being established in the various provinces; these were essentially centralized community efforts, adapted for work in cities and towns. The nurses's position in antituberculosis work was strategic. At first, graduate nurses knew little of the disease, other than the fact that it was contagious, and thus fear prevented them from working with it. Lack of adequate training for their role was a growing concern, but eventually postgraduate instruction became available in the sanatoria. With the realization that the disease was not only preventable but also curable through education, larger numbers of nurses specialized, particularly after the affiliation of some of the sanatoria with the nurses' training schools (see below).

As more nurses became involved in the battle against tuberculosis, increased attention was given to the prevention of the disease among the nurses themselves. Until the emphasis shifted to control and prevention, many nurses contracted the disease through exposure (many of them were between the ages of nineteen and twenty-five, a particularly vulnerable age for the disease). Nurses who had recovered from a bout were a source of recruitment for sanatoria as it was possible for them to resume their nursing careers on a part-time basis under medical surveillance. The residence and salary were advantages to them during the convalescence-work stage.

In the sanatoria the nurse was the only professional worker whose contact with the patient was personal and continuous. Luckily, the nurses had a versatile concept of patient care, which was free from the rigidity that came into the service some time later. The nurse fulfilled many roles in meeting the mental, emotional, and social needs of the patient and his family, and in the early stages of case-finding a clinic nurse even took the x-rays and developed the films.

In the sanatoria the morning care of patients under the method in practice in the early days, particularly during the winter months, was hard both on the patient and on the nurse, although both sympathized with the then modern method of treatment in which rest, fresh air, a balanced diet, and surgery were particularly important. In the old days at Tranquille, BC, patients had to consume raw eggs and milk at every meal and between meals, and had to go out of doors in all kinds of weather, taking exercise under the close supervision of orderlies. This could mean a walk with bare feet in the snow. The routine called for a cold chest bath at 7 am, breakfast and dinner with windows thrown wide open, though the temperature outside might be 40 degrees below zero, and open-air exercise in the cold. At mealtime, a minimum of twenty minutes had to be devoted to the first two courses in a three-course meal.

There was a close affinity between long-term illness and poverty, and resources for help were few or non-existent. Consequently, nurses became involved in attempting to bridge the gap by soliciting help from voluntary agencies and groups to provide necessities such as food and clothing. Warm clothing was needed to outfit the patient for admission to the sanatorium, where he would spend the greater part of his time on an open porch to get the abundance of fresh air prescribed by the 'cure.' There was an added complication, too, since often by the time that the patient was ready for exercise, none of his clothing would fit because of the large gain in weight from the good meals and customary between-meal nourishment of eggnogs and milk.

Many patients were loggers, fishermen, or miners, and the transient nature of their way of life meant they often had no home to return to upon discharge; nor could they, as a rule, continue to earn their living in the same occupation. On a limited scale, boarding homes provided a home base during convalescence. Nurses visited them regularly to supervise the isolation technique, check temperatures, and arrange for x-ray appointments, and to supply patients with requirements for diversionary and occupational activities to offset the boredom of illness and idleness.

EDUCATIONAL PREPARATION FOR NURSES

At first there was very little educational preparation for tuberculosis nursing. Nurses were exposed to known and unknown sources of infection in both hospitals and sanatoria. Lacking the balance of adequate instruction and supervision in a safe environment, practical nursing experience often had disastrous results, which later had adverse effects on the recruitment of nurses for expanded tuberculosis services.

In the 1930s tuberculosis programs became centralized and facilities greatly enlarged in most provinces. Case-finding clinics and beds for treatment increased in number, as did the case loads for the public health nurse. Chest surgery was also on the increase, but because of the serious shortage of nurses in all branches of the service, it often had to be curtailed and many beds left unoccupied. Some veteran tuberculosis nurses were no longer physically able or professionally competent to give the specialized and arduous care required for the surgical patients, and suitable replacements were hard to find. World War II also contributed to the shortage of nurses, but there were other factors too.

There was growing concern over the situation, which began to receive attention by various groups. In 1944 the Canadian Nurses Association arranged a conference to explore the situation and the problems of tuberculosis nursing. A subsequent survey in Manitoba provided some enlightenment by revealing that nurses avoided the specialty for fear of the disease and because of inadequate preparation, two related problems. In the spring of 1944 the Manitoba Association of Registered Nurses organized another conference to discuss the prevalence of tuberculosis and the shortage of nurses competent to undertake tuberculosis nursing, two important problems in a province with four sanatoria. In the light of the survey, the association agreed that the nurse would have to realize the importance of her own personal hygiene and the value of enforcing a good aseptic technique in all sanatoria.

At the Winnipeg conference the lack of adequate training of both nurses in the sanatoria and public health nurses who dealt with tuberculosis in the home was admitted by a number of speakers, including Miss E. Stocker, superintendent of nurses at Ninette Sanatorium, who said: 'We find the present-day sanatorium for tuberculosis a hospital where the modern and progressive scientific treatment is carried on, but we do not, in many instances, find here nurses who have had any special preparation in the field of tuberculosis nursing prior to coming on the staff.'[8] On that account she urged more and better instruction, greater clinical experience for the student nurse, and special postgraduate work for the institutional nurse and the public health nurse.

Prior to 1944, attention had of course been paid to the protection of staff in sanatoria. From 1938 BCG vaccine was administered to all nursing personnel in the sanatoria of Saskatchewan, and in 1945, it was claimed that at the Keith Sanatorium in Calgary, there had not been a breakdown in the nursing staff for seven years. The standard rules of the latter institution were as follows:

These personal habits should be developed in all staff members and strictly adhered to:

1. Hands should be kept away from the mouth, face, and hair while working.
2. Hands are to be washed frequently, and always before leaving the ward or touching food.
3. Eating in kitchens or accepting candy or food of any sort from patients should never be done.
4. Every nurse, orderly or maid should develop the habit of observing breaks in patients' technique. The nurses are responsible for correcting all such digressions.
5. Paper handkerchiefs should be used on duty. A pocket should be provided for same in gown.
6. Pencils, erasers, etc., should never be put in the mouth.
7. Patients' dishes should never be used.
8. Technique on removal of gown: Wash hands, untie strings, remove gown and hang up, then wash hands again. If hung in a clean area, such as an office or dressing-room, the gown should be hung inside out by the shoulders. If in a dirty area, a ward, it should be hung right side out.[9]

Other provinces were also concerned about the need for well-prepared nursing personnel, and in increasing numbers, to carry out expanded plans and programs for tuberculosis control with minimal hazard to their own health. In 1943 in British Columbia, the director of tuberculosis control, Dr W.H. Hatfield, with the co-operative participation of the Registered Nurses Association of the province, took action to set up a program for on-the-job training of student nurses for tuberculosis work. An organizing committee with representatives from the medical and nursing professions, the schools of nursing, the nursing department at the University of British Columbia, and the public health department of the province and of the city of Vancouver was established, but soon found that the objectives of the program would be impossible to meet without concordant changes in the hospitals and chest clinics to update the practices and isolation techniques and develop a broader scope in tuberculosis nursing. A public health nurse, Miss Esther Paulson, who had been on loan for a year to the Division of Tuberculosis Control from the Metropolitan Health Service in Vancouver for the purpose of correlating the clinic and outpatient services, was persuaded to transfer to the division's staff in January 1944 as director of nursing for the hospital and chest clinic and to assume joint responsibility with the instructor for the program.

In January 1944 the first affiliation course was given, with the participation of four of the seven nurses' training schools in British Columbia, and with financial assistance from the provincial government, which paid three-fifths of the expenses of the student nurses for the whole course and also paid for the necessary teachers. It was an intensive course of six weeks' duration (the length was reduced to five weeks to accommodate the increased enrolment when all schools became involved a few years later) covering instruction and related practical experience in all phases of tuberculosis nursing in the hospital, chest clinic, and home, and was given in a safe environment at the Vancouver unit of the Division of Tuberculosis Control. The course proved to be eminently successful and led to the initiation, by the province of British Columbia, of compulsory tuberculosis training as a requirement in the basic course for all students admitted to the schools of nursing from September 1945 on.

The British Columbia Tuberculosis Society gave substantial assistance by awarding cash prizes annually to students selected for their interest and performance during the affiliation course. Later, the society gave a sustaining grant of $2000 to the School of Nursing of the University of British Columbia to assist in preparing nurses with advanced qualifications for supervisory positions in the expanding program and services of the Division of Tuberculosis Control.

In no other province was such a comprehensive and concerted approach taken. The objectives, which were achieved in a relatively short time, justified the wisdom and the courage of the sponsors. Fear of the disease was dispelled, and recruitment of prepared personnel became a reality – at least for the tuberculosis services in urban centres, where the service was on a par with that of general hospitals in the same area.

Better preparation for students and graduate nurses was a decisive step toward recruiting and retaining qualified staff, and efforts to improve and expand affiliation courses were supported by tuberculosis authorities nationally and provincially. In the United States, the National Tuberculosis Association gave a grant to the American Nurses Association in 1947 for the foundation of the Joint Advisory Service in New York, the purpose of which was to explore the service and educational needs of the existing situation and to provide an advisory service for schools of nursing, public health agencies, and the nursing profession. Two publications were prepared, *The Instructional Plan for Basic Tuberculosis Nursing*, which dealt with the curriculum and related clinical practice, and *Safer Ways in Tuberculosis Nursing*, which dealt with technique, practices and quality of nursing care, on the premise that affiliation courses, to be effectual, must provide a good standard of patient care in a safe environment. The Canadian Tuberculosis Association accepted responsibility for the distribution of these booklets in Canada. An up-to-date textbook, *Nursing in Tuberculosis* by Louise L. Cody, was also available by this time (1947) and was widely used in Canada in student affiliation courses and for staff education. Later, the nurses in British Columbia were invited to submit material and pictures of procedures for the revised edition of the text in 1961.

Other publications and texts appeared which helped to dispel fear and stimulate interest in the clinical field of tuberculosis. *The Canadian Nurse* for November 1951 was devoted to tuberculosis and included articles by nurses from different regions of the country stressing the expanding opportunities.

Tuberculosis nursing was no longer in an isolated position. The nursing profession had become aware of and involved in the preparation of personnel and nursing service standards for the specialty. It was equally important that nurses in the tuberculosis field should participate in professional affairs in order to interpret for others the factors specific to tuberculosis nursing and the disease, and make them aware of the resources for control and prevention.

NURSING ORGANIZATIONS

In 1929, at the meeting of the International Council of Nurses in Montreal, a Canadian group of tuberculosis nurses was formed. The aims of this group were five in number: (1) to keep nurses doing tuberculosis work informed about the disease and new methods of treatment and prevention; (2) to keep all nurses in the group in touch with each other; (3) to educate members of the nursing profession generally as well as the specialists in regard to tuberculosis; (4) to study and promote the progress of affiliation between the sanatoria and training schools for nurses; (5) to advocate that all nurses should have experience with, and special instruction in, tuberculosis before graduation.

Nurses became more interested in the problems of tuberculosis as publicity increased, teaching aids improved, and the profession generally became aware of the special training and qualities needed for this branch of its work. However, because the nurses were so widely scattered and the sanatoria so far apart, it was difficult for them to meet, yet frequent contact was deemed essential. At a meeting of the Canadian Nurses Association in Sackville, NB in 1948, a group of twelve tuberculosis nurses from across Canada took the opportunity to gather and confer on mutual problems. Stimulated and reassured, they agreed to seek support from their respective provinces to obtain a means of communication and representation within the Canadian Tuberculosis Association. Inclusion of the nursing discipline in the official organization at the national level would give recognition to nursing as a key service in the control and prevention program and help to achieve greater uniformity in the standards of patient care and preparation of nursing personnel. No definite action was taken immediately on the nurses' request, but in 1950 two nurses from the western provinces were invited to present papers on nursing services and student affiliation at the general meeting of the association in Vancouver. The nurse attendance continued to be limited to those who worked in the area of the annual meeting for a few years, and there was no response to the request for greater representation until the association met in St John, NB, in 1954. That was a momentous year for tuberculosis nursing. Nurses were present from Ontario, Quebec, the Maritimes, Alberta, and British Columbia, as well as the chief nurse from the Indian Health Service in Ottawa, and there was a special program for them for the first time. Sixty-eight nurses, representing general hospitals, schools of nursing, and public health agencies as well as the tuberculosis centres attended the sessions.

The nursing section of the Canadian Tuberculosis Association was formed at that meeting, with Miss Ellen Ewart of Hamilton, Ontario, as the first chairman and Miss Louise Bartsch of Ste Agathe, Quebec, as secretary. The newly organized section submitted a resolution through the association to the Canadian Nurses Association, urging support in developing and expanding affiliation in tuberculosis nursing in all provinces.

The section has been an integral part of the parent organization and has arranged a program for every annual meeting since its inception. Some difficulty has been encountered in program planning, participation, and follow-through at the provincial level over the years, however, because representation at the meetings has been irregular and lacking in continuity. Nevertheless, communication with tuberculosis nursing sources in all provinces has been maintained with the co-operation of the staff in the national office. All program papers and section reports have been reproduced in French and English and distributed to all tuberculosis centres, the Indian Health Service, the national and provincial nursing associations, and the schools of nursing.

The program topics of the fifties dealt with student affiliations, education, and nursing techniques and standards. An annual display of ideas under the caption 'Have You Thought of This?' provided much co-operative help in improving practical procedures and routines. Other topics, centred on the interchange of pertinent information and methods of referral, helped to promote mutual understanding and better co-operation between hospitals, chest clinics, and public health nurses which carried through to the provincial levels.

Staff education was advanced further in 1963 when the Canadian Tuberculosis Association undertook to finance educational institutes for nurses, to be held annually, alternating in the east and the west. This type of project was chosen by the nursing section, in preference to fellowships for individual nurses, because of its greater benefit to a larger number. The institutes have been immensely successful, and have given added impetus to co-operative planning and participation between nurses in the clinical specialities and the profession generally.

Together with other groups, the provincial branches of the nursing section of the association, which were established in Quebec, Alberta, British Columbia, and Newfoundland after the idea was first proposed in 1964, have been responsible for the basic planning and implementation of the regional institutes when held in their areas and have undertaken other projects as well. The Quebec branch has arranged twelve study sessions for doctors and nurses; the one at Ste Agathe in 1968 had an attendance of 110 despite a hurricane-force storm. This branch also held a most successful institute in May 1972 at the University of Montreal, which was attended by over 250 nurses. In 1965 and 1966 the Alberta branch arranged for one-week programs at two tuberculosis centres for thirty-two senior and staff public health nurses and new appointees to senior positions. The British Columbia branch broadened its membership and maintained continuity of attendance, for nurses from diverse sources, at annual meetings of the Canadian Tuberculosis and Respiratory Disease Association and nursing institutes when they were held in the West. In Nova Scotia, in 1971, the 20th Annual Institute of the Dalhousie University School of Nursing, which discussed tuberculosis, was held in Halifax.

The appointment of a nursing consultant to the national office of the association was made in 1966. This has added strength to the nursing section, and has provided it with a vital link with the provincial branches. The consultant is in a key position for keeping informed about new trends and developments and is alert to the implications for nursing. Her assistance in planning the programs for institutes and in co-ordinating arrangements for the annual meetings of the section is invaluable. The recent appointment of a nurse on the board of management of the association has also provided a stimulus to the fulfilment of nursing's partnership in the objectives and goals of tuberculosis control.

CHANGING MANAGEMENT OF THE DISEASE

National and provincial programs over the years have reflected the advancement of knowledge and changing trends in the management of the disease. The increased emphasis placed on rehabilitation led to greater involvement by nurses. Formerly the idleness enforced by confinement in the sanatoria, and the uncertainty over their ability to return to their regular occupations, contributed to the restlessness and frustration of patients. New procedures called for exercise rather than bed rest, and after 1950 chemotherapy eliminated the long invalidism and distressing symptoms of cough, sputum, and haemoptysis which formerly had been an element of restraint on behaviour. In contrast, most patients were ambulant and asymptomatic, which often resulted in aimless restlessness, resistance to education, and indifference to personal responsibility for treatment and recovery.

Nurses in hospitals, chest clinics, and public health departments were of necessity involved in rehabilitating the tuberculosis patients to life outside the sanatorium. Their staff education programs, conferences, and publications were evidence of their concern and of the efforts they were making to upgrade skills and knowledge and to find new ways of helping patients. The traditional type of ward and regime seemed unsuitable for patients who were no longer on strict body rest or in hospital for prolonged treatment. Some form of reorganization seemed to be indicated in order to provide the opportunity for the patient to use his time and energy in a more constructive manner for his benefit and well-being.

One innovation, the minimal care unit, involved renovation of the ward for self-care with a minimum of staff service and supervision. Interdisciplinary co-operation and effective participation by all professional and auxiliary staff members were essential for the plan to attain its full potential. Two advantages evolved: greater incentive for the patient to become self-sufficient and better-prepared for eventual discharge, and better use of nursing staff and their acceptance of a different nurse-patient relationship with emphasis on interpersonal skill as much as on technical competence.

In the 1950s the first minimal care units were set up in British Columbia and Saskatchewan whereby patients took care of their own physical needs as much as possible.

The perplexities of the fifties were projected into the sixties. However, fewer patients in hospital for shorter periods, early ambulation, and chemotherapy did not lessen the nurse's responsibilities. Problems of a different nature emerged with the intensification of case-finding in areas of higher incidence of infection and disease and the subsequent increase in the proportion of patients in the older age group or with socio-economic or behavioural problems. The hospital nurse had now to provide time-consuming assistance to the elderly ambulant patient and nursing care for attendant geriatric conditions, but the most difficult and unrewarding task for the nurse in hospital, chest clinic, or public health service became that of handling male patients over fifty years of age, because of the variety and degree of character disorders found in the group, including alcholism and drug addiction. Many of these were homeless, or from skid-row areas or prisons. They were men for whom drunkenness could be a normal state and assault a natural reaction, and who had become elusive because of their transient way of life and difficult to instruct in new ways of living. The disease is still most prevalent in the older group, and one cannot help but feel apprehension about the future of tuberculosis nursing on this account, that again there might be difficulty in recruiting and holding nurses for around-the-clock institutional care for acute tuberculosis patients.

Nursing problems are not confined to problem people, however. The average patient, male or female, who has contracted tuberculosis in the past decade or so is not always receptive to teaching or to the regime of taking drugs. Indeed one might say more generally that it is not easy to establish rapport with ambulant patients, whatever their personalities. The shorter stay in hospital, ambulation, and leave of absence during treatment have all reduced the nurse's time and opportunity for teaching, getting to know the patient, and helping with problems. The trail of contacts with transient patients often becomes obliterated before the public health nurse is aware of the newly diagnosed case, and the patient discharged before she has had time to visit. To ensure that the nurse could make the most of available opportunities, staff education in the sixties was directed toward improving interviewing techniques and gaining a broader knowledge and understanding of behavioural attitudes, which are a determining factor of success or failure in treatment and recovery for the patient and control of the disease in the community.

Nurses have had to accept a shared responsibility for the fact that many readmissions come, not from new infections, but from lapse of drug administration and social stress. Dr. C.W.L. Jeanes, medical director of the Canadian Tuberculosis Association, made the following statement at the annual meeting in 1964: 'Some 856 re-activations have had second or third occurrences. Twelve to fifteen percent of such patients have the new resistant-type organisms for which treatment is difficult. The most urgent need is for more adequate follow-up for recently treated patients. Persuading patients to keep with their drugs and periodic check-ups is the toughest part of the current program of tuberculosis control.' The effect of our present permissive society cannot be overlooked as a factor in the situation. Indifference and resistance to self-discipline and to acceptance of personal responsibility are formidable obstacles in recovery to the patient and in the control of tuberculosis in Canada.

Nurses have persevered in their part of the program despite the difficulties and obstacles. The present trend toward domiciliary treatment has entailed continued participation and major responsibility for them, as 'it is generally agreed, [it] depends on a well-developed local health service because, in the final analysis, the day to day supervision of the patients at home and the distribution of their drugs, depend on the public health nurse.'[10]

Similar views have been expressed about the needs in developing countries as well as in Britain and the United States. In all these countries, so different in the economic sense, the eventual success of out-patient treatment plans is equated to the relative availability and adequacy of informed nursing personnel for surveillance and supervision.

WHAT OF THE FUTURE?

What, then, of the preparation of nursing personnel in the seventies? Some authorities question the need for any time to be given to the tuberculosis specialty in the basic nursing course. Affiliation programs such as were common in the 1940s to 1960s are no lónger suitable or possible because of reduced facilities and personnel in the tuberculosis centres. The diminishing nursing force cannot assume the major responsibilities for education in this specialty. However, it is still possible to arrange a good learning program despite reduced clinical facilities for student experience in the disease. Students and graduate nurses still need to be informed and prepared for tuberculosis nursing, not only in Canada but in the developing countries as well, where the disease is still a health hazard. It would seem that authorities in nursing education must assume the responsibility for preparing personnel for tuberculosis work in other parts of the world if not in Canada, and especially public health nurses at advanced levels.

Continuing education about tuberculosis for nurses working in this area in the expanded program for respiratory diseases, and for the nursing profession generally, is necessary. The annual institutes of the Canadian Tuberculosis and Respiratory Disease Association, though highly successful, are regional in scope and cannot sustain a continuity of interest unless augmented by similar programs in the provinces. The primary objective of the nursing section of the association and of its provincial branches is to foster the interest of the profession in tuberculosis and other respiratory diseases and to encourage its participation. The provincial branches should be instrumental in achieving the goal. The small force remaining in tuberculosis nursing, however, has an added obligation to remain actively involved at both the national and provincial levels to ensure that the specialty receives adequate recognition and does not become submerged in the consideration of other respiratory diseases.

Nursing has played an indispensable and steadfast role through the many stages of change and adjustment in the campaign against tuberculosis. Medical authorities throughout the world have confirmed their dependence on a stable and informed nursing force for the success of domiciliary plans and chemoprophylaxis programs. Vigilance and sustained interest of nurses and nurses' training schools are, however, essential in order to ensure that the needs of the future, whatever they might be, will be met by available nurses who are prepared to take full part in the treatment, control, and prevention of tuberculosis and other respiratory disease problems in Canada and throughout the world.

Nursing has a long history of service in the control of tuberculosis. Its contribution through the struggle has been both necessary and valuable at every stage of the campaign, first in the homes, then in the institutions, and now in the domiciliary phase. The service is still needed among segments of the population where strongholds of the disease remain. Indeed, nursing services were the first to appear on the battlefield and will be the last to leave. Theirs is the task not of 'raking the embers of old camp fires' but of maintaining an active service which is still as necessary as it ever was.

7

Tuberculosis in Native Races

THE INDIANS

The Indians of Canada do not seem to have suffered from tuberculosis before the coming of the white man; however, once encountered, the disease became a pitiless scourge which threatened to annihilate them completely. It has been estimated that when the first settlers arrived in New France in the early seventeenth century there were some 200,000 Indians and Eskimos in what we now call Canada. By the time the first census was taken in 1871 this number had fallen to 102,358 (Table 6), the drastic drop being due in large part to tuberculosis.* Smallpox shared in the devastation, but it was eventually brought under control by vaccination. It was a much longer time before effective means of tuberculosis control were found.

The onset of the disease was paced by the penetration of white settlement from east to west, the tribes living east of the Great Lakes Region being the first to suffer. Though some Indian tribes were nomadic, their villages, like those of the agricultural tribes, were discrete, with many miles of hunting grounds between them. The spread of the disease was thus slow, but it was steady. The eastern tribes were ravaged for 200 years before the prairie settlers introduced the Plains Indians to the disease. By the time the outbreak of tuberculosis was beginning in the Red River country, in 1870, the epidemic had passed its peak in Quebec and Ontario, though it continued to be the leading cause of death among the Indians there for decades to come. Even today, the incidence rates are higher among Indians of northern Quebec and Ontario than among the white populations in the same areas.

* See Appendix 4 for a graph of the mortality rate for tuberculosis among Canadian Indians.

TABLE 6
Estimates* of registered Indian population, 1871–1971

Year	Population	Year	Population	Year	Population
1871	102,358	1910	106,914	1944	125,686
1881	108,547	1915	103,774	1949	136,407
1891	120,638	1924	104,894	1951	143,983
1896	100,027	1929	108,012	1954	151,558
1897	99,364	1931	110,261	1959	179,126
1898	100,093	1934	112,510	1961	185,168
1899	98,981	1939	118,378	1966	224,164
1900	99,010	1941	122,031	1971	257,619
1905	107,637				

* Made by Statistics Canada

It seems scarcely credible today that the white population remained indifferent to the spread of the disease among the Indians, which frequently wiped out whole families. Indeed, one feels that the settlers were perhaps more fatalistic than indifferent. The epidemic among the European settlers had probably long since passed its peak, but a death rate due to tuberculosis of 200 per 100,000 was still common in 1890, and all had witnessed the disease in their own communities, where it caused the death of whole families. Familiarity had bred resignation: there was nothing the settlers could do for themselves, and so nothing they could do for their Indian neighbours.

At the turn of the century mankind was still helpless against tuberculosis, but there were factors in the everyday life of the Indians that made them particularly and devastatingly vulnerable to attack. Epidemiologists have long recognized that people who have had no previous experience with a communicable disease have no built-in immunity to it, and so it was with the Indians and the onslaught of tuberculosis. Added to their lack of immunity was the fact that they lived in crowded teepees and lodges where isolation of the sick was impossible, even if they had recognized the necessity for it. Malnutrition also aggravated the situation. The Indians depended on hunting for their food, a precarious base at best for maintaining an adequate food level for the community. As the white settlers advanced west the areas for hunting shrank, and as serious as the reduction of the hunting grounds was, worse was yet to come.

The huge buffalo herds of the Prairies had been the staple of the Plains Indians' economy. Not only did they provide a plentiful meat supply, but their skins were used for teepees, bedding, and clothing. In 1879 disaster struck. The buffalo herds moved south to their winter feeding grounds and never returned north again. The hardship which their disappearance brought about can hardly be overrated. The flour ration doled out according to treaty was hopelessly inadequate. A Royal North West Mounted Police inspector at Fort Walsh protested that he was distributing to the Indians, as their weekly allowance, two days' ration of flour![1]

Lack of sanitation also contributed to the general havoc. When the plains and forests of America were available as living space, the Indians solved their sanitary problems by moving when conditions became untenable. As settlement spread they had less and less land to move around in. Reservations were set up in an effort to provide them with land that was inalienably theirs for all time, but, as they had never worked out methods for maintaining standards of cleanliness within fixed limits, this proved unsatisfactory. The consequent insanitary and unhealthy conditions added to the nurture of tuberculosis.

The scattered locations of the reservations and the great distances between them made it difficult to bring medical assistance. Even when methods of controlling tuberculosis had been developed, it was still impossible to visit all the outposts without the help of an automobile or aeroplane. With the best will in the world, those concerned about the decimation of the Indian population were frustrated in their attempts to establish effective programs.

Superimposed on these adverse physical conditions was the hard-to-estimate part played by emotional strain. Physicians had long felt that there was a link between deep unhappiness and the progress of tuberculosis. There can be no doubt that the Indians, and in particular the Indian leaders, were very unhappy and prey to unrelenting anxiety or resentment, or both. Why should they not be? The encroachment of the white man's settlements had forced on the Indian people an unwelcome way of life. They had become displaced persons in a cramped, though familiar place. Not unnaturally they tried to escape by drowning their worries in liquor. Alcoholism, long known to be an ally of tuberculosis, became general. It remains to this day an avenue of escape, which is also a road to despair.

Was the white community horrified at the catastrophic death rates in the native population? No. It must be remembered that there were no telephones, radios, or other means of rapid communication. Outside official circles, the figures were known to few, but even if the people had known there was little they could do. They were resigned because they did not know any other way to face tuberculosis. The government's parsimony would not have shocked them either. At that time governments did little or nothing about the distress of the poor and diseased in cities all over the world; welfare allowances, as we know them today, were still hidden in the mists of the future.

As if all these factors were not enough – malnutrition, lack of sanitation, confinement on reservations, the disappearance of the buffalo, lack of immunity to tuberculosis, despair, alcoholism, and government parsimony – there was another problem. This was the assumption on the part of the white people that the Indians, seeing the settlers enjoying more material comfort and prosperity than they did, would try to achieve equal comfort and prosperity by imitating the farmers who were ploughing the fields and scattering the good seed on the land. There were no sociologists or anthropologists around to warn them that this was not going to happen. It is only in recent years, a century later, that officials dealing with native peoples have learned that the ways that have enabled a people to live for a thousand years or more satisfactorily and with dignity are not abandoned because people with different traditions have moved in on them. Pointing out the impracticability of the assumption, an Indian said to Sir John A. Macdonald, first Minister of Indian Affairs: 'We are wild animals; you cannot make an ox out of a deer.' However, officials were quite unconvinced of the validity of this comment. Far more weight was attached to the advice of persons such as Indian Superintendent Joseph Albert Norbert Provencher, who in 1873 urged that the Indians be 'instructed, civilized and led to a mode of life more in conformity with the new position of this country, and accordingly make them good, industrious and useful citizens.'

Obviously each side had a tenable point of view, and it is not strange that, allowing for certain shifts in thinking concerning the means by which their ends might be achieved, both sides still feel they have a strong case. The sad fact was that as each side tried to maintain its position, progress for the native people in general, as well as progress against tuberculosis in particular, was painfully slow.

It should not be thought that the Indians took what was handed out to them – or more correctly what was *not* handed out to them – submissively. When treaties were being arranged their demands were listened to with the knowledge that in 1870 some had joined the Metis in the Red River Rebellion and fifteen years later some of the Saskatchewan tribes had cast their lot with the Metis when they took up arms again. It is puzzling that the possibility of trouble did not carry more weight. When the Indians demanded guarantees that government aid would be forthcoming in times of need, one would have expected that as a result of apprehension, if from no more worthy motive, such guarantees would have been given promptly. But no. The government spokesman for the Department of Indian Affairs answered: 'We cannot foresee these things and all I can promise you is that you will be treated kindly.'

This did not satisfy the Indians and they persisted in their demands and won partial victory: a clause was inserted in one treaty (Treaty No. 6) which guaranteed that 'a medicine chest would be kept at the house of the Indian agent for the use and benefit of the Indians at the direction of such agent' and that aid would be given should a tribe be 'overtaken by any pestilence or general famine.' By present-day standards this effort seems about the equivalent of offering bandaids to treat cancer, but meagre as the concession was there is plentiful documentation that some thought it too much. The minister of the interior regretted one clause which 'was agreed to by the commissioners, as it may cause the Indians to rely upon the government instead of upon their own exertions.'

Lieutenant-Governor A. Morris, of the newly organized province of Manitoba and of the Northwest Territories, was even more frank. He told a delegation of Indians that to do what they wanted would take a lot of money. 'And,' he added, 'some of you would never do anything for yourselves.' He was far from alone in this view. In 1890 a report of the Indian Affairs department actually stated: 'If a man will not work, neither shall he eat!' There must have been contrary souls who asked: 'But what work is there for the Indians?' If so, their dissent has not been recorded. Before judging government spokesmen too harshly, it would be realistic to note that the same tone pervades present-day comment on unemployment payments throughout the western world.

Despite government parsimony, officialdom was trying to help the Indians adapt to a new life. There were people who felt that the soundest approach would be to concentrate on the children, that if the children were educated in the ways of the white man they would be weaned away from the lifestyle of the reservations. They believed that if the children lived in a residence, slept in beds, ate at a table with cutlery and dishes, they would prefer these things to the culture of the lodge or teepee; along with a working knowledge of reading, writing, and arithmetic such amenities would fit the young people for modern life.

To achieve this seemingly desirable end industrial schools were set up. Usually they were put in charge of missionaries who, like the rest of the population, had no idea of the difficulty of the task they were undertaking. Only in recent years have social scientists propounded the view that by the time a child is of school age he has already absorbed the ways of those around him. If the people around him are shiftless, if they do not save for a rainy day and are frequently drunk, that is the pattern the child is likely to follow tenaciously for the rest of his life. This is one reason why it is so difficult to eradicate a poverty culture. Despite other training in later years, men and women adhere to what they have seen through their first window on the world. To be sure, there are exceptions. There are millionaires who have struggled up from the slums and sons of honest parents who have turned to forgery or embezzlement, but the publicity attending such developments attests that they are rare enough to be newsworthy. However, such ideas had no currency in 1884 and the residential schools were set up. The annual report of the Department of Indian Affairs in 1891 commented that 13,430 Indian children were in these schools.

Before too long it became apparent that these schools were aggravating the tuberculosis problem. This should have been anticipated. Many of the buildings had not been constructed as schools but had been taken over because they were available cheaply. They were badly ventilated, and the dormitories were overcrowded. The per-pupil allowance was not enough to provide a balanced diet containing sufficient protein. The children did not like the schools and had to be confined there to prevent them from running away. Before the coming of the white man they had worn few clothes in summer and thus absorbed enough vitamin D to last through the winter. The missionaries persuaded parents to clothe them, and certainly in the schools they were clothed, and there was no cod-liver oil ration to replace the vitamin D they had formerly received from the sun. These adverse circumstances combined to cause soaring tuberculosis death rates. In 1896 the Department of Indian Affairs sent out a letter to its agents asking if they believed that the residential schools were contributing to the tuberculosis problem and those who answered said that in their opinion the schools did.

Among the most coherent of the critics of the residential schools was Dr J.D. Lafferty of Calgary, who was to get backing for his campaign to improve matters when Dr Peter Bryce, who had been chief medical officer for Ontario, was made the first full-time chief medical inspector of the Department of Immigration in 1902. Dr Bryce was a well-informed, energetic, conscientious, intelligent pioneer in public health. Before his appointment he was already conversant with the disastrous inroads tuberculosis had made among the Indians of Ontario, where he had endeavoured to improve sanitary conditions on the reserves. He had compiled statistical information and continued to prepare annual reports which were based solidly on facts for which he supplied data.

This appointment marked a change in the approach to Indian medical services. Among the reasons that neglect had been so flagrant was that there was no clear line of command. The British North America Act had given the provinces the responsibility for health in the areas under their jurisdiction but it was the federal government which dealt with the native population. The only government with authority to deal with the Indians in Canada was in Ottawa and it had no jurisdiction in health matters. This evasion of responsibility continued until Dr Bryce took over – a man who did not shirk responsibility.

One of the first things Bryce did was to set up tent sanatoria, with trained nurses in charge, on some of the reservations in southwestern Ontario. Sanatoria were just beginning to be opened, but it was to be many years before there would be enough of them to accommodate all the patients with tuberculosis. In the meantime, some patients were segregated in tents, sometimes in their own backyards. The tents had floors and double walls and were certainly a decided improvement on anything the Indians had up to that time, but they were still not proof against Canadian winters and the experiment was abandoned after Bryce's employment with the government was terminated.

The nursing service initiated as part of this program was a success. The nurses obviously established good relationships with their clients. Not only did they treat patients, but they also instructed the Indian women in methods of cooking on stoves rather than on open camp fires.

Yet another innovation was to have circulars on the subject of tuberculosis prepared in the Cree language by the Department of Indian Affairs so that some Indians could learn in their own language about the disease which was killing so many of them so steadily. A manual on hygiene was also prepared for the Indian agents. Health education among the Indians was thus begun.

Meanwhile, Dr Bryce kept a supply of factual information flowing into the department. He compiled statistical data on tuberculosis mortality rates by bands. When he asked for $20,000 for a program to prevent tuberculosis among the Indians he had already given the information to show that the program was needed. Parliament still did not give the money.

Among the studies instigated by Bryce was one of the occurrence of tuberculosis in the residential schools. He found that the schools were every bit as bad as the rumours and complaints about them had claimed: they all suffered from lack of ventilation, and their records of discharged pupils showed an alarming death rate from tuberculosis. An attempt was made to improve the ventilation and to give instructions in the isolation of children suffering from open glandular or pulmonary tuberculosis. In 1909, with Dr

Lafferty of Calgary, Bryce inspected seven residential schools for Indians. Their report stated: 'In no single instance in any school where a young child was found awaiting admission, did he not show signs of tuberculosis.' In two schools they found not one child with a normal temperature.

From the statistics available it appears that the death rate from tuberculosis among the Indian school children was 80 per 1000, or 8000 per 100,-000, as rates are quoted today. No wonder there were claims that tuberculosis would soon wipe out the native populations. Deaths were far in excess of births.

The solution offered by Dr Bryce to halt this tragedy was that administration of the schools should be turned over to him, and that most of them should be turned into sanatoria.

No record can be found stating why Dr Bryce's services were terminated. It may have been because his programs were considered too ambitious and too costly, but there is reason to suspect that it was a result of the hornet's nest of protest from the churches over his suggestion that the administration of the Indian schools be taken out of their hands. Certainly his services terminated in 1912, and it is a significant fact that he was not immediately replaced. Perhaps there was recognition that the conditions in the schools called for drastic action and that such action would arouse a storm of opposition from some quarters, and thus the most comfortable way out for officials and politicians was to forget the whole thing for a while. No successor to Dr Bryce was appointed for seventeen years.

In the opening years of the twentieth century, though the rate of incidence of tuberculosis among the Indians was still catastrophic, the epidemic (at least among adults) had passed its peak. Several developments made for a slightly more hopeful outlook. The most susceptible families had disappeared, and those remaining had more resistance. Also, much progress had been made in sharpening diagnostic techniques following Koch's isolation of the tubercle bacillus in 1882.

Though no director of medical services was appointed, in 1914 the Department of Indian Affairs appointed Duncan Campbell Scott to the position of deputy superintendent general, the equivalent now of a deputy minister. Dr Scott was not only a conscientious and able man, he was a philosopher, a poet of no mean ability, and a lover of music, who, it is said, maintained a piano in his spacious office. He was truly interested in the Indians and respected their culture. He wanted to preserve it and at the same time to find some compromise that would enable the Indians to keep their mode of life but at the same time have a reasonable living. He would have been quite unhappy administering the department in later years when the

Indians began to question departmental policies and express and exert themselves in deciding their own future.

Scott's faith was expressed in his report of 1920: 'Although [the Indian] has been wasted in the struggle [against tuberculosis], he has not been worsted, and the vestiges of the tribes that remain are of stronger stock as the years go by.'[2] He dedicated himself to improving services and when, a few years later, the Canadian Tuberculosis Association began taking an active interest in promoting a program among the Indians it could rely on him for sympathy and for effective presentation of its recommendations to government. Under his direction, the nursing and medical service was expanded, and the government became less parsimonious in its expenditure.

Meanwhile, discharge procedures for men returning from duty in World War I had unexpected effects on the tuberculosis program. Routine medical examination revealed that great numbers of these men had contracted the disease, and there was no other solution than to provide sanatorium treatment. Empty beds in existing sanatoria were utilized for returned soldiers, the government paying the costs, and new sanatoria were built, again at the complete or partial expense of the government. Though the Indians were exempted from military service 3000 of them had enlisted voluntarily and naturally there were Indians among the tuberculous veterans who were treated in sanatoria.

At the same time, there was tangible evidence that the Indians were adapting themselves to changed conditions and were taking an interest in medical services. The Blackfoot, one of the more prosperous and more progressive tribes, built their own hospital. Duncan Campbell Scott having loosened the government's purse strings, thirteen other hospitals were built on the reserves. These, like the residential schools, were run by the churches.

Among the doctors who came into the service following the war was Dr E.L. Stone, whose area was Norway House, north of Lake Winnipeg. He had been the youngest colonel in the Canadian Medical Corps and was awarded a CMG for his outstanding services. He brought not only medical experience to his work but knowledge of how treatment of large numbers of persons is administered under very difficult conditions. In 1927 Scott recommended that he be appointed as director of medical services for the Department of Indian Affairs, and there was finally a successor to Dr Bryce.

At Norway House, Dr Stone had recognized that not only were there several health problems with which he would have to deal but that tuberculosis was by far the most acute. True, trachoma was causing a great deal of blindness and he initiated a program to cope with it, but he knew that the most critical medical battle to be fought was against tuberculosis: 'disease here means one malady and only one for practical purposes – that is, tuberculosis. Practically nobody dies of anything else.'[3]

Regulations stated that no child who had been infected with tuberculosis was to be admitted to the schools. However, if the regulations had been strictly adhered to, Dr Stone would have been obliged to reject every child. As it was, he did reject those with active disease, but admitted those in whom the disease appeared to be dormant. Otherwise, the schools would have been empty.

Dr Stone is remembered as a keen, kindly, conscientious officer working under great difficulties with a small office staff and smothered with the job of assessing numerous financial accounts which reached his desk from the field. He had neither time nor staff to undertake much in the way of long-term planning. However, he was kindly disposed to the suggestions that reached him for a more aggressive program for tuberculosis work among Indians. As early as August 1930 he drew up a memorandum for Dr Scott outlining a program for tuberculosis control by the department with a budget for a ten-year period, rising from $100,000 to $1,000,000 over the ten years, and providing clinic service and treatment beds for 450 Indians. This was disregarded in the economy drive of treasury officials that followed in the next few years, a drive which greatly frustrated Stone. He was basically a shy man and was no match for the forcible bureaucrats whose job it was to cut estimates. He usually acquiesced to their demands although one could see that he was under considerable strain in doing so.

The organized campaign for the control of tuberculosis among the native people depended very largely on the development of a general medical service. It is not our intention to describe in detail the development of such services, but rather to focus attention on the steps by which the services for the control of tuberculosis were developed over the years. There is no doubt that the disease soon became recognized as a great and most costly medical problem. It was the one disease which at a certain stage threatened the survival of both Indians and Eskimos, and hence became a prime target.

The development of health services is well described in several papers by Dr George Graham-Cumming and Dr Brian Brett, published in the *Journal of the Canadian Medical Association,* 15 March 1969. They mention such early medical men as Sir John Richardson, a physician who accompanied Sir John Franklin on some of his polar voyages; Dr W.M. Mackay, who was perhaps the first resident physician of the western Arctic and a pioneer doctor in Alberta prior to Confederation; and Dr Leslie Livingston, who was the first resident physician of the eastern Arctic. They also enumerate the establishment of the mission hospitals, and the establishment of government health facilities from 1887 to 1967, and are generally useful historical documents.

Dr Graham-Cumming has also published a very full article, 'Health of the Original Canadians, 1867–1967,' in the *Medical Services Journal,* February 1967, which was very largely drawn on a master's thesis entitled 'Indian Health, 1867–1940,' prepared by the late Lieutenant D.R. Maundell, MARCA, for submission to the Department of History of Queen's University. Dr Graham-Cumming gives a good summary of the attitude of the federal government in regard to its responsibilities for providing health services. He points out that the government never fully recognized the provision of health services as its responsibility. It seemed to have assumed that the Indians would and could eventually provide their own medical services, as other Canadians did. This view actually persisted until the advent of medical services paid by the provinces assisted by federal subsidies, and the coming of hospital and medical programs. Then it became a problem of integrating the services for the Indians and Eskimos with the provincial ones, and of determining how these were to be financed and what arrangements needed to be made with the provincial authorities.

The approach to tuberculosis for the Indian population of southern Canada was assumed to be a public responsibility almost from the start, but it was some time before the responsibility for the cost of treating tuberculosis in Indians and Eskimos was recognized without question by the federal government, and, even then, the budget provided was far from sufficient to pay for the diagnostic and treatment facilities required.

At the outset, some Indians were treated in the provincial sanatoria already provided for other Canadians. These sanatoria and clinics had been in operation for varying periods, having been set up in the first place by efforts of interested laymen who had been stimulated by an interest in the disease or by health officers and doctors with enough vision to see that tuberculosis could be controlled.

The program of education and the mobilization of public opinion in favour of health services for native peoples have been important factors throughout the campaign and in the results obtained. As has been mentioned above, Dr Peter Bryce, who assisted in the organization of the Ontario and Canadian tuberculosis associations, at an early stage suggested a program for control among the Indians as well. Representatives of the association from Alberta, Manitoba, and Saskatchewan also spoke of the plight of the Indians.

Perhaps the first important step taken was the setting up of a committee to study the problem by the executive council of the Canadian Tuberculosis

Association in 1924, during the period when Dr R.E. Wodehouse was executive secretary. It was a deplorable fact that no definite information was available on tuberculosis among Indians. The study was financed by the Department of Indian Affairs and carried out in British Columbia by Dr H.W. Hill, Dr A.S. Lamb, and Dr C.H. Vrooman, who reported the results at the meeting of the executive committee in 1925. Dr Duncan Campbell Scott, deputy director general, was invited to attend and give his comments. He supported the reports and assured the committee of his co-operation, stating that medical officers, being usually part-time, did not have time for such detailed reports. It was then that he recommended the appointment of Dr Stone to headquarters in Ottawa to direct medical services for Indians under the authority of the superintendent general.

In 1928 the Saskatchewan Anti-Tuberculosis League, as a result of its surveys of Indian schools and the reserves of the Qu'Appelle Valley, spearheaded a research project in the Health Unit there, with the participation of the National Research Council through the Associate Committee on Tuberculosis. It was under the direction of Dr R.G. Ferguson, medical director of the Fort Qu'Appelle Sanatorium, assisted by Dr A.B. Simes, a full-time officer of the unit. The activity undertaken included tuberculin testing of school children and x-ray surveys, as well as a BCG vaccination program developed by the committee in co-operation with Dr Armand Frappier of the University of Montreal (see chapter 4). For the latter an excellent control system was set up whereby the families were divided into two groups, and the babies of only one group were vaccinated each year, the babies of only the second group being vaccinated the following year. This double system of controls continued throughout the project (to 1945), which is outlined in a report on 'BCG in Indian Babies' by Dr Ferguson.[4] The results of the BCG program were remarkable; they showed a reduction of 80 per cent in active cases of tuberculosis among those who were vaccinated.

Although the research project in the Qu'Appelle Valley continued, the economic crash of 1929 put an end to the general program of expansion, and some nursing services were discontinued after 1930.

In 1934, at a conference of provincial ministers of health in Ottawa, the problem of tuberculosis in Indians was emphasized by several of the ministers. Dr Ferguson had given to Dr J.M. Uhrick, the minister of health for Saskatchewan, information outlining the results of a number of school surveys conducted during 1933. In a thousand public school children, the percentage of positive reactors ran from 46 to 79 per cent, and 2.17 per cent had active tuberculosis lesions as demonstrated by x-ray. His recommendations were for more full-time physicians on the reserves, regular diagnostic services, and segregation of school children with active forms of the disease. Mr R.A. Hoey, the minister of health for Manitoba, presented a report on a research project on tuberculosis in Indians in Manitoba which was carried out in 1932. The death rate was 820 per 100,000 among Indians, and 1290 per 100,000 among the Metis, in comparison with 41 per 100,000 for the remainder of the population. Manitoba also recommended more full-time medical and nursing staff and advised segregation for active cases.

The annual meeting of the Canadian Tuberculosis Association in 1935, held in Vancouver, devoted a session to Indian tuberculosis. Some figures were given on the percentage of Indians in those who had died from the disease during the previous five years and the percentage of the total population that the Indians constituted in each of a number of provinces as follows: Manitoba 41 per cent of deaths, 2.2 per cent of the population; Saskatchewan 27 per cent of deaths, 1.6 per cent of the population; Alberta 34 per cent of deaths, 2.1 per cent of the population: and British Columbia 35 per cent of deaths, 3.7 per cent of the population. A strong resolution was sent to the prime minister and to the minister of health, pointing out the menace of uncontrolled tuberculosis on Indian reserves to the surrounding white population, and suggesting that more active measures be taken. This was met with the usual response of the period: sympathy with the suggestions but a stressing of the need for economy.

In 1936 the Department of Indian Affairs became a branch of the enlarged Department of Mines and Resources. The economy drive persisted and reached a climax in January 1937 when the director of Indian affairs, formerly the deputy minister of the Department of Indian Affairs, Dr H.W. McGill, the first registered physician to hold the post, sent out a directive to all Indian agents with instructions regarding the medical care of Indians. It stressed that it was their duty to keep costs at their lowest point consistent with reasonable attention to acute cases of illness and accident. Services were to be restricted to those required for the 'safety of life, limb or essential function.' This directive read, in full:

Ottawa, January 14th, 1937.

TO
All Indian Agents:

Kindly give this instruction the widest possible distribution among all concerned with the medical care of Indians. Further copies are available on request.

1. The expenditure for medical services during the present fiscal year has been much

greater than was anticipated. The prospect is that there will be a heavy over-expenditure on this account. There is little indication that additional funds will be available for next year. It is necessary that a substantial reduction in cost be made immediately and maintained until further instructions are issued.

2. Kindly instruct all personnel concerned with the care of sick Indians that their duty in the immediate future is to keep the cost of medical services at the lowest point consistent with reasonable attention to acute causes of illness and accident. Their services must be restricted to those required for the safety of limb, life, or essential function.

3. Hospital care must be similarly restricted. An immediate survey is to be carried out to discover and discharge any patients who can be maintained at home or elsewhere safely and more economically than in hospital.

4. The Department will expect a reduction in drug expenditure and demands of about 50%. The waste, if it exists, is not uniform and this paragraph must be interpreted with some discretion by the more economical.

5. There will be no funds for tuberculosis surveys; treatment in sanatoria or hospitals of chronic tuberculosis; or other chronic conditions; tonsil and dental clinics; artificial teeth and limbs; spectacles except for prevention of blindness; dental work except for the relief of pain or serious infection; nor, in fact, for any treatment except for acute illness.

6. Expenditure for the following services must be regarded as exceptional, to be authorized in advance by the Indian Agent and explained satisfactorily in his vouchers:
(a) Transportation of sick Indians – allowable only when relatives or neighbours positively have no available means of conveyance.
(b) Payment of Indians for services to their sick neighbours.
(c) Aeroplane transportation: Accounts will be accepted only when they comply with the conditions in the Regulations for Medical Services in every respect. Each must bear a certificate by the Indian Agent that he has satisfied himself that the use of any less expensive method of conveyance would have endangered the patients [sic!] life, limb or essential function.
(d) Fees claimed by Doctors on salary for extra services either for their own or other Indians.

7. Every precaution is to be taken to prevent the outbreak and limit the spread of communicable disease. Vaccination is to be kept up and inoculation against typhoid fever where that disease exists or has been a menace in the past. Quarantine for the more serious communicable diseases is to be rigidly enforced, with guards if neces-

sary, to prevent spread beyond the first households affected. The powers of an Indian Agent are ample for this purpose and delay is not kindly regarded.

8. Kindly review the Regulations affecting medical services for Indians not living on Reserves. It applies only, but very strictly, to Indians living in premises assessed for taxes.

9. While there is no occasion for over severity, the necessity is not too highly emphasized by these instructions. Indian Agents are particularly advised to inform all hospitals, specialists, surgeons, dentists, etc., that they (the Agents) are the only persons finally competent to authorize special or hospital services and that payment is not guaranteed for services rendered without their knowledge and consent, preferably in advance, if time and distance will permit.

    While these instructions apply in a general way to Departmental Hospitals and Health Units, special directions will be issued for their guidance.

Harold W. McGill,
Director of Indian Affairs[5]

This was probably the lowest point in the discouraging picture of Indian medical services. It was not an encouraging beginning for the newly set-up Department of Mines and Resources and indicated an utter lack of appreciation of the medical needs of the Indians. Although there was subsequently a change in the policy, many who were close observers of the period of the development of Indian medical services felt that not until they became a part of the Department of National Health and Welfare in September 1945 was the serious deficiency appreciated and a real effort made to correct the situation. Fortunately the decade following the above directive would see changes that led up to the excellent health service which is operating today. Prevention of the disease was a concept not taken seriously as a government policy for Indians up to this point. There seemed to be, if anything, less interest under this new set-up than when Indian affairs was a separate ministry of its own.

    On 1 March 1937 the following letter was sent to the director of Indian affairs by the executive secretary of the Canadian Tuberculosis Association, Dr G.J. Wherrett, on the direction of its executive council, suggesting that a study be undertaken of the Indian tuberculosis problem and offering the assistance of a representative committee to give advice:

As the problem of Indian tuberculosis is the most urgent one confronting not only the Department of Indian Affairs, but also the Canadian Tuberculosis Association, we would again at this time desire to offer the help of the Canadian Tuberculosis Association in working out a solution of this acute problem.

Every week the problem is brought to our attention from the provincial health department, tuberculosis officials and from the general public. The feeling is undoubtedly growing that a more aggressive policy will have to [be] adopted, not only for the sake of the Indians, but to protect the interests of the White population as well. The provincial health authorities are protesting against this focus of infection in their midst, over which they have no control. The opinion has been expressed in some quarters that there is a higher incidence of the disease in communities adjacent to Indian reserves. The problem is made even more difficult by reason of the fact that we do not know the one solution that if applied, would be acceptable to all parts of the country. We know the principles that have proved successful in combatting tuberculosis in the White population, but it is not so easy to put into practice these same principles in regard to the Indians of Canada.

It seems strikingly evident that if there was ever a time when a complete survey of existing conditions in regard to tuberculosis among the Indians in the various provinces was necessary, it is at the present time.

The Canadian Tuberculosis Association desires to offer the Department its services for this purpose. It is our belief that we can assemble a committee that would represent all interests, survey existing conditions, and lay down a policy that would be practical and desirable to follow. We believe that this policy would vary in different parts of Canada. While the general principles would be the same, certain features would need to be emphasized in some provinces, while other features should be emphasized in different parts of the country.

We would suggest that such a committee should be truly representative of the Indian Department, provincial health departments, and tuberculosis workers. In addition, it should include a professor of public health and a professor of medicine, from one of our universities, with some representation also from the general public.

The Association would undertake to asemble this committee and to secure personnel capable of undertaking the survey, under the direction of this committee. This would require an expenditure of funds on the part of the Department, but it would place in their hands valuable information from which a policy could be formulated. It would also pave the way for the carrying out of a programme that public opinion will sooner or later demand of the Federal Government.

We would desire that these suggestions be presented to the Minister. Should they receive favorable consideration, we would be glad to discuss the matter with you further at any time.

G.J. Wherrett, M.D.
Executive Secretary[6]

The minister, the Honourable T.A. Crerar, agreed to convene a conference and Dr E.L. Stone, medical director for the Department of Indian Affairs, and Dr Wherrett were authorized to organize the meeting. The conference was held in Ottawa in June 1937 with a full representation from all the tuberculosis authorities of the provinces and the medical services of the department. It was opened by the Honourable C.D. Howe in the absence of Mr Crerar. The situation was reviewed, recommendations were made, and an advisory committee was set up under the chairmanship of Mr John Mac-Eachern, chairman of the Sanatorium Board of Manitoba. An important outcome of the conference was that an additional sum of $50,000 was placed in the departmental estimates for the year, as a result of which the number of Indians under treatment in sanatoria increased to about 300. The following year, 1938, the appropriation was increased to $275,000 and the year after that to $575,000. Thus was begun a diagnostic and treatment program which was enlarged every year until treatment was available for every Indian who required it.

During the following ten years, which included the war years 1939 to 1946, the department made steady progress in its tuberculosis program, despite staff problems. It is sometimes difficult to explain the phenomenon that during wartime it is possible to increase budgetary requirements in spite of the tremendous demand for military needs. The department took every advantage of this seeming relaxation of the former economic restrictions. In 1938 Dr P.E. Moore was appointed assistant to Dr Stone and when the latter entered military service at the outbreak of the war, Moore became acting medical director of medical services. Dr Stone served as embarkation medical officer during the war and obtained a field position in Alberta at his own request following demobilization in 1945. Dr Moore was then appointed medical director.

The next twenty years probably saw the greatest progress, and much of the credit must go to the progressive policies Dr Moore introduced. He was temperamentally suited for the task before him in the department. He was outgoing and aggressive and well able to make his demands known to his minister and in turn to officials of the Treasury Board for the increased funds required. He rendered valuable service as a member of a committee dealing with the ultimate disposal of wartime hospital facilities. Many of these he was able to obtain for the treatment of Indians, such as the Charles Camsell Hospital in Edmonton, the Miller Bay Hospital near Prince Rupert, and the hospital in Nanaimo. He co-operated well with the provincial departments of health and with provincial voluntary bodies. He introduced a complete case-finding service, extended the BCG program, and strengthened the northern services by instituting the Eastern Arctic Medical Patrol – first on the ss *Nascopie* and later on the ss *C.D. Howe*. Many facilities were provided on the boats and films were developed and read at the time of the visit to each settlement.

In addition to acquiring defence hospitals, the department also built hospitals at Fort Qu'Appelle, Moose Factory, and Frobisher Bay on his advice. Nursing stations were introduced among many arctic communities. Dr Moore was a strong believer in the operation of hospitals by the department rather than by church denominations, and hence was often at odds with church authorities. Those who knew him well must testify that his criticisms of the hospital services provided by church authorities applied to all denominations alike, not to any single one as might sometimes have been supposed. This is attested to by the fact that, without exception, his ministers, of whatever religious persuasion, supported him wholeheartedly in his efforts to provide a full and efficient health program. While conscious of the great service church hospitals had rendered in the past, he felt that they had not sufficient funds to carry out the program that was required in the future.

Perhaps his greatest assets were the staff he was able to build up during his term of office. He needed the steadying influence and organizing ability of such persons as Dr Harry Proctor, who was his assistant throughout and was largely responsible for the form of organization which emerged in the national office and in the regional and subregional offices, and who later succeeded him. The set-up of medical directors with lay administrative and nursing assistants proved a sound basic structure. It is interesting to note that while some 300 Indians were reported to be under treatment in 1936–7, ten years later the number had increased to 990 and by 1953 it had risen to 3,200. The number of Indians and Eskimos treated in institutions between 1953 and 1964 is given in Table 7.

Dr Moore also made efforts to interest agencies outside the department in the problems of the Indian and Eskimo. A study was made on health conditions in the James Bay area in 1947 by a group interested particularly in nutrition, financed by the Canadian Life Insurance Officers' Association and sponsored by McGill University, which included Dr Fred Tisdall of the University of Toronto, an authority on nutrition. Another group made a survey of the nutritional conditions at Norway House, Manitoba, in 1945. Dr Moore also organized a study of nutrition in Newfoundland in 1944 and 1948, and a study of health and hospitals in the Mackenzie River district in 1944 in co-operation with the Northwest Territories Council, carried out by Dr G.J. Wherrett, executive secretary of the Canadian Tuberculosis Association, under the auspices of the Social Science Research Council. It was evi-

TABLE 7

Registered Indians and Eskimos in tuberculosis institutions, calendar years 1953–64

Year	Indians		Eskimos		Total	
	Registered in at end	Patient days	Registered in at end	Patient days	Registered in at end	Patient days
1953	2627	965,593	348	125,875	2975	1,091,468
1954	2380	978,285	344	144,185	2724	1,122,470
1955	2284	879,454	698	183,336	2982	1,062,790
1956	1894	770,842	703	231,425	2597	1,002,267
1957	1602	640,588	535	206,551	2137	847,139
1958	1375	528,129	450	186,264	1825	724,393
1959	1209	465,876	345	153,598	1554	619,474
1960	989	410,375	295	111,277	1284	521,652
1961	899	366,923	279	109,043	1178	475,966
1962	753	306,805	292	104,478	1045	411,283
1963	664	270,369	331	130,744	995	401,113
1964	639	244,459	221	107,375	860	351,834

SOURCE: Systems and Statistics Division, Medical Services, Department of National Health and Welfare

dent that tuberculosis was the first health priority in the area, and these findings led to a definite policy for dealing with the disease in the north.

Local hospitals that were empty at the time of the survey were used for initial treatment of patients with open active cases and those recommended for long-term treatment were sent to hospitals in the south. Actually, with the acquisition of the Charles Camsell Hospital, it was possible to treat everyone from Alberta and the western Arctic who required treatment. It was because of the attention focused on these areas that the department was persuaded to build the hospital at Moose Factory on James Bay.

Dr Moore's period of administration was characterized by bold, progressive steps that changed almost overnight the situation in regard to tuberculosis care of Canada's native peoples. At the same time, it should be noted that he was fortunate to work under such outstanding ministers as the Honourable Brooke Claxton and the Honourable Paul Martin. Mention should also be made of deputy ministers such as Charles Camsell of the Department of Mines and Resources and Dr Brock Chisholm and Dr Donald Cameron of the Department of National Health and Welfare, which embraced the Indian medical services in 1957. At this time the Honourable Waldo Monteith was serving as minister of health, and through his ministry and later that of the Honourable Judy LaMarsh and of the Honourable John Munro, the program became a popular one, not lacking in support by either the government or the opposition.

The Advisory Committee on Indian Tuberculosis was formally set up by order-in-council in 1946. In effect, it had the same personnel as the management committee of the Canadian Tuberculosis Association. The subject of Indian tuberculosis was routinely put on the agenda of the annual meeting of the council of the association until about 1960. After that date the committee was convened irregularly at the request of the director of medical services for Indians and Eskimos.

THE ESKIMOS

The epidemic in the Eskimo population seems to have followed a different pattern than that among Indians. It was not so acute in onset or so long in duration. Although miliary and meningeal forms were common, glandular and non-pulmonary forms were not often observed. Along with a seemingly high incidence of the disease, evidence of chronicity and the tendency to calcification were noted. There has been no evidence of acute outbreaks in settlements of the north, although Vilhjalmur Stefansson speaks of an outbreak of 'lung disease' in the area of Coronation Gulf in 1921 and Dr Otto Schafer was told of a period of 'coughing sickness' within the living memory of the inhabitants of Pangnurtung when he served there as medical officer during the 1950s.

Opportunity for universal infection was greater with the Eskimos than with the Indians, confined as they were in igloos and tents, and as they are even now in government housing. How could they have survived without a good deal of natural resistance? The theory is advanced that not only has the Eskimo powers of resistance not enjoyed by the Indian, but that the epidemic followed a slower course, or that there were a series of epidemics by which the Eskimo was exposed to infection over a longer time. It is possible that the first explorers who went into the Arctic, as early as 1576 in the case of Martin Frobisher, took with them individuals who had tuberculosis, some of whom died during the voyages, which often lasted a year or longer. All these men had been in contact with the Eskimos.

The first x-ray survey was carried out in 1947 on the ss *Nascopie* by Dr H.W. Lewis, Medical Services, Department of National Health and Welfare. The medical party took x-ray films of the Eskimos along the Hudson Straits and Southampton Island. These films were developed in Ottawa and read by Dr G.J. Wherrett and further checked by Dr E.J. Lehman of the medical staff of the Ottawa Sanatorium and by the Dr E.L. Ross, medical director of the Sanatorium Board of Manitoba. From the reading of the films alone it was considered that 5.9 per cent had active tuberculosis and 4.7 per cent were considered inactive. Much evidence of calcification was also noted. Similar findings were noted in the films taken at Pangnurtung by Dr J.A. Bildfell in the 1940s during a two-year service at the Anglican hospital there.

During the 1950s the western Arctic was covered by surveys travelling by aeroplane from Edmonton. The eastern Arctic was later covered by the ss *C.D. Howe* of the Eastern Arctic Patrol until 1969, when the aeroplane took over. In the meantime, however, some of the northern hospitals and many of the nursing stations acquired x-ray facilities, and so carried out their own regular surveys.

For nearly twenty years an extensive program of segregation and treatment was carried out, and this became more effective with the development of the newer drugs and the use of chemotherapy. Regular case-finding surveys, including tuberculin tests and x-ray and sputum examination, have also been conducted. All active cases were treated with the new drugs – first in the institutions in the south and later in the settlements of the north where supervision was possible. Deaths declined to the point where in 1969, 1970, and 1971 there was not a single death from tuberculosis among the Eskimos. There has not been the same decrease in morbidity, however, and the incidence on Baffin Island is still in the vicinty of 1 per cent, perhaps the highest morbidity rate anywhere. During the years 1950 to 1971 the Eskimo population increased from 6,680 to 12,080, indicating the effectiveness of the program (see Table 8).

TABLE 8

Eskimo population of Northwest Territories, 1950–71*

Year	Population	Year	Population	Year	Population
1950	6,680	1958	7,814	1965	9,492
1951	6,822	1959	8,058	1966	10,225
1952	6,963	1960	8,337	1967	10,278
1953	7,016	1961	7,977	1968	10,726
1954	7,102	1962	8,316	1969	11,175
1955	7,277	1963	8,615	1970	11,100
1956	7,437	1964	9,064	1971	12,080
1957	7,625				

* 1951 and 1961 are Census figures; remaining years are estimates by Statistics Canada

In 1965 the northern zones were amalgamated into the Northern Region Medical Services of the Department of National Health and Welfare with administrative offices at Yellowknife, and the medical services were centralized in Edmonton. Dr G.C. Butler was appointed regional superintendent and Dr J.D. Galbraith director of chronic disease control.

THE FUTURE OF TUBERCULOSIS CONTROL FOR THE NATIVE PEOPLES

Successive programs in tuberculosis control have followed those elsewhere in Canada. The policy of early diagnosis, prompt treatment, and segregation has been most effective. The advent of modern drug treatment has had miraculous results, and the number of deaths has been drastically reduced, but the disease still occurs with a higher incidence in the Indian population than among the population generally and with an even higher incidence among Eskimos. Awareness of this problem has led to the introduction of a program of prophylaxis whereby drugs are given not only to those with active disease, but for a period of time to those groups where the incidence has been particularly high and the disease prone to develop. In many places native workers have been hired to supervise the administration of drugs at home. In a research project at Frobisher Bay in 1971, for example, native workers were employed in this way, and this ensured that the drugs were taken regularly. It was suggested that through the use of native workers further progress could be made in the control of the disease among the original Canadians.

The target for complete x-ray coverage of all Indians and Eskimos at least once a year has been attained partly because the Indian population was largely concentrated in reservations and hence easy to reach. Mortality and morbidity rates were so high that the mass survey approach was a wise one. Now there are areas where the survey approach has become unproductive and tuberculin testing and sputum examination are receiving more attention and emphasis. They are also much less costly, and perhaps as effective.

In the Arctic nursing has become an important part of the medical services, and nursing stations have been set up throughout the region, usually equipped with x-ray facilities. The nurses have an important role in the control of tuberculosis there, being responsible for the supervision of drug treatment, the examination and supervision of contacts, including tuberculin testing, and the giving of BCG vaccine. In the newer program of prophylaxis they supervise the native workers who are concerned with the day-to-day administration of drugs.

During the years when long-term treatment was the norm and later when the newer drugs were used for treatment great progress was made in reducing the number of deaths and the mortality rate. The policy of prolonged segregation had its effect in lowering the number of new cases, though at the expense of curtailing the liberty of the individual member of the family and of increasing the incidence of family and social problems brought on by the lengthy absence of a member of a family. The present policy of domiciliary care, whereby the patient is treated in the home environment, has made the long periods of exile unnecessary. This policy will be successful just so far as we are able to ensure that the drugs are taken regularly and over a sufficient period of time. There will be disappointments but it is hoped that eventually the disease will be gradually eliminated without too many relapses and fresh outbreaks. It is believed that domiciliary care will lead to greater freedom and happiness for all patients and their families, even though it increases the risk of breaches in our control of the tubercle bacillus in the many communities in Canada.

8

War and Tuberculosis

Although it is questionable whether war influences the incidence of tuberculosis, there is no doubt that other factors associated with war have a great bearing, for good or ill, on the control of the disease. Information obtained from experience in World War I was put to good use during World War II and after.

During the two world wars there was a marked increase in mortality and morbidity in countries in Western Europe directly involved in the war. In Canada the incidence of tuberculosis was not greatly increased in civilians, although it did increase in Ontario during World War I.[1] During that war, the incidence of tuberculosis among the troops on active service was much higher than among a similar group of civilians, however. This was probably due to the close association of young people in army life with unknown infectious cases of tuberculosis, either in barracks, or trenches, or among civilians in the countries where they were stationed. This phenomenon was also observed in naval ratings confined on board ship and exposed to infectious cases. Deleterious effects of the disease, however, were offset by a number of developments which favoured the success of the campaign for early recognition and prompt and adequate treatment not only for the soldier but for the civilian as well.

There were practically no sanatorium facilities for soldiers at the beginning of World War I but the government was subjected to pressure from many sources to deal adequately with the veterans' problems. Commissions and committees discussed the question of pension regulations and responsibilities. Veterans' organizations came into existence, and eventually united to form the Canadian Legion. A subdivision was the Tuberculosis Veterans' Section, which was instrumental in getting useful legislation with regard to the disease on the statutes. The section, formed entirely of tuberculous veterans, had good leadership and sound medical advice, and was instrumental as well in bringing the problem of the tuberculous veteran before the Canadian Pension Commission and its appeal courts.

CARE OF WORLD WAR I TUBERCULOUS VETERANS

The agencies for the medical care of veterans during and after World War I developed slowly. The Military Hospitals Commission and the Department of Soldiers' Civil Re-Establishment were set up after 1917, and later the Department of Pensions and National Health. (The Department of Veterans Affairs and the Department of National Health and Welfare were set up after World War II.) As early as 1916, the soldier suffering from pulmonary tuberculosis had become a problem as far as treatment facilities and rehabilitation were concerned. The Military Hospitals Commission considered the situation and reported on it in two editorials in the *Canadian Medical Association Journal* that year; one dealt with treatment and the other, 'The Tuberculous Soldier,' described the development of facilities for treatment. The latter is so important that it is reproduced here in full:

The Tuberculous Soldier
The tuberculosis problem in connexion with the soldiers of the Canadian Expeditionary Force has been of late carefully considered by the Military Hospitals Commission. On September 15th, a meeting of experts, consisting of Dr Baldwin of Saranac Lake, Drs Parfitt and Elliott of Muskoka, and Dr Byers of Ste. Agathe, met some of the Commissioners. Dr F.J. Shepherd, of Montreal, was in the chair and Lieutenant-Colonel A. Thompson, medical superintendent of all the hospitals under the Commission, was also present. It was reported that at present there are some three hundred and ninety-seven patients under treatment in the various sanitaria for tuberculosis throughout the country. Nearly sixty per cent. of these soldiers have never been overseas. Many of these cases should never have enlisted but having accepted them the country must provide for them. It is anticipated that some thirty patients monthly may be expected from overseas and these with the cases which develop here in the various camps, it is estimated, by the spring will amount to over four hundred cases. These will have to be arranged for. The experts advised making temporary arrangements immediately with existing sanitaria for the treatment of these cases for the coming winter and indicated methods by which inexpensive temporary buildings could be provided. They also advised the purchase of property in localities suitable for the treatment of tuberculosis and erecting thereupon permanent buildings of the most modern type. Already the West is provided for to a great

extent by securing the use of the sanitarium at Frank, Crowsnest Pass, Alberta. This commodious building will hold one hundred and twenty patients and, with the already existing sanitaria at Tranquille, Kamloops, British Columbia, Ninette, Manitoba, and Calgary will afford sufficient accommodation for the present. Quebec will be provided for at Lake Edward and Ste Agathe. The Lower Provinces will be accommodated partly in Quebec and also at the sanitaria already existing at St. John, New Brunswick, Kentville, Nova Scotia, and Charlottetown, Prince Edward Island. In connexion with the sanitaria workshops and recreation rooms will be provided, and occupation suitable to the patients' condition will be insisted upon. The great difficulty is keeping the patients under treatment when they are progressing favourably as after six months they can demand their discharge and go upon a pension. The discipline will be maintained by returned combatant officers who will take military charge of the men.[2]

The next important development after hostilities ceased was the setting up of long-term plans. In April 1920 the director of medical services of the Department of Soldiers' Civil Re-Establishment appointed a board of tuberculosis consultants from the sanatoria consisting of the following specialists in the treatment of tuberculosis: Dr C.D. Parfitt (chairman), medical director, Calydor Sanatorium, Gravenhurst, Ont; Dr W.M. Hart, formerly oc Special (Tuberculosis) Hospital, Lenham, Kent, England, and Saskatchewan Sanatorium, Fort Qu'Appelle, Sask; Dr J.R. Byers, medical superintendent, Laurentian Sanatorium, Ste Agathe des Monts, PQ; Dr A.F. Miller, medical superintendent, Nova Scotia Sanatorium, Kentville, NS; and Dr D.A. Stewart, medical superintendent, Manitoba Sanatorium, Ninette, Man. This board reported on all aspects of the problem of tuberculosis in veterans, and from their reports[3] the department enunciated a policy regarding the treatment of tuberculosis in veterans, covering all aspects of diagnosis, treatment, and follow-up. The report contains valuable information on the incidence of tuberculosis in the Canadian, British, and American expeditionary forces, but perhaps the most beneficial aspect of the report was its recommendation that the veteran should be treated in civilian institutions. This policy was subsequently maintained, with the one exception that if in some provinces civilian sanatorium beds were not available the department was required to provide them. It had to do so in Quebec, but in most other provinces the department assisted in the building of additions to existing institutions.

The rehabilitation and re-establishment of veterans was a matter of great concern after the war, and many excellent reports[4] were prepared, one of which was made by a committee under the chairmanship of Mr J.R. Pyper of Tranquille Sanatorium and the Tuberculosis Veterans' Section of the Canadian Legion. Perhaps the main benefit derived from these reports was the realization that adequate pension benefits were necessary to avoid relapse and that the veteran should not be required to undertake work beyond his capacity.

The board of tuberculosis consultants had recommended that all veterans with open active cases of tuberculosis, and those in which 'the disease was moderately advanced and clinically active' during treatment, should be placed on full pension for two years and subsequently never reduced below 50 per cent pension. This regulation remained in force until after the new drugs became available following World War II.

Reporting in 1921, the Committee on Pensions, Insurance and Re-Establishment of the Department of Soldiers' Civil Re-Establishment concluded the following in regard to the problems facing the tuberculous ex-service man:

As a rule he is hopelessly handicapped and not infrequently permanently so. The tuberculous veterans are probably more or less mutilated for life, whereas a soldier with partial destruction of limbs can be rehabilitated by intensive training in some fit occupation.

Part-time jobs are few and far between, and are generally reserved for old employees. Business men cannot be expected to take into their factories, shops or offices, new employees who are unable to do a full day's work, and who are liable to lie off from time to time. As the war recedes further into the past those who from a patriotic motive made exceptions in favour of ex-soldiers are becoming less numerous. The suggestion that two men, each working half a day, take over one fit man's job is found to be unworkable ...

Even if employers could be found who would take on the average tuberculous patient with all his limitations of service, they not likely would long retain him. The concessions as to hours, etc., which would have to be made, would soon create a great measure of discontent amongst fellow employees ... Indeed it has been found that actually the great majority of employers would far rather be called upon for a direct financial contribution than be asked to find employment for the sub-standard tuberculous man.[5]

Not only was the lack of available jobs a problem, but the working environment of the rehabilitated patient was of paramount concern. Unfortunately, one of the greatest difficulties was that most of the patients belonged to the working classes, and so suffered from the acute problem of how their families would be supported while the veteran patient remained in the sanatorium. It was, therefore, of the utmost urgency that patients be supervised after leaving the sanatorium and helped to secure a suitable means of livelihood when they were unable to return to the heavy work in factories, the impure air of workshops, or the overcrowded, dark, airless, and dusty conditions that would further endanger their health.

By 1921 the recognition of the fact that many tuberculous ex-service men required suitable accommodation, sheltered working conditions, and sympathetic employers, during both treatment and training, resulted in calls for a government agency which would provide such conditions.

Meanwhile, help for those patients still too sick to work was on its way. Through the co-operation of the Tuberculosis Veterans' Association, the Military Hospitals Commission, and the Department of Soldiers' Civil Re-Establishment, a pension plan was devised to aid the patient when he left the sanatorium. With soldiers blending back into the civilian population, however, the suggestion that facilities and treatment be available to everyone was not long in coming. *The Hamilton Times,* in 1917, was quick to remark upon not only the shift in government policy, but also the implications: 'Up to the present the anti-tuberculosis movement in Canada has been entirely voluntary; the work done, assisted more or less by the various governments, has been initiated, may we repeat, by private endeavours; but the time has come when the people as well as the Federal Government should recognize their responsibility to the tuberculous civilians as well as to the soldiers, and from these war emergency measures some permanent institutions and much good should result.'[6]

Continuing along similar lines, Dr D.A. Stewart told the Anti-Tuberculosis Society of Winnipeg:

Among new interests aroused by the war, a renewed interest in tuberculosis is certainly one. It has resulted in the expenditure of large sums of public money in buildings for the care of tuberculous patients, and for the cure of these patients. It has established the treatment of tuberculous patients to an extent that it never was before as a public duty, and a matter of concern to governments. The war has led us to the verge of a new conception regarding illness, its care and cure. If the wounded or tuberculous soldier be cared for until he is well, or helped indefinitely if he should not return to complete health, it is not difficult to argue that the soldier of commerce, or industry, or of agriculture, when disabled, should be cared for in the same way. If the man who fights abroad is to be provided for in illness, why not the woman whose work and child-bearing have broken her down at home; and why not the child, the worker, or, if a stern need should arise, the fighter, of the future?[7]

Most emphatic was the secretary of the Canadian Association for the Prevention of Tuberculosis when commenting upon the work of the Military Hospitals Commission:

With this effective organization of treatment for military consumptives before our eyes, it will be absolutely inexcusable if the country fails to organize an equally efficient campaign against the 'white plague' among our people as a whole ...

When a soldier is found to have tuberculosis, he is given the most scientific treatment in a sanatorium, for as long as his case requires. And he is taught not only how to conquer the disease in himself, but how to avoid spreading it to others. If the same systematic care was applied to civilian consumptives, the gain in health and wealth to the country would be simply enormous.

We must never forget that these soldier patients in the various sanatoria will themselves be civilians again in a few weeks or months. Instead of being a source of infection and danger, as they would have been without the treatment they are now receiving, their return to civil life will be an actual gain to the community; for, by preaching what they have practised, they can do much to arouse us from our lethargy and start a vigorous offensive against this ravishing foe.[8]

Valuable lessons had been learned through the wartime experience. The basis of the sanatorium movement was being laid and it was widely agreed that 'he who can direct wisely ... can treat tuberculosis.'[9] Organization had occurred on grander scales than ever before and optimism was the keynote of the day. Dr Stewart spoke of making the world 'safe for life as well as for democracy,' and envisioned a new era: 'The war has brought to light in all countries undreamt of resources of man-power, woman-power, money-power, enthusiasm, patriotism, self-sacrifice, altruism, organizing ability. If even a tithe of this great stream can be directed into the problems of reconstruction of our social fabric, the world should be a better world for the next generation, almost, than we have ever dreamed of.'[10]

Unfortunately, progress did not reach such ecstatic heights. Enthusiasm waned as time went on and a further hindrance appeared in the form of the Great Depression. Of great value, of course, was the march of medical science and the specific studies which were carried on during these years. After studying the World War I experience, the Canadian Tuberculosis Association estimated in 1940 that for every 100 men killed in action, six had died of tuberculosis, while for every 100 pensioned, twenty-four were pensioned as a result of tuberculosis; the estimated cost to Canada was approximately $150,000,000.[11]

Although there have been separate medical services for veterans ever since World War I, the tuberculous veteran was treated in provincial tuberculosis hospitals along with civilians, except for areas where facilities were lacking. This policy was a rational one because the veteran wanted to be on an equal footing with other citizens. Also, tuberculosis tends to be a family disease and there was no reason why all members of a family should not be treated in the same institution. In retrospect, there is no question but that the policy was a wise one. It assured the veteran of the best tuberculosis services that existed at the time and assisted in his rehabilitation and re-establishment.

TUBERCULOSIS WAR PENSIONS

Pensions were awarded to veterans for tuberculosis after World War I and subsequently if it could be demonstrated that the disease 'arose on service' or was 'aggravated by service.'

Looking back on the way in which the Canadian government dealt with the problem of pensions for tuberculous veterans, one must say that every attempt was made to deal with the matter fairly and generously. There were many difficulties during and after World War I due to the lack of proper examination on discharge, particularly the lack of x-ray reports. Following the armistice of 11 November 1918, the great desire of most members of the armed forces was to get back to Canada quickly and to obtain as speedy a demobilization as possible. The result was that when tuberculosis developed in subsequent years there was no concrete evidence as to whether it had 'arisen on service' and was a 'direct result of service as such.' This posed a great problem for the Pension Commission which had been set up by the government, but through the efforts of the Canadian Legion and the Tuberculosis Veterans' Association, the Pension Commission set up machinery whereby every veteran's claim received careful consideration. In addition, appeal boards were established which met in many centres of the country.

Both the Pension Commission and the appeal boards have been active over the years in considering some of these problems, as indeed they still are. In general, the commission requires evidence that the disease was present on discharge or arose within a year of discharge, which is obtained from a history of continuing symptoms or x-ray evidence of tuberculosis. After World War II the task of the commission was made easier by the information obtained from the x-rays of members of the armed forces on enlistment and discharge.

WORLD WAR II

At the outbreak of World War II in 1939, the Canadian Tuberculosis Association, following the advice of Dr F.S. Burke, made a strong recommendation to the government that all recruits should be x-rayed. Earlier in the year Dr Burke had published an exhaustive study on 'Deaths among War Pensioners'[12] in which he pointed out the extent of tuberculosis in that group. He explained the lengthy treatment that was often necessary, as many pensioners had far advanced disease when diagnosed, and the cost to the treasury for treatment and pensions for such cases. The report also emphasized the necessity for a careful examination of recruits, including an x-ray examination. The association's recommendation was sent to the prime minister, the minister of defence, and the minister of pensions and health. It received a sympathetic response from all, and the machinery was set in motion immediately to have the Canadian army x-rayed before the first contingent proceeded overseas. It was a gigantic task on the part of the newly reorganized Army Medical Services.

Dr G.J. Wherrett, as executive secretary of the Canadian Tuberculosis Association, was in close contact with the officials responsible, who performed outstanding work. They were: Sir Frederick Banting, who had been appointed to the position of consultant on research; Dr W.A. Jones, consultant in radiology; and Dr Duncan Graham, Professor of Medicine, University of Toronto, who had been appointed consultant in medicine. Much of the actual work in setting up standards and supervising the taking and reading of films was done by Dr W.P. Warner, Dr A.C. Singleton, and Dr J.D. Adamson.

Dr Adamson published a paper describing the results of these examinations in 1945.[13] He was instrumental in persuading Dr Brock Chisholm and the Medical Services Directorate to set up the present 'Pulheems' system[14] for the methodical examination and classification of recruits. This received favourable comments from other countries and was an important contribution to military medicare.

As a result of the x-ray examinations, 1 per cent of the recruits were rejected because of tuberculosis. Of this number about one-third were considered to have active disease and were reported to the public health authorities. This was the greatest demonstration of case-finding and early diagnosis that had been made in Canada up to that time and was instrumental in the development of mass community surveys after the war. By the end of the war, army surveys and community surveys in general, together with an awakening of the need for facilities for diagnosis and treatment of

Indians, underlined the shortage of treatment beds. This need was supplied in large measure by utilizing the military hospitals which had been established in various parts of Canada during the war. Many of these were converted to civilian use and were the basis of the greatly expanded Indian Medical Services that later developed.

Although the important question of the x-ray of all recruits had been settled soon after the outbreak of war, other questions involving veterans arose during the war, and these were considered by the Interdepartmental Committee of the departments of National Defence and Pensions and Health, with the executive secretary of the Canadian Tuberculosis Association as consultant and liaison officer with the provincial tuberculosis services.

The experience of World War I provided valuable lessons on how problems should be handled. The advisability of having all recruits x-rayed on enlistment has been mentioned. The problem of x-ray on discharge soon arose. In the first few months of the war this seemed of little importance but when it was realized that a number of men with minimal cases of tuberculosis had enlisted and been discharged after a short service, the need for an x-ray on discharge became apparent in order to determine whether the disease had arisen on service or had been aggravated by it. The Interdepartmental Committee approved a decision to x-ray all members of the armed forces on discharge.

As the war progressed, the problem of supplying medical and other personnel to man the tuberculosis and general medical services in Canada became acute. As part of the larger survey of medical services generally which was then in progress the executive secretary of the Canadian Tuberculosis Association was asked to make a survey of the tuberculosis services and report to the Interdepartmental Committee who, in turn, would make recommendations to the Committee on Manpower. Details of this study are covered in a memorandum, 'Summary of Personnel and Services of Tuberculosis Institutions in Canada (1942).'[15] This study was helpful in allotting manpower to institutions which had lost staff to the services and whose patient load was now increasing by reason of the arrival of the tuberculous veterans.

The facilities of some of the provinces were already overtaxed and unable to handle the additional problem of veterans. The situation was particularly acute in the province of Quebec, where even in peace time the Department of Veterans Affairs had had to operate its own hospital at Ste Anne's because there was not space in the civilian sanatoria.

The Department of Defence authorized Colonel J.C. MacKenzie, hospital consultant, to make plans and specifications for the building of a 600-

bed institution at Senneville at an estimated cost of $6,000,000. By the time plans were completed (1946), the war had ended in Europe and the department began to have second thoughts about the necessity for expending so large a sum. Dr W.P. Warner, director of treatment services, requested Dr G.J. Wherrett and Dr R.A. Benson, superintendent of the Peterborough Veterans Hospital, to make a study of the facilities for the treatment of tuberculous veterans in the province of Quebec and to estimate the future needs and to report to the department.[16] The committee reported that, in the light of experience following World War I, the patient-load would fall rapidly and that not more than 300 beds would be required instead of the 600 planned. The department decided to seek another solution. The Air Force Hospital at Ste Hyacinthe, which was vacant, was found to be sufficient and was acquired, and Dr A.D. Temple was made medical superintendent. As it happened, the new drugs for the treatment of tuberculosis were beginning to take effect at this time, and fewer and fewer beds were being required. The abandonment of the building proposal for a hospital at Senneville represented a saving of $6,000,000.

Factors arising out of two world wars had a favourable influence on the control of tuberculosis, not only in the soldier but also in the civilian. World War I saw the increase in treatment facilities to a much more acceptable level than had hitherto existed. Governments agreed that the veteran who had offered his services in the defence of his country was entitled to the best care which a grateful country could provide. This was the first time that the federal government agreed to provide all the services required for a group of citizens. The facilities were extended sharply in all provinces, and when they were no longer required for veterans, they were made available to civilians. Provincial governments and the public recognized that if the tuberculous veteran who broke down in defence of his country was entitled to care and treatment, so also were the civilian men and women who were doing their share at home. Thus responsibility by provinces and municipalities was more readily accepted after the war.

9

The Effect of Immigration on
Tuberculosis

At the time of the great wave of immigration into Canada before World War 1 voices were raised concerning the magnitude of the problem of tuberculosis not only among citizens of Canada but also among the immigrants who were continually arriving. One voice was that of Dr T.G. Roddick (later Sir Thomas), who made this subject the topic of his maiden speech in the House of Commons in 1899. From 1882 to 1912, 80,673 had died of tuberculosis in Ontario alone; among these were many who came as immigrants.

For information on this matter we are indebted to the excellent papers prepared by Dr Peter H. Bryce when he was medical officer of the interior. In a paper published in *The British Journal of Tuberculosis* in 1908,[1] he lists the number of immigrants entering Canada from 1901 to 1908, a total of 1,097,689:

1900 – 1	49,149
1901 – 2	67,379
1902 – 3	128,364
1903 – 4	130,331
1904 – 5	146,266
1905 – 6	189,064
1906 – 7 (9 months)	124,667
1907 – 8	262,469
Total	1,907,689

He discusses the problem of tuberculosis in these immigrants and gives some figures for the year 1907 for the numbers rejected at seaports and the number who died after admission, as well as some estimated figures for the possible number who were 'tuberculized' at time of entry:

Rejected at seaports	16
Died after admission	12
Evidently tuberculized at time of entry	25
Probably tuberculized at time of entry (not dead)	17
Not tuberculized according to history	15
No particulars as to history	58

Dr Bryce also comments on the attitude of British physicians who had advised a change of climate for patients suffering from chronic diseases, notably tuberculosis:

For many years it has been the custom for physicians everywhere to recommend change of climate, and often of occupation, for their patients suffering from chronic disease, and notably from tuberculosis; and in these days, when Canada has been so advertised, and is so popular a place for emigration as a British land of new opportunities, nothing can be more natural than for British physicians to advise their young and likely patients to come to Canada. And there can be no logical reason why they should not come and enter upon a new life in the Laurentian Mountain area, with its forests, in the north central part of Canada, with their equable climates, and, if cold, yet reconstructive to a remarkable degree, and of thousands of miles in extent, yet everywhere traversed by great rivers and pierced by railway lines. Or, if with family and capital, such a one chooses the illimitable prairies and plateaus to the east of the Rocky Mountains, and takes up farming; he goes where the dry air, bright sunshine and cool breezes, and outdoor life will often restore him to health. But yet, again, should he require the milder influence of the Pacific slope, he may find in British Columbia climates with an annual mean temperature not lower than the Isle of Wight, and yet be in inland valleys or on benchlands from 500 to 2,000 feet in altitude, but so dry that not more than 10 inches is the amount of rainfall, and irrigation of the orchards is a necessity. Such, summed up, is Canada and its relation to the tuberculous immigrant. Remembering all the difficulties of distance from friends, the need for a strong spirit, an initial stage of the disease, and funds adequate for maintenance for some time, it is apparent that the medical profession of England will advise only such patients to come to Canada as will be likely to benefit themselves, and not create a sentiment – to some extent perhaps excusable – that Canada has at times in the past been made the refuge where especially some of England's physical derelicts have been sent with the pious hope and prayer that they may recover, but, if not, then that they may be kindly assisted by some good Samaritan to a peaceful euthanasia. The writer can conceive of no more natural enterprise than that some English enthusiast should go to the valleys of British Columbia, and there, with English capital, English ideals, and English methods, establish a colony in some one of her dry and pleasant valleys. Here, while the tuberculized are worshipping at the shrine of Hygeia and bespeaking her favours, the development of the *rationes vitae* may proceed at the same time on the cattle-ranch or fruit farm.[2]

Provincial authorities deplored the fact that many of these people had not been recognized as tuberculous on entry, although they had been examined for quarantine in inspection services and by the medical examiners of the Department of Immigration. It is quite understandable, however, considering the methods of examination of that day and the great numbers involved, that many cases of tuberculosis were missed.

It was not that the country lacked legislation to reject those with tuberculosis. For instance, the Immigration Act of 1906 prohibited entry of 'persons afflicted with loathsome, contagious and infectious diseases.' Also, there were regulations that provided that people could be deported if, within five years of admission, they had acquired such diseases and had become public charges. This became a serious matter during the depression years of the early 1930s when the case of each immigrant who had become a public charge became a concern of all governments. Many complaints were received by the federal government because recent immigrants had become public charges as inmates of sanatoria and other public institutions. During the years 1930–5 actual proceedings were undertaken to deport immigrants who had become a public charge and it was necessary to report to the Department of Immigration patients in sanatoria who were undergoing treatment at public expense.

Although there were some immigrants who were glad to be returned to the country from which they had come, many of them did not wish to be deported. Furthermore, most sanatorium authorities were in sympathy with the tuberculous immigrant and assisted in making arrangements for treatment outside the institution. Actually, very few tuberculous patients were deported and after 1935 no deportations were carried out.

Some studies of the problem were made, such as that of Dr C.F. Bennett, published as 'Tuberculosis in Recent Immigrants' in the *Canadian Journal of Public Health* in 1940,[3] which showed that the rate of incidence of tuberculosis was higher in immigrants than in native-born Canadians. The Department of Immigration was urged to provide an x-ray examination for all persons applying for immigration to Canada, but it was not until after

World War II that x-raying of all immigrants became mandatory and part of routine procedure. This was an important step because the policy of the department was to preclude the entry of people with active tuberculosis but to allow entry of people with inactive disease because those people whose x-ray showed signs of inactive disease could be supervised and treated, if necessary, by the services of the province in which they were domicilied. In spite of the screening procedure the incidence of tuberculosis has been high among immigrants, and indeed similar to the rate in the country of origin, from which it might be assumed that the infection with the bacillus has been accomplished before entry to Canada. A study carried out by the Ontario Department of Health covering the years 1947–52 showed that the rate of admissions to provincial sanatoria was considerably greater for immigrants than for Ontario residents (see Tables 9 and 10).[4]

Further studies made by the Ontario Department of Health in 1961 and

TABLE 9
Population of Ontario, less immigrants, 1947–52

Year	Population in 1000s	Admissions	Rate per 1000
1947	4042	3086	0.76
1948	4063	2919	0.72
1949	4122	2911	0.70
1950	2197	2905	0.68
1951	4193	2801	0.66
1952	4193	2824	0.67

TABLE 10
Immigrant group in Ontario, 1947–52

Year	Arrivals	Total immigrant population	Cases admitted to sanatoria	Rate per 1000
1947	35,543	65,147	88	1.35
1948	61,621	126,768	159	1.26
1949	48,607	175,378	194	1.10
1950	39,041	214,416	236	1.10
1951	104,842	319,258	278	0.86
1952	86,059	405,317	323	0.79

1971[5] showed the rate for Indians, foreign-born, and Canadian-born, per 100,000, as follows:

	1961	1971
Indians	243.4	105.5
Foreign-born	46.8	30.3
Canadians	19.7	9.1

The improvement over the years is obvious.

TABLE 11
Tuberculosis morbidity rates by country of birth: active tuberculosis in Ontario, 1969–71

Country of birth	Estimated number of cases*			Estimated average annual rate, 1969–70†
	1969	1970	1971	
Austria	11	6	6	30
British Isles	81	79	89	13
Canada				
Non-Indian	605	587	546	10
Indian	90	78	65	140
China	43	39	36	276
Czechoslovakia	14	7	11	53
Finland	11	14	8	56
Germany	12	12	14	11
Greece	25	29	22	84
Hungary	27	10	18	48
India and Pakistan	34	31	23	405
Italy	95	72	69	40
Poland	39	25	21	38
Portugal	36	25	32	130
Russia and Ukraine	23	27	28	38
USA	16	16	13	15
Yugoslavia	32	34	20	84
Other European	55	37	43	29
Other Asian	20	32	38	171
Other countries	17	20	14	35
Total	1286	1180	1117	16.4

* With the exception of Canadian Indians, the estimated number of cases includes a proportional distribution of 137, 78, and 31 cases in 1969, 1970, and 1971 respectively in which the country of birth was not known.

† 1971 Census data were not available at time of preparation. Rates per 100,000 for 1969 and 1970 are based on estimated 1969 and 1970 population figures calculated from the 1961 Census and adjusted for immigration trends.

Other interesting morbidity rates by country of birth are given in the 1971 report from Ontario (see Table 11).

In the first generation of immigrants from many countries, generally the incidence of tuberculosis is higher than for other Canadians, but in subsequent generations the rate falls rapidly to the average rate for Canada. The city of Windsor, which has a high percentage of foreign-born, has a low record in mortality and morbidity, however.

Canada admits many people from other lands which still have a high rate of incidence of tuberculosis. Some of these people may break down with the disease; hence the tuberculosis control program of the provinces places a high priority on the surveillance of the immigrant groups. All those with inactive disease are reported to the province in which they take up residence. This further stimulates our interest in tuberculosis as a world-wide problem.

10

Bovine Tuberculosis

Today it is hard to think of cow's milk as anything but the nourishing, refreshing liquid that dietitians tell us to drink every day, and which the government, via television, encourages us to consume for its numerous health-giving qualities. However, in Canada it is really only relatively recently that milk has been made safe to drink, and in many areas of the world the cow's milk is still unclean and pasteurization unheard of.

Some 2500 years ago Hippocrates described human tuberculosis, but until the turn of the present century there was still considerable controversy over the cause of the disease in its various forms, other than pulmonary, and the method for its cure. For some time the dairy cow was thought to be the villain in the piece. 'The unsuspected but dangerously tuberculous cow'[1] was busily infecting children and adults, urban and rural, rich and poor, by transmitting her disease through her milk used for human consumption.

As time went on the evidence that bovine tuberculosis was an important factor in the tuberculous infections of childhood increased to the point where it could no longer be ignored, and the necessity of undertaking preventive measures became evident. Of the non-pulmonary forms of tuberculosis in Canada, such as glandular disease and disease of the bones and joints, much was of bovine origin. These forms resulted in prolonged ill health and crippling, and often required surgical treatment, which left unsightly scars.

The only son of Dr John G. Rutherford, the veterinary director general, Department of Agriculture in Ottawa in 1902, was weaned at the age of three weeks, and fed thereafter on the milk of a fine Jersey cow purchased especially for that purpose. Only a short while later the child developed a 'peculiar obstinate and intractable diarrhoea.'[2] Though everything possible was done for the boy, he weakened and died. Eventually suspicion fell on the cow. She was slaughtered, and a post-mortem showed her udder to be a 'mass of tuberculous disease.' Some time later, when Dr Rutherford was lunching with a physician friend whose two children consumed large quantities of milk, he questioned the doctor about the wisdom of the practice. The doctor replied that he knew the herd that was the source of the milk and felt quite sure the cows were healthy, and he scoffed at the idea that the children's health could be affected by them. Not long after the doctor's little daughter developed diarrhoea, which was diagnosed as 'consumption of the bowels,' and died within a short time. Later a tuberculous swelling appeared on the doctor's son's neck. 'The matter forced its way up through the eustachian tube to his ear'[3] and pierced the drum. Somehow the matter also reached the boy's eye, which had to be removed to save his life. He lived, but continued in a 'weak and delicate condition.' Too late, the doctor admitted 'his grievous error,' and that tuberculous cows had caused the children's diseases.

Bovine tuberculosis, before pasteurization of milk, was often the cause of death in children up to five years of age. It frequently infected the children between five and fifteen years of age, too, and was the cause of much crippling at these ages though it was not usually fatal. In adults the disease was rarely fatal. Pulmonary tuberculosis was not often found to be caused by the bovine bacillus.

Even as late as 1901 Robert Koch, who had discovered the tubercle bacillus in 1882, was insisting that bovine tuberculosis was only very rarely communicated to man,[4] but in 1908 M.P. Ravenel and Theobald Smith proved him wrong.

Besides being a menace to man, bovine tuberculosis was an expensive proposition to farmers, and caused the ruin of many. The prevention of the disease was a national matter, but because of its widespread prevalence it was deemed unwise, in the first decade of this century, to undertake any program of universal and compulsory testing and slaughter of cattle; not only was there a lack of adequate trained personnel to carry it out, but the economic implications were enormous. It was thought that only a small community or area to which the disease might be restricted could undertake any such program.[5]

It was found in 1910 that the frequency of the occurrence of the disease in cattle was increasing rather than declining, but it was generally believed that eventually the suppression of the disease would be possible.[6] Eradication of tuberculosis from a pure-bred herd was felt to·be 'of even greater importance from an economic view than that of cleaning up the milk supply, although it does not touch so closely the question of public health.'[7] An infected pure-bred bull could contaminate a whole herd, and the disease would be carried through the herd's milk to the farmer's family or others using the milk. For many years, however, owners of pure-bred stock were strongly antagonistic towards any positive action to combat the disease.[8]

By 1925 it was thought that the incidence of bovine tuberculosis in North America did not exceed 12 per cent, and therefore that it was practical to adopt preventive measures.[9] In Canada in 1924 there were 483 herds receiving attention under the supervised herd plan (see below) and by the 1970s bovine tuberculosis was at its lowest level in history. Today animal to man infection is a rare occurrence.

THE ROYAL COMMISSION ON TUBERCULOSIS

In 1901 the Parliament of Great Britain appointed a royal commission of inquiry into tuberculosis which was to report on such aspects as:

1. Whether the disease in animals and man is one and the same;
2. Whether animals and man can be reciprocally infected with it;
3. Under what conditons, if at all, the transmission of the disease from animals to man takes place, and what are the circumstances favourable or unfavourable to such transmission.[10]

The royal commission, called as a result of Dr Koch's pronouncement at the International Congress on Tuberculosis in 1900 against the transmissibility of bovine tuberculosis to human beings, took ten years to deliberate, and presented its final report in 1911, after submitting several interim reports. By 1907 the commission had proved that the bovine bacillus could 'infect children and produce in them the most severe forms of tuberculosis – namely, meningitis and general tuberculosis with ulcerating lesions in the lungs.'[11] Cow's milk containing the tubercle bacillus was found to be clearly a cause of tuberculosis – and fatal tuberculosis – in man. The commission also found that in many cases the human disease was identical with the bovine disease, which could be communicated to man via infected milk and meat. The whole of Dr Koch's theory was thus upset, and the commissioners made the statement that 'after much disputation we are back at the standpoint of 20 years ago.'[12]

Without hesitation the commissioners reported: 'First, that man must be added to the list of those notably susceptible [sic] to tubercle bacilli; second, that mammals and man can be reciprocally infected with the disease; third, that the disease may be communicated from different mammals to man from infected cows' milk, it having been clearly shown that a large portion of the tuberculosis of childhood is due to infection from this source and from tuberculer [sic] meat.'[13]

The royal commission urged: 'That existing regulations and supervision of milk production be not relaxed; that, on the contrary, the Government should cause to be enforced, throughout the kingdom, food regulations planned to afford better security against the infection of human beings from the medium of articles of diet derived from tuberculous animals. More particularly we would urge action in this sense in order to avert or minimize the present danger arising from consumption of infected milk.'[14]

THE INTERNATIONAL COMMISSION ON BOVINE TUBERCULOSIS, 1909

At its annual meeting in Chicago in 1909, the American Veterinary Medical Association appointed the International Commission on Bovine Tuberculosis. Members of the commission came from the United States and Canada, and meetings took place in both countries. The chairman was Dr J.G. Rutherford, the director general and live stock commissioner of the Canadian Department of Agriculture. The Canadian and United States departments of agriculture, other government bodies, university authorities, and private individuals all contributed to the work of the commission.

Although the international commission's work was concurrent with that of the British royal commission, its deliberations on the various aspects of the disease, including eradication and prevention, were more exhaustive.

There was a widespread grievance on the part of the farmers of the day about bovine tuberculosis and the dangers that threatened them. Since seeing was believing, demonstrations showing the diseased parts of a slaughtered seemingly healthy animal, especially chosen to show the ravages of the disease, were organized, which were far more effective than merely telling farmers about the disease or handing out literature. The commission did, however, promote other educative measures as well. It encouraged the publication of authoritative articles in agricultural, dairy, veterinary medicine, and sanitary journals and in newspapers; gave lectures to agricultural societies, farmers' institutes, and unions, especially those interested in creameries and cheese factories; urged veterinary schools to put special emphasis on courses in bovine tuberculosis and its control; requested agricultural departments and veterinary and livestock sanitary boards to promote prevention; and especially recommended that a pamphlet be written in 'language intelligible to the layman'[15] and be distributed free. This pamphlet, entitled *Tuberculosis; a Plain Statement of Facts Regarding the Disease; Prepared for Farmers and Others Interested in Live Stock,*[16] appeared in 1911. It proved to be a most informative and valuable publication, worthy of consideration at some length here. The following sections are based on the publication.

The Tubercle Bacillus

The germ which causes tuberculosis, the tubercle bacillus, is quite invisible to the naked eye. It is tiny, thin, and rod-shaped. Seen through a powerful microscope, one would need several thousand to measure one inch. However small it may be, the bacillus grows longer and multiplies rapidly, by dividing crosswise, once it has gained foothold inside an animal. Under favourable conditions only a few hours are necessary for the production of a new generation. Before long, the natural body forces begin to battle the army of invaders. The white cells of the blood endeavour to destroy the bacillus, and sometimes they are successful. More often they fail, and are themselves destroyed. In the second phase the cells of the invaded tissue arrange themselves in a circle around the germs and try to form a living wall between the germs and the rest of the healthy body. This wall becomes thicker and thicker, eventually forming a hard lump, called a tubercle. If successful, the bacilli imprisoned in the tubercle die, and the disease in that particular spot is then arrested.

Unfortunately, more frequently than not, both the blood and the cells are unsuccessful in their efforts, and the bacilli are carried through the blood stream, or lymph channels, to infect other parts of the body. As each new process begins the animal loses some of its resistance, the tubercles increase in number, and eventually the animal succumbs to the disease.

The tubercle bacillus can flourish only within the body of an animal, though, if conditions are favourable, it can live for some time outside, for instance, in a dark, dirty stable. It is destroyed by sunlight; freezing temperatures do it no harm, but a moderate amount of heat will kill it. If the bacillus is protected by a layer of dried mucous, coughed up from a diseased lung, it can readily withstand light, drying, or disinfectants, though steam or boiling water will kill it quickly enough. Germs can escape from a diseased cow by the mouth, nose, bowels, in the milk, or in discharges from the genital organs; and when this is the case it is generally referred to as 'open tuberculosis.' When a cow's udder is infected her milk contains vast numbers of the germs, but still looks and tastes perfectly good. Therefore, unsuspectingly, the disease is transmitted to young animals, and 'it is very dangerous to children' (p. 20).

Herd Infection

The booklet made clear the various ways a herd could become infected: (1) by the purchase of an infected animal, usually thought to be healthy; (2) by feeding calves with milk, buttermilk, or whey from an infected cow (it was recommended that milk purchased from a dairy should be boiled or pasteurized); (3) by showing cattle at fairs, where no proper care is taken to keep out diseased animals, or to keep sanitary, disinfected stables; (4) by shipping animals in railway cars that have not been disinfected, and which may have recently carried diseased animals; and (5) by allowing healthy cows to come into contact with infected ones.

Though the tubercle bacillus itself multiplies quickly, tuberculosis as a disease develops slowly. A cow can be infected for months, and sometimes years, and still look perfectly healthy. The only way her condition can be detected is to submit her to a tuberculin test.

Tuberculin is a fluid containing the products of the tubercle germ without the germs themselves. As it contains no living germ, it cannot convey the disease. Great skill is required in its preparation. A special fluid (or culture medium) is prepared and the tubercle bacilli planted in it, great care being taken to keep all other germs out. The fluid is then placed in a special kind of incubator and kept at the temperature of the animal body. Under these conditions, the germs grow and multiply. Gradually the fluid becomes filled with the products of the germs. When the right point is reached the fluid is heated sufficiently to kill the germs which are then strained out. The remaining fluid is tuberculin. (p. 22)

Tuberculin is not harmful to a healthy cow, even in large doses. However, within eight to twelve hours a diseased animal will develop a feverish attack, which lasts a few hours before subsiding. The fever is evidence of infection and called a 'reaction,' and the animal is said to be a 'reactor.' Healthy animals do not react.

The tuberculin test, when done by a competent and experienced practitioner, is more accurate than any other method of detecting tuberculosis. Its accuracy is 90 per cent with a 2 per cent margin of error, which can be lessened by taking more care while making the test. Any animal reacting to the test is therefore considered tuberculous. There are a few precautions that should be considered: a cow who has recently calved should not be given the test as her temperature may not be normal at that time; the test should not be given to an animal who is already obviously feverish; also, an animal who has only recently been infected will not react, as incubation takes from ten days to two months. If an animal is so far gone as to be obviously already wasting from tuberculosis, the test will fail – and is unnecessary.

Pasteurization
The milk from tuberculous cows need not be wasted, the booklet goes on to say, even though it contains germs. By the simple method of pasteurization, that is, by heating the milk to 149°F for five minutes, the germs are killed, and the milk is made safe. It is not necessary to boil the milk.

Eradication of Tuberculosis in a Herd
If more than half of a herd is found to be infected, it is a pretty safe assumption that many of the other animals are in a state of incubation, and so, if an animal does not react to the first test, it will probably do so at the second six to twelve months later, in the meanwhile probably developing enough disease to infect several of her otherwise healthy fellows. It is therefore easier in such a situation to consider the whole herd diseased, and so commence building a new and healthier herd. This can be done by removing newborn calves immediately from their diseased mothers and allowing them to be raised by a healthy mother, or by feeding them exclusively on pasteurized milk. Calves should be tested at six months, and if non-reacting should be kept apart to become a member of a healthy herd.

Dark, dirty byres afford tuberculosis germs the most favourable conditions to spread rapidly, and make it almost impossible to keep them out. On the other hand, byres that are clean, airy, well-drained, and well-lighted are unfavourable and germs brought in do not spread quickly and are reasonably easy to get rid of. The ideal byre has lots of light, a high ceiling, roomy stalls, and wide passages, as well as some form of ventilation so that foul air can be replaced by fresh.

Keeping a Healthy Herd
The booklet suggests three methods of establishing and maintaining a healthy herd: the Bang system, Ostertag's method, and the Manchester method.

The Bang system necessitates the keeping of two herds, one consisting of reactors to the tuberculin test and the other of animals which have proved to be healthy. Each herd is kept quite separate, where possible even in different buildings. Each has its own attendants, who use different utensils. Calves born to the diseased herd are moved immediately to the healthy herd. As a result the healthy herd increases as the diseased one decreases, the infected animals being disposed of as quickly as possible. Ultimately, there will be only one completely healthy herd, which should be tuberculin tested regularly, annually or semi-annually, so that latent cases or recently infected animals can be detected and removed.

Ostertag's method is a variation of the Bang system, which demands only the clinical examination of the original herd and the elimination of all open cases. Calves of diseased mothers are immediately removed, and the herd tuberculin tested at stated intervals.

Both the Bang and Ostertag methods were not too popular in Canada as they necessitated a great deal of time and care; nevertheless, the use of both methods was encouraged as of unquestionable economic value in purebred beef or dairy herds.

The Manchester method was simply either of the two above-mentioned methods applied to local areas, or even individual farms, from which centres the work could progress into the surrounding or neighbouring districts and farms.

ERADICATION OF BOVINE TUBERCULOSIS

All efforts to eradicate bovine tuberculosis needed the co-operation of the livestock owners. Tuberculin, discovered in 1890, came into use in Canada in 1894, when it was applied to experimental farm herds; animals who reacted were kept for experimental tuberculosis work. The test was officially recognized in Canada and the United States a few years later, and in 1897 an agreement between the two countries was signed, requiring all cattle to be used as breeding stock and all milk products imported from either country to the other to be subjected to, and pass, a tuberculin test made by federal government veterinary inspectors.

The first tuberculosis control policy was adopted in 1896, and consisted of free testing of herds by government officials. The testing was not compulsory, and no compensation was paid for the slaughter of infected animals.

In 1903 an order was passed providing for the permanent marking of cattle reacting to official tests. This consisted of punching a letter 'T' through the animal's right ear. The same year a regulation was passed prohibiting the export of cattle so marked. As the demand for tuberculosis-free cattle increased, more modern policies were adopted. By 1905, a supervised herd plan was made available to livestock owners, whereby the animals were tested without charge to the farmer. A national meat inspection program was introduced in 1907. This provided reliable statistics on the incidence of tuberculosis in animals slaughtered, which, in turn, provided impetus for the development of programs aimed at the control and eradication of the disease. The next important advance was the Municipal Tuberculosis Order, which was passed in 1914, the first tuberculosis compensation policy of the Department of Agriculture. It provided for the licensing of all milk vendors, for clean and sanitary dairies, for the prohibition of the sale of milk within two years of the testing of a cow, and for the appointment of a municipal inspector. Though a popular measure, it was discontinued in 1923, because it proved impossible to control bovine tuberculosis under its provisions and, it was recognized, Canada could not develop its foreign markets without such controls.

Accredited Herd Plan

In 1919 an Accredited Herd Plan was instituted in Canada to meet the insistent demands of livestock breeders for action in the control of the disease. This plan was optional, but immediately won the support of the 'purebred breeders.'

In order for a herd to be fully accredited it had to pass two or three semi-annual tests without a reactor. Very few herds were 'clean' when first tested but after two years of operation of the plan there were only eighteen herds on the list with reactors. At least one-third of a herd had to be made up of registered cattle.

Between 1 April 1924 and 8 January 1925 under the accredited herd plan 116,572 tuberculin tests were given and 5790 reactors found; under the restricted area plan (see below) 45,553 tests were given and 3106 reactors slaughtered; under the Municipal Tuberculosis Order 61,889 tests were made and 2030 reactors found. Therefore, 223,994 tuberculin tests were made, 10,566 infected cattle found, and $537,688 paid out in compensation.[17] Compensation was paid to owners of reactors on a varying scale: half the value of the animal if it was slaughtered as an open case of tuberculosis, and one-third the value if it was slaughtered at the owner's request. However, if the dairyman was not co-operative in trying to clean up his herd, no compensation was paid at all.[18] By 29 October 1925 there were 1989 fully accredited herds in Canada, which meant that there were more than 69,000 cattle certified as being free of tuberculosis. Another 2217 herds were in the process of accreditation, and 234 were awaiting action.[19] Farmers whose herds did not qualify for accreditation could receive similar services under the 'supervised herd' plan, which, however, was not too popular as no compensation was paid for reactors.

Restricted Areas

In 1922, another step was taken in passing restricted area regulations which provided for the eradication of bovine tuberculosis in definite areas. Several townships around Carman, Manitoba, were the first to take advantage of them. All the cattle were tested three times, and those on infected premises even more often. Of 16,500 cattle tested, approximately 5½ per cent reacted and were slaughtered on the first test, 0.5 per cent on the second, and 0.3 per cent on the third. Almost $38,500 was paid out in compensation for the slaughtered animals. This demonstrated, beyond question, that satisfactory progress could be made in controlling the disease if cattlemen were interested and co-operative.

Restricted areas provided 'clean areas' for 'clean herds.' They also permitted the use of common pastures, thus doing away with double fences and the other inconveniences of keeping the animals apart, as well as lessening the restrictions on the services of valuable herd sires and so facilitating breeding operations, the improvement of stock, and the elimination of scrub bulls.

The restricted area regulations also promoted better accommodation for the cattle and better general sanitary conditions. Community support and co-operation were encouraged as general interests were protected. The regulations also provided safer milk supplies, thus reducing the incidence of tuberculosis in children. Herd profits increased and active markets at higher prices were created because of the great demand for 'area cattle.' They also provided the most practical and economical method for the Department of Agriculture and livestock owners to test systematically the greatest number of cattle in a given period, and reduced the shipping costs of reactors since they could be consigned in carload lots. 'Outside cattle' were not allowed into restricted areas, except to be slaughtered at suitable points, unless they showed satisfactory tuberculin tests.

The Department of Agriculture maintained constant supervision over the restricted areas, and their policy represented the most efficient method for eradicating bovine tuberculosis.

Because of the natural isolation and the remarkably low incidence of bovine tuberculosis there, the whole of Prince Edward Island was declared a restricted area in 1922. In 1925, 95,298 cattle were tested and 559 reactors found (0.5 per cent), and in 1929 fewer than 0.2 per cent of cattle tested reacted.

By 1954 there were 503 restricted areas in Canada, which included about 80 per cent of the country's 8½ million cattle. By 1959 Canada had some 11 million cattle, fewer than 2000 of which reacted and were destroyed. The whole country is now considered a 'restricted' area, and all reactors are automatically destroyed. Fewer than 0.1 per cent of Canada's cattle are infected,[20] but total eradication remains the goal of the Department of Agriculture. Even with such a superb record, Canadian farmers cannot relax. Vigilance is still necessary. Testing must continue on a routine basis; one infected animal can spoil a whole herd, as indeed can the farmer himself if he has unwittingly contracted the disease.

In June 1961 the first general test of all cattle in Canada was completed. All in all, some 50 million tuberculin tests had been done, 400,000 reactors ordered slaughtered, and approximately $15 million paid out to owners from the inception of the plan.

PASTEURIZATION OF MILK

Pasteurization of milk is the process by which milk is heated for a definite length of time at a moderate heat, usually about 30 minutes at 60°C (it being essential that the liquid be kept in motion), to kill any pathogenic bacteria that may be present and discourage other bacterial development. This process was discovered by (and so named after) the French chemist and father of bacteriology, Louis Pasteur (1822–95). At first, pasteurization was often confused with the boiling of milk, and since boiled milk was considered hard to digest, the method was looked upon askance in some quarters. The initial denials were not sufficent to outweigh the obvious benefits to be gained, however. Pasteurization of milk is now a generally accepted method of purification, and the milk so treated is both wholesome and suitable for feeding to infants.

Pasteurizing milk has three objectives: '1) to reduce the diarrhoeal diseases of infants; 2) to control epidemics of typhoid fever, scarlet fever, septic sore throat and other communicable diseases of human origin; 3) to guard agaist the dissemination of bovine tuberculosis.'[21]

In Ontario, the first ordinance requiring the pasteurization of milk for sale was passed in Toronto in 1918, and compulsory pasteurization throughout the province followed in 1938, despite the violent opposition of many dairy farmers. The bill was sponsored by Premier Mitchell Hepburn, who had become convinced that pasteurization would eliminate bovine tuberculosis in children when he heard that since 1915 no child born or raised in Toronto had been admitted to the Hospital for Sick Children suffering from the disease,[22] but met with much opposition, even in caucus. Only after a member of the house, a hunchback, rose to his feet and said 'Gentlemen, if you have any doubts about the wisdom of this bill, look at me. I am the victim of dirty milk,' did the bill pass without a dissenting vote.[23]

In the province of Quebec, the city of Montreal had a by-law relating to milk dating back to 1890, and in 1907 a pasteurization plant was opened, the first in the province. Sale of the pasteurized milk progressed slowly, however, since the price was higher than for raw milk – ten cents a quart rather than eight. By 1912 only about 30 per cent of all milk sold was being pasteurized. By 1920, 55 per cent of all milk sold was pasteurized, but there was still much opposition to the by-law. A revised by-law passed in July 1925 requiring pasteurization only for milk which did not meet the requirements for what was then called 'special (raw) milk,'[24] reduced the opposition somewhat, though not entirely, and by 1945, 98.17 per cent of all milk sold in Montreal was pasteurized, the remaining 1.83 per cent being the 'special (raw) milk.'[25] Legislation in other parts of the province came much later. Indeed, it was not until 1943 that a campaign was launched by the Quebec Division of the Health League of Canada for pasteurization throughout the province. In the next two years sixteen cities, as well as a few townships and villages, passed legislation for compulsory pasteurization of all milk and cream in their localities; and in 1945 there were 138 pasteurization plants, eleven more were under construction, and six were awaiting government endorsement.

The story of the introduction of the pasteurization of milk in the rest of Canada is a long and drawn-out one, and will not be told here. Though advocated in Quebec and Ontario as early as the 1890s, it took some time for other parts of the country to adopt the two measures that were to prove so useful in the control of bovine tuberculosis, namely the pasteurization of milk and the elimination of the disease in dairy cattle by the use of the tuberculin test and the destruction of those cattle which gave a positive test. In a resolution passed by its executive committee in June 1935, the Canadian Public Health Association stated: 'The necessity for general pasteurization is amply demonstrated every year in our high death-rates from diarrhoea and enteritis, in our milk-borne typhoid epidemics or septic sore throat epidemics, the increasing cases of undulant fever, and our cripples from bovine tuberculosis. Our objective must be safe, clean, wholesome milk. Proper pasteurization is the only means of assuring protection against milk-borne disease.'[26]

It has been a long struggle to get these measures universally adopted, but it is interesting to note that the control of bovine tuberculosis formed part of the early general campaigns and that in some instances more attention was paid to the problem of the bovine disease than to the human.

11

The International Picture

Tuberculosis is still a tremendous health problem when viewed in global dimensions. It is estimated that, of the three and a half billion inhabitants of this earth, twelve to fifteen million have active cases excreting tubercle bacilli. Tuberculosis has always been associated with poverty and it is therefore not surprising that it is very unevenly distributed among the people of the world. In wealthy countries it has declined to low levels although even in such countries it still presents a substantial problem among the less privileged groups in the community, such as among the native people of Canada and the negroes in the ghettos of the cities of the United States. The vast populations of Asia and Africa, however, with their low economic status, still experience incidence rates which are ten to twenty times higher than those observed in Canada.

The decline of tuberculosis in Canada and other developed countries was at first achieved by costly case-finding procedures such as mass radiography, by long treatment in hospital, and by improved standards of living, better nutrition, and a better understanding of the disease and the dangers of infection from open cases. It was soon realized that a similar program of case-finding and long periods of hospitalization for tuberculous patients in developing countries would not be possible, because of the prohibitive cost. A new approach was needed.

When the World Health Organization came into being in 1948, two new weapons to fight the disease had become available: the miracle drugs and BCG vaccination. Under the leadership of Dr Johannes Holm (the tuberculosis consultant for WHO) and later Dr Halfdun Mahler, now director general of WHO, the newer program of using drugs on a domiciliary basis and vaccinating with BCG was undertaken. Dr Holm had organized an international BCG program in 1947, which was sponsored by the Danish Red Cross.

It has been known for a long time that the most important sources of infection are persons suffering from advanced pulmonary tuberculosis, whose sputum contains enough bacilli to be visible on microscopy. These can be identified easily by technicians who are specially trained to make smears of sputum, stain them, and recognize the bacilli. In most developing countries microscopy technicians are available at even the lowest level of the health service, such as in village health centres. In India it has been shown that 11 per cent of patients complaining of a productive cough of more than two weeks' duration have tuberculosis with a positive sputum smear. The cost of finding such a case in India is approximately $3.40. Once the diagnosis is made the patient is treated by simple, cheap, ambulatory chemotherapy regimens, which have been thoroughly tested by the Tuberculosis Chemotherapy Centre in Madras. The current recommendation is to treat tuberculous patients on a daily basis with three drugs – streptomycin, isoniazid, and thiacetazone – for an initial period extending for several weeks; this is followed by at least 12 months' chemotherapy with two drugs, the two being either INH and thiacetazone given daily or streptomycin and a larger dose of isoniazid given twice weekly, the latter having the advantage that it is given completely under supervision.

In most developing countries the antituberculosis program has been conducted by specially trained workers in health units. The success has been remarkable. Without chemotherapy approximately half of the patients with pulmonary tuberculosis would be expected to die within two years of the onset of the disease but under the program the fatality rate has been reduced to at least a fifth, only about 10 per cent of such patients dying from the disease. In addition there has been a considerable reduction in human suffering, though this is difficult to measure. When no drugs are given for tuberculosis only about 25 per cent of patients manage to overcome the disease and become cured, but with the simple chemotherapy given under the program the proportion rises to at least 66 per cent. Unfortunately, some patients fail to become cured by chemotherapy and become chronic cases having positive sputum for many years. Little is known as yet about the quality of life of such chronic cases, or of their importance as sources of infection to others. Such sufferers usually harbour tubercle bacilli which are resistant to the drugs and they may pass on the resistant infection to others.

The problem of resistance of tubercle bacilli is much greater in many developing countries than in Canada or in other wealthy countries. The actual extent of the problem is not known, but in some countries it is suggested that as many as one-third of newly diagnosed patients may be infected with resistant bacilli. The true figure may be lower, however, because of the difficulty in checking whether patients have had chemotherapy previously, for some deny this lest an admission will mean that they will not receive further treatment. Nevertheless the problem of resistance in developing countries does exist, as is demonstrated by recent immigrants to Canada from Asia who have developed tuberculosis following their arrival but been found to have resistant organisms. The causes of high rates of bacterial resistance in these countries are irregular taking of drugs and poorly prescribed treatment. Unfortunately in many developing countries it is possible to obtain antituberculous drugs from a druggist without prescription and consequently self-medication is fairly common. Furthermore, some patients receive the correct treatment from private physicians but discontinue it, for economic reasons, as soon as they feel better, long before any permanent cure can have been achieved. Lastly, the treatment prescribed under the program, although generally good now, has been sometimes inadequate. For example, in India many years ago, due to shortage of drugs, isoniazid alone was used in certain parts of the country. This saved lives but was the cause of a lot of bacterial resistance.

At present, the antituberculous drugs used in the program of any one country are purchased by the government of that country; previously UNICEF supplied drugs to a number of countries on the recommendation of the World Health Organization.

BCG vaccination is used extensively in all developing countries and constitutes the second of the two prongs in the fight against tuberculosis. A Medical Research Council trial in the United Kingdom has shown that BCG vaccination is 80 per cent effective, i.e., the tuberculosis incidence rate in the vaccinated is reduced by 80 per cent over a period of more than ten years. Other trials have been carried out, but the results have been less spectacular. So far no trial of BCG in tropical or subtropical countries has been completed, but one is currently being undertaken in South India; its results are eagerly awaited as they will reveal the effectiveness of this measure under conditions vastly different from those of previous trials.

The BCG program varies from country to country. In some, only the newborn are vaccinated; in others, BCG is applied exclusively to the adolescent group; and in others the policy is still to vaccinate at birth and revaccinate at school age. Although it is unlikely that the 80 per cent efficacy shown in the British Medical Research Council trials will be achieved by any of these vaccination programs, there is little doubt that this simple and cheap measure has prevented many deaths from tuberculosis and much tuberculous disease, particularly in the form of tuberculous meningitis, which occurred frequently in recently infected children, often leading to death or giving rise to permanent disability.

The incidence of tuberculosis in the world is declining, and the decline is to a great extent due to the program developed by the World Health Organization. Its program of treating the disease on a domiciliary basis in the community rather than by costly institutional treatment is the only one possible for poorer countries with high incidence rates.

Many features of the antituberculosis program in developing countries are changing, partly because a number of these countries can now afford to allocate more funds to it. In particular, we can look forward to integration of the tuberculosis program within a broader program oriented towards public health generally. Improved diagnostic procedures are also being introduced, as well as better treatment programs for those patients who fail on initial chemotherapy. Effort is being made, too, to avoid unnecessarily prolonged treatment for patients who either have already been cured or who have become chronic and resistant cases and can no longer benefit from drugs offered in the program. The antituberculosis programs in developing countries will probably have to remain essentially oriented toward public health in the foreseeable future, with individual treatment of patients remaining the exception rather than the rule. Nevertheless an increased sophistication in diagnosis and treatment and the stratification of patients into groups requiring different management will undoubtedly become possible, leading in turn to improved results.

INTERNATIONAL UNION AGAINST TUBERCULOSIS

With the arousal of interest in the prevention and cure of tuberculosis around the turn of the century came the realization that the problem was worldwide. Many attempts were made in different parts of the developed world to organize a concerted attack on the problem and explore what could be done to fight the disease. Congresses and conferences were held, and voluntary associations with an international interest were set up. The result of these first assemblies was the formal organization, in 1920, of a body called the International Union against Tuberculosis.

The purpose of the union was twofold: to provide a forum where doctors and scientists from many countries could meet and exchange information and ideas on the most modern methods of fighting the disease, and to encourage the formation of voluntary associations aimed at stimulating people and governments to undertake active tuberculosis programs.

The Health Section of the League of Nations, which was formed after the First World War and succeeded by the World Health Organization after the Second World War, welcomed the union as a partner. Over the years there has been close co-operation between the two organizations.

The international union was officially organized in 1920, but before that a Congress for the Study of Tuberculosis in Man and Animals had been held in Paris in 1867, at which fifteen countries were represented by physicians and veterinarians (there is no record of Canada being represented). Four more congresses were held, also in Paris, in 1888, 1891, 1893, and 1898. At the last initial steps were taken to form an international association at the suggestion of a Viennese professor of medicine. This association, a forerunner of the union, was called the International Anti-Tuberculosis Association. These congresses sparked the formation of a number of organizations in Europe and America as well, such as a society for the establishment of sanatoriums for the consumptive poor organized in 1890 in Vienna, which was the earliest recorded national association in the tuberculosis field. In 1891 a French league against tuberculosis came into existence, and about the same time the National Association for the Prevention of Consumption was organized in London, England. The Ligue National Belge contre la Tuberculose was organized in Belgium in 1898, an association known as Assistencia nacional aos Tuberculosos was established in Portugal in 1899, and a national organization in Italy was also reported. The Canadian Association for the Prevention of Consumption and Other Forms of Tuberculosis, later to be renamed the Canadian Tuberculosis Association, was organized in Canada in 1900, an organization was formed in Denmark in 1901, and what is now the National Tuberculosis Association in the United States was established in 1904. These may not have been the only national organizations to combat tuberculosis at the turn of the century, but they show that Europe was then leading the way in tuberculosis control.

The First International Tuberculosis Congress, sponsored by the International Anti-Tuberculosis Association, was held in Berlin in 1899, under the auspices of the German committee. This congress was recognized as the first truly international gathering in the field of tuberculosis, with official representatives appointed by governments and voluntary associations. It was also open to the public. Two thousand people attended the meetings at the Berlin Reichstag, and the Empress Augusta Victoria opened the proceedings. A prize for the best essay given at the meeting was won by Dr S. Adolphus Knopf, a tuberculosis specialist of New York City. His essay, on 'Tuberculosis as a Disease of the Masses and How to Combat It,'[1] was published in 1901 and may have been the first piece of educational material on tuberculosis to circulate around the world. By 1913 it had been published in thirty-four editions and twenty-four languages.

The Second International Congress was held in 1900 in Naples, Italy, and was graced by the presence of King Humbert I and Queen Margherita. The Third Congress was held in London in 1901, with Robert Koch, discoverer of the tubercle bacillus, in attendance. It was notable for the heated discussion which arose over Koch's beliefs regarding the possibility of man being infected by the bovine bacillus and cattle being infected by the human variety. Sir William Osler was listed among those present.

At the 1902 meeting in Berlin the double-barred cross, or Lorraine cross, was adopted as a badge of the conference, and so became the symbol of the voluntary movement against tuberculosis in many countries. Another event of great importance at that meeting was the introduction, by Dr Karl Turban of Switzerland, of an international uniform nomenclature or classification of tuberculosis. Also, great improvements were made in organization, memberships were set up, and a constitution was drafted. At the fifth conference, held in Paris in 1905, about 4000 delegates were registered and 1000 papers listed in the program. An international committee of the association was set up at this meeting with Dr William Osler as chairman. Twenty-one national associations were reported as having been organized and were accepted as members of the association.

The Sixth International Congress was held in Washington, DC, in 1908. Theodore Roosevelt accepted the presidency of the congress and addressed the last session. This was the first meeting to be held outside of Europe. The attendance was over 6700, and thousands more visited the large exhibit which had been prepared for the occasion. Foreign delegates included Dr Robert Koch, Sir Robert Philip, Dr Albert Calmette, and other distinguished people. Canada was represented by Dr J.H. Elliott and Dr George Porter; Dr C.J. Fagan of British Columbia also attended. Their reports are in the records of the Canadian Tuberculosis Association.[2] It was at this meeting that the 'Christmas Stamp' was first mentioned, and delegates were informed that the stamps would be sold 'for the benefit of the Red Cross anti-tuberculosis work.'

International meetings continued to be held every year, either a large 'congress' of members and delegates from governments and national associations or a smaller 'conference' or closed meeting of members. (Today the international union holds conferences only.) Prestige was given to the meetings by the interest and actual presence of royalty or heads of state, who testified to the importance of tuberculosis in the national life of every country. The gatherings generated great enthusiasm in many countries, and included discussion on medical procedures and techniques which today we take for granted.

But the clouds of war were closing in on Europe, and the conference in Berlin in 1913 was the last to be held by the International Anti-Tuberculosis Association which had done so much to stimulate the organization of national associations. Credit must be given to Germany for its work in organizing the first international conference on tuberculosis.

Seven years later, in 1920, after the close of hostilities and the collapse of Germany, representatives of thirty-one countries met in Paris and established the International Union against Tuberculosis with Sir Robert Philip of Edinburgh as president. Paris was chosen as headquarters. Tuberculosis incidence rates in all the European countries had risen sharply during the war, a natural result of lack of food and the breakdown of medical services, so help on an international level was needed more than ever. At this organizing meeting Canada was represented by Dr J. Odilon Leclerc who, on his return, gave a masterly report to the Canadian Tuberculosis Association on the 'Organization of Anti-Tuberculosis Campaigns.'[3] The minutes of these early meetings are sketchy indeed. Each year a conference was held in various capitals of Europe until 1926, when the conference took place in Washington, DC. This was a great event for this continent, and twenty-nine foreign countries were represented by 101 delegates, not a large number by today's standards, but large for the time given the facilities for travel, the difficulties of foreign exchange, and the limited budget of the organizations of that day. Canada was well represented; indeed the annual meeting of the Canadian Tuberculosis Association was held in Washington at the same time, the only one ever to be held outside of Canada.

At the conference in Rome in 1928, 1160 delegates representing forty-four nations attended. Benito Mussolini, then on his meteoric flight to fame and eventual extinction, officially greeted the conference. The group of thirty-three Canadian physicians and laymen chosen by the Canadian Tuberculosis Association to represent Canada at this conference, with financial assistance from the Sun Life Assurance Company of Canada, also toured Great Britain and other European countries studying tuberculosis problems.

At this meeting a resolution was passed urging member organizations to adopt a standardized model of the double-barred cross in accordance with the proportions of the design in the United States, that is, with both bars of the same length. Through some error, the reproduction of the cross shown in the union's *Bulletin* pictured the upper horizontal arm shorter than the lower one, and so, unfortunately, the standard adopted was not that used by the National Tuberculosis Association (American). Canada uses a cross with the same proportions as that registered by the National Tuberculosis Association. In recent years, some countries which are not Christian by tradition have raised objection to the use of the cross and as a result the crescent is occasionally used instead.

It is of some wry interest that there was considerable criticism of the Rome meeting because of the organization of the program. At each session, for example, thirty persons were listed to discuss the first paper, thirty-two the second, and forty-two the third, each having been told he or she would be allowed twenty minutes. At this time there was no simultaneous translation of papers, and delegates had to make do with what high school interpretation of other languages they could muster.

In spite of the lack of instantaneous translations, programs improved from year to year, but there were always political rumblings in the background. The conference in Lisbon in 1937, which had been delayed one year because of the Spanish Civil War, was perhaps the most disruptive. Fred Hopkins of the National Tuberculosis Association reported that 'unfortunately, the banquet developed into an uproarious demonstration by the delegates from Nazi Germany and supported by an impassioned political speech by a delegate from Spain.'[4]

These biennial conferences continued until the outbreak of World War II in 1939. That year the conference was to be in Germany and a special Christmas Seal had been designed by the German organization. But the conference was cancelled. Obviously, Hitler had other plans as was evident when September came.

It is of historical interest and not generally known that, following the fall of France in World War II, a representative from Berlin called at the office of the International Union against Tuberculosis in Paris and inferred that it was the intention of the German organization to take the union back to Berlin and 'right the old wrong' whereby the International Anti-Tuberculosis Association (the original association) had been taken from Berlin following World War I. However, there is no record of any follow-through on this visit.

It was again seven years before the threads of the international program against tuberculosis were gathered together at a meeting of the council of the union in Paris in 1946. Leadership in the work of the union now definitely passed to North America. Indeed it is only through the generosity and industry of the National Tuberculosis Association that such great steps have been taken in reorganizing and establishing the union on a sound footing. Canada followed the lead of the United States and has generously supported, financially and morally, the promotion of the union's work.

The union's office in Paris was run by Professor Fernand Bezançon and a part-time assistant from 1934 to 1948, and the union was operated mainly as a scientific society. At the council meeting in 1948, in Paris, a number of countries such as Great Britain, the United States, and the Scandinavian countries urged that the program be broadened and more interest shown in countries and continents outside Europe. They also suggested the organization of voluntary national associations in different countries. The United States agreed to contribute a special grant of $10,000 if such a program was undertaken, and Canada, as well as other countries, agreed to contribute on the same understanding.

In 1948 Dr Etienne Bernard was appointed secretary general of the union, following the death of Dr Bezançon. He instituted simultaneous translation at both council and conference meetings, which was a tremendous boon and a great booster of the calibre of the meetings. Previously, although the contribution of the reporters was of high order, the following discussion by delegates from many countries became long and boring and often policies were misunderstood.

Dr William Gelner was appointed executive director in 1952. He successfully established a budget and quota system for contributions to the finances of the union by member countries. He set up a committee to study and report on scientific problems of tuberculosis, and also organized a conference at council meetings, composed of representatives of the national voluntary associations, which made it possible for lay members to participate. He set up regional sections of the union for Latin America and the Far East, the Near Middle East, Africa, and Madagascar, to arouse interest in these areas.

The union promoted the use of the Christmas Seal as a means of fund raising. The seal has been used in the United States since 1907 and in Canada since 1908, and many other countries have since adopted its use. At the conference in Copenhagen in 1950, the first one after World War II, a moving tribute was paid to Einar Holboell, originator of the Christmas Seal:

The idea of the Christmas Seal having originated in Copenhagen, the program of September 4 included the ceremony of laying a wreath on the statue of Einar Holboell, a Danish postmaster and founder of the Seal, in the little park in front of the railroad station of Charlottenlund, a suburb. The post office, above which the Holboell family had lived, was across the square. At one end of the square the bust of Holboell, an excellent likeness, is on a pedestal and below are the figures of two children partaking of the stream of water that comes out of the pedestal, symbolic of the healing of children provided by Christmas Seal funds.

Mr. J.B. Nikolaisen, postmaster at Aalborg, presided over the brief ceremonies. Several tributes were paid to Holboell in the presence of Mrs. Holboell, three of the children, other members of the family and a delegation of postal employees in uniform. At the request of Professor Jensen, President of the Conference, Mr. Hopkins, who was representing the NTA, spoke of the tremendous value of the Christmas Seal to the anti-tuberculosis movement. He recalled the warmth of the reception given Mr. Holboell on his visit to the United States in 1924. 'No words of ours', he concluded, 'will ever express adequately our gratitude to Einar Holboell but he is enshrined in our hearts and we shall always remember him as one of the great men of Denmark and a contibutor to the welfare of mankind.'5

Later, at the conference in Toronto in 1961, a handsome and extensive exhibit of Christmas seals from around the world was featured. The exhibit was sponsored by the National Tuberculosis Association, and arranged by Charles Lorenz, owner of the collection.

Conferences continued to be held biennially. The conference in India, in 1957, was an important one in the history of the union because it was the first to be held in the Far East. An eastern section, which has been active ever since, was organized to deal specifically with eastern problems. This meeting coincided with a project which had been organized under the auspices of the Colombo Plan, whereby four Canadian doctors would visit India, Hong Kong, and Japan, in order to consult with health officials and exchange ideas. The doctors were: Dr Hugh Burke, Montreal; Dr Armand Frappier, Montreal; Dr Cecil Shaver, St Catharines; Dr G.J. Wherrett, Ottawa.

That the work of the International Union against Tuberculosis was gathering momentum and still had a world of problems to face was indicated by the resolution sent to the World Health Organization from the conference in Istanbul in 1959: 'That the International Union Against Tuberculosis recommends to the World Health Organization that it now accept as another target, to receive top priority in emphasis, the elimination of tuberculosis as a public health problem throughout the world.'6 Dr Wherrett was elected president of the union at this meeting, and Canada was chosen as the country to host the conference in 1961 in Toronto.

In 1960 Dr Gelner was made executive director emeritus and Dr Johannes Holm was appointed executive director. Dr Holm had previously been consultant in tuberculosis to the World Health Organization. His wide knowledge of the world situation and his organizing ability enabled the union to make great progress during his period of office (1960–71).

At the conference of the union in Toronto in 1961, the mutual assistance program of the union was adopted, out of which a number of projects (case-finding and treatment) were organized in Africa and the Far East. In the fifty years' review prepared in 1971,[7] Dr Holm gives high praise to Canada's contribution and mentions specifically Dr Jeanes, medical director of the Canadian Tuberculosis Association, and Mr E.J. O'Brien, executive director of the Ontario Tuberculosis Association, for their efforts on behalf of the union.

The Moscow 1971 meeting was the end of an epoch in that it saw the resignation of Professor Etienne Bernard, secretary-general of the union since 1948. His medical statesmanship was a great influence in creating the necessary co-operation and goodwill which has characterized the development of the union. His classical and scientific reviews at the conferences of the union were enthusiastically received and appreciated for many years and will be sadly missed in the future. The Moscow meeting was significant in that eighty-seven countries participated.

As this was the last meeting of the union that the author attended, the following impressions may be of interest. It was the impression of the Canadian group that many more sanatoria were in use in Russia than in Canada and that domiciliary care had not reached the stage it has here. Our delegation found some difficulty in reconciling themselves to a society in which no mention was made of inflation or unemployment and which was also devoid of the many forms of advertising with which we are so familiar. Delegates were given a cordial welcome to the Soviet Union by the president of the union, Dr Philip Chebenov, and the minister of health for the USSR, Mr V. Petrovsky, who outlined the great progress made in health matters and particularly in tuberculosis. While no long-term figures were given, it was estimated that deaths from the disease in the USSR had been reduced to one-seventh during the Soviet regime.

Looking to the future, there is no doubt that there is still a great task for the union in controlling tuberculosis in the underdeveloped countries of the world. The problem will be that, with the decline in tuberculosis in western countries such as Canada, great difficulty is apt to be experienced in maintaining interest in the union. Indeed, Canada's interest is now mainly a financial one, supporting the union itself and contributing to the union's Mutual Aid Programme in the Far East and Africa. The union is now ready to undertake a wider program for respiratory disease, as is being done by the associations in Canada and the United States.

12

Retrospect and Prospect

Despite all the advances made in the conquest of tuberculosis in Canada, and they are impressive (see the Appendices), one has a lurking impression that the complete disappearance of the disease is still a long way in the future. Noting the current upsurge of venereal disease, one wonders whether the same could not happen for tuberculosis, and whether we are fooling ourselves in believing that the disease is all but conquered.

To paraphrase the opening paragraph of Charles Dickens's *The Tale of Two Cities,* the present situation is the 'season of hope but it is also the season of despair.' *Hope* because deaths from tuberculosis are rapidly disappearing from the records and are now confined mainly to people over fifty. *Despair* because morbidity remains at a comparatively high level. In 1972 there were 4339 notifications, of which 15 per cent were reactivations which, we are told, will require treatment with drugs for eighteen months if the disease is to become inactive and reactivation prevented. We are also learning that comparatively few patients are treated in institutions but most are, instead, receiving drugs on a domiciliary basis. Studies indicate that very few of these are taking the drugs for the required eighteen months and that only the innate resistance of the individual patient produces a state of arrest of the disease. We also believe that many among them are a source of infection in the community. These are factors which should be kept in perspective as we recount the spectacular advances made over the past 100 years in the organized attempt to combat tuberculosis.

The conquest of tuberculosis can rightfully be said to have begun with the researches of John Antoine Villemin in 1865, which clearly indicated that the disease was communicable. The discovery of the germ by Robert Koch opened the way for a scientific approach to the problem. The introduction of the stethoscope by Rene Laennec around 1800 led to an interest in the clinical diagnosis of the disease, and many clinicians became expert at recognizing even small lesions in the lung. When the x-ray first came into use, however, films were so poor that often a physician's evaluation of history, symptoms, and physical signs was of greater value in giving an accurate diagnosis than an unreadable radiograph. Later, as techniques improved, the x-ray reached its full status as a help in diagnosis. The laboratory added to greater accuracy in diagnosis, first by the identification of the acid-fast germs in the stained specimen of the patient's sputum under the microscope; and later in refinements whereby the sputum was concentrated and cultured from the few bacilli lurking in the sputum which had been missed in the stained film. Then came the inoculation of guinea pigs and the demonstration of the disease in laboratory animals.

The tuberculin test became useful in determining who was infected and whether or not the disease was active, and in excluding those in whom there was no suggestion of disease. In earlier years infection with the tubercle bacillus was so general that practically all adults gave a positive reaction to tuberculin. As infection declined, the number of individuals who were uninfected, and hence gave no reaction to tuberculin, increased and this was helpful in confining the search to likely suspects; also, the widespread use of case-finding procedures made it possible to recognize the majority of cases of tuberculosis in the community.

Methods of treatment improved as the number of sanatoria in Canada increased and the value of rest treatment became recognized. Greater and greater use of sanatorium treatment was advocated, a major objective being the provision of enough sanatorium beds to accommodate all patients with active disease who required treatment. This was the sanatorium era and it reached a greater peak in Canada than in most countries.

Not only did more and more patients recover by rest alone as the years went by but other improvements were added, such as the use of collapse therapy either by pneumothorax (introducing air into the pleural sac) or the surgical procedures for partial or total collapse of diseased lungs by removal of ribs and finally the resection of lobes and even entire lungs.

Although the use of the sanatorium as a means of isolation affected the incidence of the disease in the community, mortality was high and over 50 per cent of those who were afflicted died within ten years' time. Frustrating also were efforts at rehabilitation and resettlement of ex-patients. Despite all efforts, the rate of relapse was high.

In Canada, as elsewhere, the care of tuberculosis at the outset was an individual matter between the patient and his physician. As public health services developed, various health programs became the responsibility of the local and provincial departments. Tuberculosis was one of the first of these services. Possibly most important was the reporting of the disease to the health departments, and then the setting up of dispensaries and clinics for supervision, diagnosis, and treatment, which had been spearheaded by Dr R.W. Philip of Edinburgh.

From an early period the place of the public health nurse was of the greatest importance. She supervised the care of the patient and the family. In the absence of social services, which came later, most of this work fell on her shoulders.

BCG, the vaccine produced by A. Calmette and C. Guérin of France, was introduced in Canada in the 1930s. The vaccine was developed by the successive inoculation of some 230 strains of bovine tubercle bacilli in a glycerin-ox bile medium. The result was an organism which had lost its virulence but was still capable of producing a reaction to tuberculin. Studies proved that it had immunizing properties which many observers believed to be about 80 per cent effective in comparison with unvaccinated negative reactors. The vaccine was used in Montreal by Dr J.A. Baudouin on those who had been in contact with open cases and by Dr R.G. Ferguson of Saskatchewan on nurses in training and Indian babies in the Qu'Appelle Valley. Later, a general program for children and teenagers was developed in Quebec and Newfoundland, and it was used in other provinces for persons unavoidably exposed to tuberculosis, such as contacts, nurses in training, and medical students. In some areas of high incidence a general vaccination program was introduced.

The search for a cure went on for years in many countries of the world and numerous remedies were suggested only to prove disappointing. Wandering patients failed to find the ideal climate for treatment of the disease and many there were who, disappointed and frustrated, died in exile. Hence it was a miracle when, through the efforts of research workers in drug laboratories, streptomycin appeared in 1944, and in less than five years two other useful drugs, para-amino-salicylic acid and isoniacid were discovered. The introduction of these drugs led immediately to increased recoveries and a decline in the number of deaths. However, resistance to the drugs appeared, but it was found that this could be avoided by using two or more drugs at a time. As additional drugs, such as ethambutol, ethionamide, and rifampicin, came on the market, the likelihood of resistance to any one drug became even less. Optimum duration of drug therapy was ascertained, and there are few cases today that will not respond with proper therapy. The greatest problem has been that of keeping the patient on the drugs as long as necessary to secure the greatest benefit, usually about eighteen months to two years.

While there were local case registers for the clinics, the provincial departments gradually assumed a greater role with the setting up of provincial case registers and the appointment of full-time directors of tuberculosis control. This position entailed an important over-all function of directing all facilities necessary for diagnosis, treatment, and follow-up, including supervision, if not always direction, of the x-ray surveys that had been developed as early diagnosis became the goal.

The provincial budgets became greater, and the total cost of the treatment of tuberculosis in Canada reached $33,000,000 by 1962, exclusive of the administrative costs of operating clinics and dispensaries, case-finding services, and nursing services, which would probably add a further $10,000,000 as a conservative estimate. In 1948 the federal government became more actively involved with the introduction of the Federal Health Grants. For tuberculosis alone, the grants reached $4,000,000 per annum, a large sum in those pre-inflation days.

The success of the campaign has been referred to as the 'miracle of the empty beds' because the population in the sanatoria decreased until these institutions were finally empty and were converted to other uses. With this optimistic picture one wonders whether it might not be only a matter of time until the disease is completely controlled. There are, however, disturbing features that make the total picture disappointing and frustrating.

Even in our own country, Canada, there are ethnic groups, such as Indians and Eskimos, in whom the incidence of the disease is what it was in other groups fifty years ago. There are immigrants coming to Canada with a higher incidence of disease than Canada's own population, and there are centres of poverty to be found in every province where there are nests of the disease.

Reports of an upturn in the annual crop of new cases keep coming and, although these are usually followed by a compensatory fall, they do entail extra supervision on the part of the public health staff in investigating the outbreak and instituting a drug routine for those who are found to be infected.

The public has lost its fear of the disease and become complacent, and the knowledge we have gained is not always being used in an intelligent approach to the problem. There is the fear that this complacency will lead to toleration of the disease and that it will remain for many years to come a source of infection, with its ups and downs, and at best there will be only a truce with the disease rather than a victory over it.

Health department officials and administrators are placing tuberculosis on a lower list of priorities than other public health problems. General hospital care and medicare have become the important factors in health department budgets and, in fact, a declining problem, such as tuberculosis, goes lower on the list of important health demands and priorities. Other disease entities are occupying the centre of the stage, such as cancer and heart disease, and mental health is beginning to occupy the place of tuberculosis in the public consciousness.

Physicians can no longer look upon tuberculosis work as a career, as they did twenty-five years ago; more than ever it is now looked upon as a narrow medical specialty. Non-tuberculosis chest diseases are appealing more and more to young physicians and, even though tuberculosis is at present treated in university hospitals, it does not occupy an important place in teaching and treatment. There is still lack of recognition of the need to impart knowledge of the clinical and public aspects of the disease, and the importance of the preventive aspects is not clearly emphasized to students. In short, both the public and public health and other professional personnel believe that tuberculosis is beaten and no longer requires the attention it once deserved.

This philosophy has permeated the thinking of the voluntary associations that once found their greatest satisfaction in pursuing an energetic campaign against tuberculosis. One has only to attend the meetings of the Canadian Tuberculosis and Respiratory Disease Association to realize that tuberculosis receives less and less attention, while other important respiratory diseases, such as emphysema, bronchitis, and asthma, get the attention of chest physicians. At a conference of chest diseases in North America, held in Toronto in 1973, there was only one paper on tuberculosis in a week's sessions!

What then is the future of tuberculosis and what is the program that should be pursued? My considered opinion may be summarized as follows:

1 / The present tuberculosis control program should be maintained with whatever modifications are necessary in the light of changes in recent years. The first essential is the maintenance of case registers and figures which can be used to direct efforts to areas and groups where the disease is still found. Sanatoria can be closed in most provinces and treatment carried out in hospital units in general hospitals when institutional treatment is required. The clinic services need to be maintained so that facilities are available for ready diagnosis. Drug treatment, which is now mainly on a domiciliary basis, should be adequately maintained and supervised wherever the disease exists. It is essential that the public health aspects of the problem continue to receive attention, especially the follow-up of ex-patients and the supervision of contacts. More selective use of survey programs, tuberculin testing, and

BCG vaccination should be considered. Suggestions for the elimination of all x-ray chest surveys, as now advocated by some authorities, while accepted in principle, may require modification in certain instances. The BCG program should also be carried out under the clinic services.

2 / More attention to research is called for if Canada is to play its full part in the control of tuberculosis throughout the world. There are still many unsolved problems in diagnosis, treatment, and prophylaxis. There is also a place for research in certain laboratories where young investigators can pursue a program in bacteriology, biochemistry, and immunology. A successful search for a more practical vaccine than BCG and the discovery of drugs effective without the necessity of months and years of administration would do more to control tuberculosis than all our efforts so far in the long struggle against the age-old problem.

3 / Teaching of medical students and senior hospital staff physicians must be undertaken with an over-all appreciation of clinical and public health aspects of the disease, as treatment and diagnostic services become integrated with general hospital services. This requires that they be brought under the direction of an associate or assistant professor in the department of medicine who has a wide knowledge of respiratory disease, including the management of tuberculosis.

4 / The voluntary associations should not relinquish their interest in the residual tuberculosis program, even though it has not the appeal of former times. The associations should see that a due proportion of the funds raised is spent on the tuberculosis program and not diverted entirely to other aspects of the total respiratory diseases problem. The international program should be considered carefully to determine where available funds might be put to the best use.

At the time of writing (1973), the status of BCG needs further consideration. Although its effectiveness has been demonstrated, as outlined in records of the British Research Council and studies by R.G. Ferguson and Armand Frappier, the difficulty of administration has proved a great handicap. An excellent summary of the present problem of tuberculosis is to be found in an editorial, 'Tuberculosis Returns to the Fold,' in the *Canadian Medical Association Journal,* 9 October 1971. Further research on the methods of administration of the vaccine is needed, such as by inhalation, the scratch, intracutaneously, or the much abused and discarded oral method. The use of the vaccine in malignancies will arouse considerable interest in the whole matter of BCG vaccination.

At present there is a sharp division between programs in western countries and those in the underdeveloped countries of the Far East and Africa, where there is a great gap between the technical knowledge available and the means of putting it to practical use. Better co-operation between all categories of health personnel would help – that is, between clinical specialists, general internists, medical practitioners, public health officials, technicians, nurses, and social agencies. Consideration should be given to the employment of local citizens as monitors in drug taking. This procedure was successfully demonstrated in 1972, in an experiment on Baffin Island, when Eskimos supervised the taking of pills.

More and more it becomes evident that the key to the eradication of tuberculosis in the world may be found in the control of the disease in underdeveloped countries and particularly those of the Third World. There the disease is as great a problem as it was in the western world at the turn of the century. The World Health Organization and the International Union against Tuberculosis are both keenly interested in the tuberculosis problem, but their work so far has only scratched the surface. We in Canada have also a deep concern since immigrants from these countries continually reach our shores, and reports from health departments tell us that the incidence of the disease in these people is greater than the total for the remaining population on the tuberculosis registers of the provinces.

PART II

PROVINCIAL SERVICES

13

Introduction

This part of the book covers the development of both voluntary and government tuberculosis services in the provinces. When the government health departments were organized, they usually assumed direction of the tuberculosis program and took over the provincial responsibility for the financing of the services, as was their duty constitutionally. Often insufficient credit has been given the provincial governments for their part in the battle against tuberculosis, perhaps because these services had developed as a result of stimulation from voluntary associations and those who directed the associations sometimes overplayed their importance in their zeal to arouse public interest. Not that one should ignore the contribution of the volunteers either.

Outstanding physicians who had sparked the development of dispensaries and sanatoria (see the chapter on the Canadian Tuberculosis Association) were also the moving spirits in developing the provincial programs, both voluntary and official. Two of the more noteworthy were Dr Peter Bryce in Ontario, who was secretary of the Board of Health from 1882 to 1904 and chief medical officer for the Department of Immigration until 1912, and Dr Emmanuel Persillier-LaChapelle, who organized the Medical Faculty of Laval University in 1879 and headed the Provincial Board of Health as president of the Royal Commission to Prevent the Spread of Tuberculosis. Others are mentioned in chapters on the individual provinces below.

The development of a complete program for the control of tuberculosis came gradually in the provinces but it is of interest that as early as 1912 Dr Herman Michael Biggs of New York City provided an outline for the administrative control of tuberculosis and discussed the development of such a program in that city in terms of developments in other cities.[1] This report was a far-reaching one for its time and had a great influence on the development of programs elsewhere. It covered the whole field of diagnosis and reporting, the various institutions for treating all stages of the disease, and the machinery for supervision of patients whether in institutions or at home. It was also concerned with the steps being taken to supervise and rehabilitate ex-patients, and measures for the care and supervision of children of tuberculous households by treating them in open-air homes and schools as well as summer camps. Canada with its far-flung areas was slow in developing all these refinements but nonetheless kept them in mind.

There is much history bound in the evolution of the early voluntary agencies that played a pioneer role in the control of tuberculosis. The physicians were always aware of the seriousness of the disease and, in their attempt to inform the public, they made studies and presented papers to learned societies as well as to the public. In so doing they inspired many people, particularly prominent laymen, to associate themselves with the work of treatment and prevention.

There was always some opposition by the medical profession to the development of public health measures. Although the medical associations supported the early efforts for better health, the conservative body of the profession dubbed the development 'socialistic' and considered it the opening wedge for 'state medicine.' An example of this attitude was their opposition to the reporting of infectious diseases, such as tuberculosis, though in the case of this disease they may have felt reluctant to label an individual with a diagnosis that carried a certain social stigma. The setting up of clinics, dispensaries, and other diagnostic services was also considered an invasion of the domain of the private practitioner. The practice was tolerated, however, because these aids were necessary for the poor and destitute, and it was even accepted when the services were seen to be helpful to the practitioner and not in competition with private practice, and when those responsible seemed to have no axe to grind.

The author speaks with some personal knowledge in this matter. In three provinces it was his task to organize a free consultation service for general practitioners for the diagnosis and treatment of tuberculosis. As he was paid by the Department of Health, he was clearly participating in 'social medicine.' The author made it his practice to discuss the proposed service with every registered physician with whom he was likely to come in contact. The reaction ranged from an offer of full co-operation to open opposition to any such 'socialistic measures,' though in virtually every instance the opposition was eventually withdrawn and pleasant relations established once the purpose and advantages of the service were realized.

Perhaps the work of the visiting nurses has been of the greatest value in the public health work that was undertaken, and yet the Ontario Medical Association placed on record its opposition to the proposal for the founding of the Victorian Order of Nurses by adopting the following resolution in 1897: 'After careful consideration of the scheme for the founding of a Victorian Order of Nurses, so far as its details have been made public, the Ontario Medical Association desires to express its full appreciation of the kindly motives that have prompted the movement, but feels that it would be neglecting a serious duty if it failed to express its most unqualified disapproval of the scheme, on account of the dangers which must necessarily follow to the public should such an order be established.' Like so many of these services which at first were criticized, the work of the Victorian Order of Nurses was eventually appreciated and the medical profession became the first to give it the highest praise.

It could have been anticipated that Koch's discovery would bring renewed hope to physicians in their centuries-old struggle against tuberculosis. What was not anticipated and was to become a phenomenon of the twentieth century in the western world was the emergence of a new force – the volunteer, the lay component of the voluntary association. Some were rich, some were poor, some were men and women of great prestige, and others were humble folk. What they had in common was the conviction that tuberculosis, the world's leading cause of death, could be vanquished. Such was their dedication to the cause that their progress was commonly spoken of as a crusade.

Nowadays volunteers are no rarity. The western world has become accustomed to their faces, their voices, their efforts. Sometimes it is a neighbour, sometimes a celebrity, whose voice comes into the living room by radio or television asking for help against lung disease, diabetes, arthritis, cystic fibrosis, blindness, deafness, cancer, asthma, mental illness, or mental retardation. Their friendly tones come over car radios asking the driver or his passengers to give of their time or energy, or both, to help in hospitals, read to the blind, teach a skill to the handicapped, or assist in the rehabilitation of criminals. Over a bridge table or at a chance meeting in a supermarket, these enthusiasts recruit their friends or even strangers to deliver hot lunches to shut-ins or provide transportation for someone who has no way of getting to a hospital or recreation centre unless some kindly soul will drive him. It seems incredible, now that they undertake thousands of tasks, that not so long ago health and welfare organizations lacked the support of such individuals, who bring not only cheerfulness and industry but a variety of talents to bear in both the promotion of programs and the raising of money for the causes they espouse. The greatest gift of all is the stimulus of their conviction that the distressed of the world have a right to help from those who are more fortunate. First in dozens, then in hundreds, and now in tens of thousands the volunteers have changed the public's idea of social responsibility. It was the enormous challenge of tuberculosis, coupled with the vision that it was possible to conquer it, that revealed to the western world the great potential for good that exists in almost any community.

It is difficult to analyse the motives that activated many of these people, but we should and must be generous and believe that they were mainly altruistic even though through hindsight one knows that sometimes selfish motives influenced their activities. Many had personal experience with tuberculosis, having either suffered from it themselves or seen another in the family smitten. Some who made great contributions had strong personalities in which power complexes operated, and these aroused opposition and animosity in others of different views. Such differences did harm to the movement and produced bitterness that was only forgotten as a new generation succeeded the old in the march of time. Difficulties sometimes arose between laymen and medical personnel. Having raised the money the former felt they should direct the program, under the maxim 'he who pays the piper calls the tune.' In time the importance of the cause overcame all difficulties.

In some organizations it was the executive officer who became the dominating personality. He was usually a strong, capable, commanding person, whose experience in office made him seem indispensable. These individuals were able to keep out any dissenting opinion on the board of directors and continued for years to hold undisputed sway over an entire organization. They accomplished much, but did much harm through the ill will created in other well-intentioned people, who either lost interest or dissipated their efforts in unnecessary controversy.

A fault of some organizations was the tendency to retain programs that should have been handed over to official agencies. An example of this was the allocating of funds for relief. The function of the association was to direct the individual to the appropriate welfare agency, or if none existed to try and have them developed, but many lay members felt strongly that funds should have been given directly for relief.

Another fault was the tendency to retain such services as 'specialized nursing services,' case-finding services, and even treatment services when all had become clearly the function of the official agency. While all these services at one time or other fell within the purview of the voluntary association, the time came for them to be handed over, leaving the association with the funds necessary for its chief function, a broad educational program. Fortunately, the experience with the campaign against tuberculosis was not repeated later, when voluntary societies concerned with cancer, mental health, arthritis, and many other problems came into existence. The pattern then was to organize the service part of the program under official auspices while the voluntary counterpart devoted its activities to fund-raising for education and research.

There is a great need today to educate the public and the medical profession on the most economical and efficient use of hospital and medical services; otherwise their staggering cost could bring us all to the brink of disaster. Such a task requires the attention of the best brains of medical, welfare, and government departments as well as voluntary associations, and it is hoped that they will put forth the necessary effort.

14

British Columbia

Efforts to control tuberculosis in British Columbia began around 1900. The belief that a dry climate was beneficial to consumptives brought many people with the disease to Kamloops, the centre of the dry belt. In fact the old Fortune Ranch at Tranquille (near Kamloops) boarded some of these health seekers in shacks adjacent to the farm house so it is not surprising that it was here that the first sanatorium in the province was built.

A noteworthy event was the appointment of Dr Charles Joseph Fagan as secretary of the Board of Health in 1899. He is credited with initiating the first steps to control tuberculosis in the province. As a result of his efforts the legislature passed an amendment to the Health Act in 1901 prohibiting the use or sale of milk from tuberculous cows, and requested that all cases of tuberculosis in humans be reported to the board. Thus the first move was made by the official health services.

Dr Fagan continued his campaign by calling a public meeting in Victoria City Hall in 1904, with the mayor, Dr G.H. Barnard, the premier of the province, Richard McBride, and other prominent citizens in attendance. The result of this meeting was the formation of the British Columbia Society for the Prevention and Treatment of Consumption and Other Forms of Tuberculosis (incorporated in 1907 as the British Columbia Anti-Tuberculosis Society). Dr Fagan agreed to act as secretary of the newly formed society, and stated that its first tasks should be to raise money to build a sanatorium, and to form local societies in every town and village, that being, as Dr Fagan said, 'the kernel of the whole work in educating the public on this question.'[1]

In August of the same year a rally was held in the portion of the legislative grounds known as Bird Cage Walk for the purpose of demonstrating to the public the use of 'tents' for patients undergoing treatment. Samples of these specially made 'tents,' with double walls six inches apart to allow free circulation of air, were actually erected on the grounds. It was intended they be used until sanatoria could be built.

Plans for raising funds received a great stimulus when in 1906 the Honourable James Dunsmuir, lieutenant governor of the province, offered to subscribe $10,000 for a sanatorium if the society could raise $50,000. This was accomplished during the next two years. In the meantime, a site had been acquired at Tranquille on Kamloops Lake along with the Fortune and Cooney farms, which were adapted for use as a sanatorium. Dr R.W. Irving was the first medical superintendent of this modest institution, which could treat ten patients.

Under the act to incorporate the British Columbia Anti-Tuberculosis Society, passed in the legislature in 1907, the objectives of the society were to be 'the prevention and treatment of tuberculosis, including the establishment and maintenance of hospitals and sanatoria throughout the Province for the reception and care of persons afflicted with the said disease.'[2] Branch societies were formed in Victoria, Vancouver, New Westminster, and Penticton, and soon there were nearly 2000 members. The local societies were urged to collect money for the support of indigent patients and to study the needs of the tuberculous in their areas. In addition they were to interest educational authorities in teaching public health in the schools, with emphasis on tuberculosis, and to urge municipal authorities to pass and enforce health laws, in particular one with regard to indiscriminate spitting. They were also to seek the co-operation of teachers as well as ministers of religion, who should be asked to make tuberculosis the subject of one Sunday sermon a year.

The fund-raising objective for the building of the new sanatorium at Tranquille was met, and the lieutenant governor laid the foundation stone on 11 November 1908. Dr Irving continued as medical superintendent until his resignation in 1910, when Dr C.H. Vrooman was appointed.

During the next few years the board of governors of the society met annually and the executive committee, which had become the administrative body of the sanatorium, met more frequently. This task became a heavy burden for the committee, who requested the provincial government to take over the administration and financing of the sanatorium (the request was not granted until 1919).

Meanwhile a new problem arose as a result of the 1914–18 war, that of the returned soldier with tuberculosis. Where was he to be treated? In 1915 an arrangement was made with the Military Hospitals Commission to treat all veterans at Tranquille. In his annual report in 1917 the president of the society stated that this arrangement was satisfactory. He also reported that hospitals in Victoria, Kamloops, and New Westminster had set up wards for the treatment of civilians with tuberculosis.

In 1918 the Department of Soldiers' Civil Re-establishment was created in Ottawa and it was agreed to build a new infirmary and service building at Tranquille. Assistance was also received from the provincial government. As a result facilities for treatment were doubled.

In 1919, by mutual agreement, the provincial government took over the sanatorium from the society. The $100,000 Greaves bequest, which had been donated to the society in 1915, was also given to the government.

The British Columbia Anti-Tuberculosis Society could look back with satisfaction on what had been accomplished since its founding by Dr Fagan in 1904. It had aroused interest in tuberculosis throughout the province, it had set up branches in the major cities, and the membership had reached 3000. It had instigated the building of the first sanatorium in the province and the setting up of wards in hospitals for the treatment of tuberculosis. When the sanatorium was handed over to the province, the society had planned to devote itself to the educational part of its program but unfortunately this good resolution was never fulfilled and the society lay dormant for many years.

In 1925 Dr A.D. Lapp, who had become medical superintendent of Tranquille in 1921, in co-operation with Mr J.R. Pyper, a veteran who had recovered from tuberculosis, set up a new society, The Tranquille Tuberculosis Publicity Society. The three objectives were: to carry on a publicity campaign against tuberculosis, to stimulate public interest in the prevention and treatment of the disease, and to disseminate information on prevention. In 1927 the name was changed to the Tranquille Tuberculosis Society (and in 1936 to the British Columbia Tuberculosis Society). Its magazine, *The Tranquillian,* published monthly, contained useful information for patients and public alike. The society also organized and conducted the Christmas Seal sale when it was introduced in 1927 except in Vancouver and Victoria, where it was conducted by local service clubs or the IODE.

Dr A.S. Lamb, a member of the Tranquille staff, was appointed travelling medical health officer in 1927. His duties included inspection of hospitals, the organization of travelling clinics, particularly in remote areas, and the provision of consultant services for family physicians in these areas. Christmas Seal funds provided a portable x-ray machine and a nurse technician for this most valuable service.

At this time the tuberculosis program in the province lacked central direction. A number of services were operating with little co-ordination.

Tranquille was the main treatment centre, as well as the base of operation of the travelling clinics under Dr Lamb, but there were also tuberculosis wards and clinics in the Vancouver General Hospital and in the Jubilee Hospital in Victoria. The Rotary Institute for Diseases of the Chest, which had been set up in Vancouver in 1918, was also operating as a clinic. An effort to co-ordinate the services in Vancouver was made when Dr J.W. MacIntosh was appointed medical health officer for the city in 1933 and set up a Division of Tuberculosis in the Health Department. Dr W.H. Hatfield was appointed director of the division and concentrated services at the Vancouver General Hospital in the chest clinic on Willow Street (part of the hospital). The services of the Rotary Club clinic were taken over and the public health nursing service was also directed from this centre.

In 1933 Dr G.M. Weir, the newly appointed provincial secretary, whose portfolio included the provincial Board of Health, proceeded to investigate the whole health program in order to improve and reorganize it. He invited Dr Grant Fleming, professor of public health at McGill, to make a study of the program and also to make recommendations for improved services. In the field of tuberculosis Dr G.J. Wherrett, executive secretary of the Canadian Tuberculosis Association, was invited to give a report on tuberculosis services for the province. The report recommended that a division of tuberculosis control be set up for the province and a director be appointed, that the number of treatment beds be increased, and that clinic services be strengthened.

The Division of Tuberculosis Control was set up in 1935, with Dr Hatfield as director. A temporary structure at the Willow Street Chest Centre was built to accommodate the new division, which developed an active program. The Chest Centre was further extended, ninety additional treatment beds being added, and a chest surgical service was introduced with Dr W.E. Harrison in charge. A new sanatorium, the Pearson Hospital, was constructed at 57th Street in Vancouver. Together with the hospital units in Victoria, Vancouver, and Tranquille the bed capacity for the province reached 850.

In addition to the clinic centres in Vancouver General Hospital and the Jubilee Hospital in Victoria, clinics were established at Trail, Rossland, Prince Rupert, and Kelowna. Dr Lamb, who had introduced the travelling clinic service in 1927, was attached to the Vancouver unit until his retirement in 1938, when Dr G.F. Kincade was appointed director of clinics and later assistant director of the Willow Chest Centre.

In the early 1940s the tuberculosis services for Indians in the province were improved. The Indian industrial school at Sardis was converted into a sanatorium and Dr W.S. Barclay was appointed medical superintendent. His duties included the direction of a tuberculosis program for Indians of the province. After the war, defence hospitals at Nanaimo and Prince Rupert were also taken over by Indian Medical Services for treatment of tuberculosis, thereby rounding out the treatment services for the province.

The setting up of the Division of Tuberculosis Control in the Department of Health brought about a change in the provincial voluntary society. With the official agency directing and co-ordinating all activities in the province it dominated the picture and for a time supervised the program of the voluntary agencies. It became obvious that as the official program was centralized in Vancouver through the Division of Tuberculosis Control, it would be preferable to operate the voluntary effort from Vancouver rather than Tranquille. The Tranquille Tuberculosis Society was therefore reorganized and its scope of activities broadened. The name was changed to the British Columbia Tuberculosis Society in 1936, and Mr J.R. Pyper became the chairman. In the same year *The Tranquillian* was renamed *Your Health.*

The new society undertook to assist the work of the division in a variety of ways, including the provision of operating room and x-ray equipment at Tranquille. The Kiwanis Club in Victoria instituted rehabilitation work in that city. In 1938 the society provided a nurse for the Fraser Valley area on the understanding that the municipalities would assist at the end of one year.

When the society was moved to Vancouver Mrs V.M. McGeer was employed as full-time executive secretary. Later, as an active program developed, a health educator, a Seal sale organizer, and a mass survey organizer were added to the staff.

Thus a well-balanced program with a strong official tuberculosis division and an equally strong voluntary society took form. The society operated as an independent voluntary body with the function of education in its widest sense. Not only did it undertake the education of the public, but it also assisted in the education of professional groups, such as physicians, nurses, and health educators, by arranging meetings and congresses.

In 1944 the health education program of the society was enlarged. A health education director, Mr Harold C. Huggins, was appointed and received the assistance of a $600 grant from the Canadian Tuberculosis Association.

In May 1949 the British Columbia Tuberculosis Institute was opened in Vancouver as a part of the Willow Chest Clinic. The building cost of approximately $400,000 was met by contributions to the Christmas Seal campaign, and the furnishing and equipping of the building were provided by a health grant from the federal government. It formed a valuable addition to the buildings and offices of the Division of Tuberculosis Control, and provided library and research laboratories as well as a 300-seat auditorium. The division now had medical facilities for all kinds of chest work and could act as a centre for many public health activities.

Since 1954 the British Columbia Tuberculosis Society has assisted in the expansion of public health services and facilities by providing grants in the amount of 10 per cent of the total construction costs of community health centres, which serve as headquarters not only for the official agency but also for the volunteer organizations.

In 1958 Mr Huggins resigned and Mr Douglas A. Geekie was appointed health educator for the society. That same year the society gave $100,000 towards the construction of a building in Vancouver to accommodate seventy children and a further $9000 to furnish a lounge where the young patients could entertain their friends and relations.

Surveys continued to be of prime importance. Vancouver's 'Operation Doorstep,' conducted by the British Columbia Tuberculosis Society under Mr Geekie in 1959 for the Metropolitan Health Committee in co-operation with the Division of Tuberculosis control of the provincial Department of Health, was a large-scale tuberculosis case-finding survey in a concentrated community. Two x-ray vans travelled from block to block throughout the city, and community organizations provided volunteer clerks and canvassers to supplement the professional staff. The program was essentially of the 'crash' variety, lasting ten to twelve weeks in any one area, and providing a screening service for some 5,000 people a week, based on 75 per cent of total population participation. Communities with the highest prevalence and incidence rates were served first.

The program, which was conducted under the name of the local health service, included a tuberculin test for all pre-school children from the age of six months up, a similar test for all school children, and a tuberculin test and x-ray for all adults. About a month before the survey would start in an area a survey physician would attend local medical society meetings to explain the project and enlist support, and to make arrangements to handle any cases discovered. At the same time the society's executive secretary would attend local municipal council meetings to explain and demonstrate the service to be provided. A prominent member of the council would be given a tuberculin test and the meeting covered by radio, televison, and the newspapers. Before the start of the program every school child would be given a 'parental consent card' and a letter explaining the program and a pamphlet describing the tuberculin test. Parental involvement was an important part of the educational program designed to obtain 100 per cent participation of the general public. The media were used extensively in education and promotion, arrangements being made for advertisements, feature articles, pictures, and weekly reports. The survey staff would give talks to local service clubs who had offered to help. The most important factor in public participation was involvement of members of the community on a voluntary basis. The volunteer would canvass door to door as the mobile clinic served in the neighbourhood, advising the people to attend and have their free skin test and x-ray, and sometimes even baby-sitting so that mothers could attend.

In 1961 the society organized and constructed the School of Rehabilitation at the University of British Columbia to train both physio and occupational therapists. Several other voluntary health agencies helped with the renovation of existing university buildings for this purpose, among them the Cancer Society, the Canadian Arthritis and Rheumatism Society, and the Mental Health Association. Another research project that year was the experimental production of pulmonary insufficiency and control in animals conducted at the G.F. Strong Rehabilitation Centre under the direction of Dr P.G. Ashmore by the University of British Columbia Department of Surgery.

In 1962 Mr Geekie became executive secretary of the British Columbia Tuberculosis Society, which became known as the British Columbia Tuberculosis–Christmas Seal Society. A policy decision was reached to extend its area of interest to the general field of chronic chest diseases, with priority to be given to medical research and professional education. The society's major accomplishment in this field was the establishment, in 1966, of a respiratory disease section within the University of British Columbia's School of Medicine, the first such in Canada. The society agreed to pay $5000 annually for three years to support the section's program, which comprised the following: continuing education in the field of respiratory diseases, including a major symposium on respiratory diseases for medical practitioners and specialists which featured outstanding speakers, all experts in their own fields; a conference on community health problems in respiratory diseases and tuberculosis; organization of teaching clinics throughout the province to disseminate knowledge about chest diseases to physicians and other health workers; and co-operation where possible with the society in its public health education program.[3] The original three-year agreement with the university was renewed for another five-year period in 1969, with the society providing a minimum of $10,000 annually towards the appointment of Dr Stefan Grzybowski as Associate Professor of Medicine of Respiratory Diseases, University of British Columbia.

In line with the continued expansion of the society between 1962 and 1964, a senior fellowship was granted to Dr Gordon Pirie, at the University of British Columbia Faculty of Medicine, Department of Pediatrics, to further research in paediatric pulmonary diseases, and the Pediatric Pulmonary Laboratory was equipped as the health centre for children. A conference was also held for the Vancouver Department of Public Health staff members 'to restate and clarify public health goals regarding tuberculosis, to determine what threat tuberculosis poses in communities today and what it means in terms of public health programs and personnel,'[4] the Christmas Seal Auditorium was renovated at a cost of $28,000 and rededicated on 6 November 1964, and 'Operation Doorstep' was greatly expanded.

In 1964 the constitution of the British Columbia Tuberculosis–Christmas Seal Society was amended to give the society authority to widen its program to include all forms of thoracic disease in addition to tuberculosis, which remained its primary interest. These newer objectives were in line with the program of the Canadian Tuberculosis and Respiratory Disease Association. The society continued to publish *Your Health* six times a year as part of the education campaign and to distribute public service material to radio, television, and the newspapers; it also sent abstracts and clinic notes on respiratory diseases to all physicians in the province. It gave financial assistance to the British Columbia Thoracic Society (the medical section within it) in 1965, and established a special nursing section as well.

Today the society still continues to work to fulfil its objectives.

15

Alberta

Early days in the antituberculosis campaign in Alberta were vigorous ones. People who were concerned about the disease held meetings, formed associations, and presented petitions to the provincial legislature. As early as 1907 a petition was made requesting that money be given to set up a system of tuberculosis prevention among the indigent, that competent people be employed to search out all cases of tuberculosis in the province, and that no known sufferer from tuberculosis be allowed to enter the province without special permission and without reporting immediately to the secretary of the Board of Health. The petition contained other interesting clauses as well, such as that no carpets be allowed on the floors of a public house; no dry sweeping be allowed in public buildings; no one suffering from tuberculosis be allowed lodging in a hotel, boarding house, or private home without making his condition known; spitting be prohibited in all public places; and the government be requested to ask the Railway Commission to disinfect all railroad cars and replace the dust-collecting upholstery with washable materials.[1] The reason for these drastic demands was the position which the climate of Alberta occupied in the minds of tuberculosis pilgrims who came to the province in search of the elusive cure.

Early associations were formed in Calgary, Lethbridge, Medicine Hat, and Red Deer, but only the Calgary Tuberculosis Association endured, mainly through the efforts of two women, Mrs William Carson and Mrs Harold Riley. In 1910 they supplied sixteen beds in a building and four tents for use as a tuberculosis hospital.

When the need for a sanatorium for the treatment of tuberculosis 'returned soldiers' from Alberta became acute following World War I, an agreement was signed in 1919 by Sir James Lougheed, representing the Department of Soldiers' Civil Re-Establishment of the Government of Canada, and the Honourable A.G. MacKay, representing the Department of Public Health of the Government of Alberta, whereby each party consented to the payment of a sum of $200,000 to be used to acquire a site and to erect a sanatorium. The 210-bed institution, at Bowness near Calgary, was opened in 1920, with Dr A.H. Baker as medical superintendent. For the first five years of operation, it was administered by the federal government, and administration was then transfered to the provincial department of public health.

The first tuberculosis clinic was opened by Dr Baker in Drumheller in 1925, and in 1927 a follow-up service was organized and the clinic service extended. In 1928 tuberculosis clinics were established in both Edmonton and Calgary.

The Tuberculosis Act of Alberta, proclaimed in 1936, made available free institutional treatment and clinic diagnostic services to those persons who had resided in the province for the previous twelve consecutive months. Preference in accommodation was given to people with pulmonary and other infectious forms of the disease.

A branch administration and tuberculosis clinic were opened in the Edmonton General Hospital in 1936, under the direction of Dr G.R. Davidson, formerly travelling diagnostician attached to the sanatorium staff in Calgary. This service was transferred to the Aberhart Sanatorium when it opened in 1953.

In 1939 the need for a rehabilitation service to assist sanatorium patients and for a program of mass surveys became acute. To meet the challenge, service clubs in Medicine Hat, Lethbridge, High River, Edmonton, and Drumheller and the Calgary Tuberculosis Association formed a permanent council, called the Alberta Tuberculosis Association. Dr Baker and Dr Davidson acted as ex officio members. The new association channelled its initial energies into education, x-ray surveys and rehabilitating patients in whom the disease had been arrested, by setting up suitable training programs in trades and crafts, using funds from the Christmas Seal sale to pay for staff. To develop these programs Mr C.R. Dickey, a former tuberculosis patient, was engaged as executive secretary in 1940 and a miniature chest x-ray machine was purchased for $15,000 using proceeds from the Seal sale. Mr Dickey was a superb organizer and, with the crusading spirit of an ex-patient, turned his talents to organizing the Seal sale, the mass x-rays surveys, and the educational program. When he resigned in 1955, and Mr Cecil Crooks assumed the position, these services were well developed.

In 1945 the Alberta Tuberculosis Association gave the Calgary General Hospital and the Edmonton Royal Alexandria Hospital a grant of $1500 each for the x-ray of all patients on admission, which stimulated the hospital x-ray admission program in the province.

Alberta had by this time four major organizations working in the tuberculosis program: the provincial Department of Public Health, which provided free diagnosis and treatment; the Alberta Tuberculosis Association, which assisted in diagnosis by paying for equipment, provided a rehabilitation service, fostered education, and assisted in occupational therapy; the Indian Affairs Branch, which provided free diagnosis and treatment for Indians; and the Department of Veterans Affairs, which took care of the service pensioners by maintaining them in the Charles Camsell Indian Hospital in Edmonton and conducted rehabilitation and follow-up services for veterans.

In 1946 the Canadian Tuberculosis Association held its first full-scale post-war annual meeting in Calgary. The general session outlined the postwar program and stressed the importance of the attention being given to the rehabilitation program and to tuberculosis in Indians. It was at this meeting that the medical section of the association was recognized as a separate section with its own program.

In 1965 the Alberta Tuberculosis Association set up the first diabetic detection survey in Canada, in co-operation with the Edmonton District Branch of the Canadian Diabetic Association. The interest in diabetics stems from the fact that the incidence of tuberculosis is greater among people with diabetes than among the general public.

In 1968 the association changed its name to the Alberta Tuberculosis and Respiratory Disease Association and extended its program to include all forms of these diseases.

In 1973 the annual meeting of the Canadian Tuberculosis and Respiratory Disease Association met in Calgary. There was great interest in the program of the Canadian Thoracic Society, and the nurses' section had the largest attendance in history. An excellent phase of the latter's program was the attention given to the domiciliary program for the treatment of tuberculosis and the place of the nursing profession in the education of tuberculous families and the general public. Another exceptional event was the demonstration of the use of 'Youth Councils' in carrying out the society's program.

The 1973 program brought out the great progress that had been made in Canada and Alberta since the first post-war meeting in 1946 in Calgary, which had also represented a milestone in initiating the post-war program.

16

Saskatchewan

Dr Maurice Seymour, commissioner of public health for the province of Saskatchewan, discovered in 1906 that his son had tuberculosis, and promptly took him to the sanatorium at Saranac Lake, NY, one of the few institutions at that time where sufferers could get treatment. Dr Seymour was so impressed by his meeting with Dr Edward Livingstone Trudeau, the founder of the sanatorium, and by the methods used to control the disease that in 1907 he recommended the establishment of a sanatorium in Saskatchewan so that early cases of the disease could be cured, and advanced and incurable cases isolated. He also recommended that hospitals set up isolation wards for the tuberculous, and strongly emphasized the importance of educating the public. In February 1910 the secretary of the Canadian Association for the Prevention of Tuberculosis (as the Canadian Tuberculosis Association was then called), Dr George D. Porter, visited Saskatchewan and together with Dr Seymour lectured and organized local antituberculosis associations (leagues were formed in Estevan, Candruff, Wapella, Grenfell, and Lumsden, but none of these continued after the provincial league was formed the following year). That summer the two doctors carried out an educational program throughout the province to inform the people of the necessity of preventing the disease.

The Saskatchewan Anti-Tuberculosis League was founded in Regina on 17 February 1911 as a result of a meeting held by 18 leading citizens. The mayor of Regina, Mr Peter McAra, was elected the first president. The real purpose of the league was to find ways and means of building a hospital for advanced tuberculosis cases and a sanatorium for early cases When approached, the provincial government promised to provide $25,000 when the trustees could provide a similar sum. In March 1911 an act of the legislature gave the league official status, and constituted it a corporate body, empowering the trustees to establish hospitals and sanatoria, and to appoint medical and other employees for these institutions.

The league immediately set forth on an educational program, and local organizations set out to raise funds by holding tag days and making other appeals. The required money was soon raised and a site was chosen at Fort Qu'Appelle in the Qu'Appelle Valley. When plans were drawn up and it was discovered that the buildings would cost $93,000, the provincial government agreed to change its grant to $60,000 if the league could raise the additional $15,000. Through tag days and canvasses between 1911 and 1914, $97,000 was raised. By 1914 the government had generously given a total of $104,125 so that the league could commence construction.

Dr Seymour, who had acted as secretary to the league up to this point, asked to be allowed to resign, urging that a full-time paid secretary be appointed. The league then drafted a five-year plan and the provincial government agreed to see the project through. By July 1914 the work of construction was well under way, but at the outbreak of war all activities of the league ceased, including the completion of the partially finished buildings.

Dr Wm M. Hart had been appointed medical superintendent for the as yet unfinished buildings in 1914, but at the outbreak of the war he enlisted. On his return to Canada he remained in Ottawa with the Department of Soldiers' Civil Re-Establishment, and so in June 1917 Dr Robert George Ferguson was appointed to the position. At this time the return of numbers of tuberculous ex-servicemen provided the impetus to complete the sanatorium. A loan of $150,000, secured by a first mortgage on the property, was obtained from the federal government for furnishings and equipment, and the sanatorium was officially opened on 10 October 1917. The following year two additional pavilions of forty-five beds each were financed by the federal government to accomodate more veterans. In February 1919 the sanatorium's first x-ray machine arrived, and a month later the Red Cross Society built and furnished a comfortable lodge for the accommodation of visitors, which was presented to the Saskatchewan Anti-Tuberculosis League. A growing interest on the part of the public was shown, both by the large numbers of visitors who came to see the institution at Fort San (as the Fort Qu'Appelle Sanatorium postal station was known) and by the increased number of gifts and contributions for the recreation and comfort of the patients. In 1920 the Independent Order of the Daughters of the Empire presented $75,000 to the league for the purpose of adding accommodation for seventy children. The following year the Local Council of Women formed an endowment of $50,000, called the 'Everywoman's Fund,' to provide sanatorium care for mothers of families who were unable to secure treatment at the expense of any other fund.

On 22 July 1921, the provincial legislature passed an Order-in-Council appointing a commission to inquire into the problem of tuberculosis. Their report listed as the most urgent requirements: hospital and sanatorium accommodation for those considered 'spreaders of the disease'; provision for children from homes where tuberculosis was found; improvement in the methods of financing treatment so that all who needed it would get it as quickly as possible; improved and extended diagnostic facilities; and extended nursing services and follow-up work for all ex-patients.[1]

In 1921 the first tuberculosis school survey in Canada was conducted by the Saskatchewan Anti-Tuberculosis Commission to determine the incidence of infection among school children, to discover the source of the disease, and to ascertain the conditions – pathological, economic, and social – which would tend to encourage the disease. Of some 170,000 school children in Saskatchewan, 1346 were surveyed. A second survey, in Weyburn, of 500 children, showed the incidence of tuberculosis at one per cent.[2]

Mr Andrew B. Cook, sheriff of Regina and the second president of the Saskatchewan Anti-Tuberculosis League, initiated in 1922 the idea of free treatment for tuberculosis sufferers by the pooling of facilities in the various municipalities of the province. Mr Robert D. Roberts, as secretary, was for many years a power behind the throne in the league. A returned soldier and ex-patient, he was prominent in the Tuberculosis Veterans Association and as such participated in the struggle for the pension legislation for veterans. His work with the civilian forces bridged the gap between soldiers and civilians, and he organized the Christmas Seal sale and veterans' Poppy Day campaign.

In 1926, at a meeting of the Association of Rural Municipalities, only about twenty out of some 600 delegates voted for free treatment. A similar resolution was passed at the meeting the following year, but the majority was too small to warrant government consideration. In March 1928, however, the resolution was passed unanimously. The Association of Rural Municipalities and the Association of Urban Municipalities were two of the most influential bodies in the province, and when they both presented resolutions to the provincial government favouring free treatment of all tuberculosis cases, an immediate amendment was made to the Sanatoria and Hospitals Act, effective 1 January 1929. Saskatchewan thus became the first province to treat all tuberculosis patients without charge to the individual, the cost being met by taxation.

The Saskatoon Sanatorium had opened in 1925 and two years later the Preventorium at the Fort Qu'Appelle Sanatorium. In 1930 the Prince Albert Sanatorium opened. *The Valley Echo*, which had originally started as a project of ex-servicemen at Qu'Appelle in December 1919 but was now published by the patients and staff of all three institutions, became the connecting link which bound them all together. Most issues were read thoroughly by the patients and then passed on to families and friends for their comfort and education.

By 1927 research in tuberculosis was being given full consideration.[3] One of the most important studies was on the state of the disease among the Indians living in the Qu'Appelle Valley. It was found that five per cent had evidence of active disease, and even more showed evidence of past infection.

A province-wide Christmas Seal campaign was conducted by the league in 1928. The money collected was spent on a number of programs: consultation services, permanent and travelling clinics, mass x-ray surveys, special surveys and tuberculin tests, and the Fort San Preventorium.

The Saskatchewan program was gaining world-wide recognition. The December 1932 issue of the *Canadian Tuberculosis Association Bulletin* reported: 'The Saskatchewan Anti-Tuberculosis League has created for itself a most remarkable field of activity and an equipment and programme unequaled anywhere, unless it might be in Denmark ... The various medical services of the League, include treatment, diagnosis, follow-up, Indian research, examination of Normal School students and Battleford School children, and the maintenance of a Preventorium at Fort San for the care of new born infants whose mothers are undergoing treatment in the sanatorium.'[4]

In 1932 volunteer teachers were enlisted to provide instruction in various subjects to patients in sanatoria so that their education would be continued, and in the fall of 1934 a sanatorium school was organized based on the provincial government correspondence school courses.

In 1934 the Associated Canadian Travellers pledged their support in the fight against tuberculosis. During the ensuing thirty years their clubs in Saskatchewan raised a million dollars in support of the preventive campaigns of the league. Education of the public remained an important objective. In a paper on 'Minimum Requirements for a Provincial Tuberculosis Programme,' presented at the annual meeting of the Canadian Tuberculosis Association in Montreal in June 1934, Dr Robert G. Ferguson stated (pp. 7–9): 'However fundamental the facilities for treatment, diagnosis and follow-up care, of equal importance and much more difficult of attainment, is the education of the mass of the people.' He stressed publicity by the sale of Christmas Seals, education of the board of directors, the need for annual meetings, the benefit derived from giving talks to conventions and various groups and from showing movies in the theatres, and professional education. In 1935 he stated: 'The first step in a provincial programme for the control of tuberculosis is a publicity campaign. This campaign, making known the facts relative to the unnecessary loss and suffering from the disease, should be aimed at a public demand for action. Such a demand is created by the championship of the press and the backing of leading citizens popularly known to have the public welfare at heart. A humanitarian appeal on behalf of the unfortunate sick is the foundation upon which a successful campaign rests.'[5]

In 1936 a concerted effort was made to publicize tuberculosis. All the newspapers printed editorials about the league's program, and advertising material was accepted by many, thus making the public more aware of the facilities freely available to them. Staff members of the Saskatoon Sanatorium designed and constructed a float which was placed on view at both the Regina and Saskatoon industrial exhibitions. It is impossible to estimate its publicity value in that year's Christmas Seal campaign.

The occasion of the twentieth anniversary of Saskatchewan's first sanatorium was celebrated in 1937. Newspapers told again the story of the province's fight against tuberculosis. Some 200 towns observed the occasion by organizing dances at which special speakers made an appeal for the year's Christmas Seal fund and pointed out important features of the league's programs.

The history of tuberculosis in Saskatchewan seems to be one of 'firsts.' Another occured in 1938 when Dr Ferguson introduced BCG to protect student nurses at the Fort Qu'Appelle Sanatorium. In recognition of this pioneer work and its great success, in 1948 Dr Ferguson was appointed a member of the World Health Organization's Sub-Committee on Tuberculin and BCG. In 1930, Ferguson, under the auspices of the National Research Council, had begun the BCG vaccination of Indian infants. Because this project was so successful and the results so conclusive, it was adopted by the then Department of Indian Affairs, later the Indian and Northern Health Services of the Department of National Health and Welfare.

In 1941 Saskatchewan conducted the first mass survey in Canada, examining approximately 75 per cent of the resident population of the town of Melville. After this initial survey more and more were carried out in other parts of country. Moose Jaw was the first city in Canada to institute an x-ray examination of all residents. Local organizations canvassed the city urging everyone to attend the clinics. Children were sent in groups from school to be x-rayed and the whole city council turned up one evening after a regular meeting. Dr Ferguson continued to urge that the educational campaign be continued and enlarged and carried on 'vigorously' at all school and university levels, as well as among families.

Nurses' training in sanatoria began in 1948, with the approval of the Saskatchewan Anti-Tuberculosis League in affiliation with the nursing schools and the Fort Qu'Appelle Sanatorium.

1947 was a year to be remembered, for on 1 August of that year the province completed a once-over photofluorographic survey of its population, another 'first' for Saskatchewan. Some 677,651 persons were examined, constituting 75 per cent of the estimated 818,000 non-Indian population. That same year, at the suggestion of Dr Ferguson, the provincial government and the hospitals set up a system of x-raying all persons entering hospital, as a result of which an estimated 80,880 persons would be examined each year.

Radio gave the league invaluable aid. The Associated Canadian Travellers in various towns organized a series of two-hour amateur programs on their local stations on Saturday nights, each program coming from a different community. In 1946 alone they collected some $70,000, and over the years the stations donated four to five thousand hours and thousands of contestants took part.

With the decrease in the number of patients following the advent of the drug era, the Prince Albert Sanatorium closed in April 1961. The revised Tuberculosis Sanatoria and Hospitals Act of 1968 stated that the objects of the league would be the care, conduct, and management of the sanatoria and tuberculosis hospitals, the establishment of clinics for examination and diagnosis, and the adoption of measures and the promotion of works necessary to prevent the development and spread of the disease in Saskatchewan.

In their 1966 *Report and Recommendations on Tuberculosis Control in Saskatchewan* Drs G.J. Wherrett and S. Grzybowski stated: 'The unique character of the League, when compared to other organizations in Canada, should be realized. It shares with the Sanatorium Board of Manitoba the distinction of being a semi-official body, mainly lay and voluntary in its composition and operation, given the specific task of organizing all facilities for the diagnosis, treatment and prevention of tuberculosis in the province.'[6] Their study also outlined the many firsts enjoyed by Saskatchewan, and which bear repeating. The province was 'the first to provide sufficient sanatorium beds to treat all tuberculosis patients ...; the first to provide free care for the tuberculous, financing this in the beginning from voluntary funds ...; the first to set up group surveys, commencing with school children, and later with community surveys ...; the first to undertake a BCG vaccination programme for the Indian population; the first to do a BCG vaccination programme for nurses-in-training.'[7]

In a letter dated 1 September 1965 to Dr A.A. Bailey, Professor of Medicine at the University of Saskatchewan, Dr Wherrett wrote: 'would the university be prepared to appoint or accept an associate professor of tuberculosis and respiratory disease? His chief function would be to co-ordinate the outpatient work, treatment and teaching at both University Hospital and the sanatorium. I would see this position being financially supported by the League and the university. It could work in with the desire of the League to honour the memory of Dr R.G. Ferguson by the implementation of an "R.G. Ferguson Associate Professorship." '[8]

The Wherrett-Grzybowski report gave impetus to this proposal by pointing out that the day was coming when separate tuberculosis services could no longer be justified since the disease was becoming less common, that the medical profession would eventually have to be able to deal effectively with the residual problem and so should become thoroughly familiar with the disease, and that in future medical education in the field of tuberculosis would become increasingly important. The report also recommended integration of the program at the Faculty of Medicine and the Saskatoon Sanatorium and the appointment of a member of staff responsible for the teaching of tuberculosis and other respiratory diseases. Tuberculosis should be brought back into the main stream of medicine, he said, becoming a matter of regular concern, rather than being segregated in out-of-the-way places; modern methods of treatment made the treatment of tuberculosis feasible in regular hospitals.

Following the Wherrett-Grzybowski report, on 14 June 1973 representatives of the University of Saskatchewan, the University Hospital, and the Saskatchewan Anti-Tuberculosis League met in Saskatoon to sign an agreement establishing a respiratory unit and research laboratory for chest diseases at the University Hospital in Saskatoon. Funds were to be allotted for a second physician, and the league agreed to support the chest physician as director of the unit, with the title of 'The Dr George Ferguson Professor' in honour of the great pioneer in tuberculosis work in Saskatchewan.[9]

17

Manitoba

The first antituberculosis campaign in Manitoba was launched in 1904, when twenty-four prominent Winnipeg citizens banded together to form the Sanatorium Board of Manitoba. They set, as their first goals, the building of a sanatorium at Ninette and the education of the public, and became, in fact, the first provincial organization which combined the functions of an official agency and voluntary association, being constituted by a provincial act. The Winnipeg Anti-Tuberculosis Society, organized as a direct result of the Ninth World Congress on Tuberculosis held in Washington in 1908, was the only other voluntary tuberculosis association. It does not seem to have persisted in its operations, however, since its functions were carried out by the Sanatorium Board, but it did maintain two visiting nurses and ran a dispensary aided by the Women's Auxiliary for a short time until absorbed by the city's Health Department.

Dr David A. Stewart was appointed medical superintendent of the Ninette Sanatorium and, with the admission of the first patient on 20 May 1910, the pioneering efforts in tuberculosis control in Manitoba began. Pamphlets were distributed and lectures given to school children and other audiences. Articles were prepared and published in the daily papers. A demonstration of charts and models about the disease was carried on at the Winnipeg Exhibition. There was no provincial association, and, though people in other parts of the province were interested, there were no associations outside Winnipeg. The sanatorium at Ninette became an official military centre during the war years of 1914-18, when its capacity was doubled and the available equipment became greatly improved.

Early in the history of the sanatorium, programs were developed for the training of undergraduate medical students in tuberculosis work. The program, which was one of the first of its kind in the world, was most successful and a fine spirit of co-operation was established between the Sanatorium Board and the doctors of Manitoba.

Dr Stewart was 'a man of great vitality of mind and had a physical vigour almost incredible in the light of his physical history. This tremendous vitality found expression in amazing industry.'[1] He also 'brought life, comfort and healing to thousands of patients who passed through the Sanatorium in twenty-seven years; he trained hundreds of medical students and doctors in physical diagnosis and fitted many for positions of trust and responsibility as tuberculosis leaders.'[2] He once stated: 'Our first big job is to find diseased people and make them safe by treatment, by segregation, by education, safe for themselves, safe for their families, safe for their communities, safe anywhere and at all times ... The whole field should be mapped out, the whole need envisioned.'[3]

During the 1930s a number of developments took place in the tuberculosis program in Manitoba. The Union of Manitoba Municipalities instituted a levy to be paid by the various municipalities on a pro rata basis so that all tuberculosis patients who were unable to pay the costs of sanatorium treatment would be automatically looked after. New treatment facilities were added in 1930 when the Central Tuberculosis Clinic was opened in Winnipeg, adjacent to the Winnipeg General Hospital; in 1931, the St Boniface Sanatorium, operated by the 'Grey Sisters,' was opened at St Vital with Dr J.D. Adamson as medical superintendent. The King Edward Hospital had been built in 1912 and operated by the city of Winnipeg for the treatment of tuberculosis.

On the death of Dr Stewart in 1937, Dr E.L. Ross became medical superintendent of the Manitoba Sanatorium at Ninette.

The 1940s saw many changes in the administrative set-up and in the treatment and preventive programs of the Sanatorium Board. Perhaps the most important was the institution of a rehabilitation program organized by Mr T.A.J. Cunnings, the recently appointed director of the board's new Division of Rehabilitation. The purpose of the program was to assist all patients in re-establishing themselves in self-supporting, productive positions in industry or business. Mr Cunnings's career as a banker had been cut short by tuberculosis of both the pulmonary and non-pulmonary forms. After a long fight to overcome the disease, he became the outstanding proponent of rehabilitation as, having lived through the ordeal, he knew the value of the measures used to reinforce sagging morale in patients and for successful and practical planning for their rehabilitation. Dr Ross believed that the community had a responsibility in this matter, for if difficulties were too great and the patient relapsed, he would again become a source of infection and would have to undertake another long and costly course of treatment. Consultations were made through regular visits to the sanatoria and the division's office of consultation, both of which offered vocational counselling and training, as well as guidance and assistance in employment. Prospective employers were provided with specific information on the expected work capacity of the patients, or ex-patients, many of who were prepared to offer special skills to compensate for their physical handicaps. Courses available by correspondence included air-conditioning, aircraft materials and processes, aircraft construction and design, bookkeeping, blueprint reading, civil engineering subjects, commercial law, economics, fiction writing, shorthand and typing, and watch repairing. Regular public and high school subjects were available too. Also, the excellent vocational and academic courses offered by the Canadian Legion War Services Committee on Education were made available to the members of the armed services in sanatoria.

In 1943 industrial surveys were started in Winnipeg in conjunction with the city Health Department. In the same year, the Winnipeg City Council made the decision to provide *free* treatment for all citizens suffering from tuberculosis, another milestone in the campaign to eradicate the disease.

In 1944 miniature chest films became available, which made it possible to x-ray entire communities. The surveys and travelling clinics were continued and regarded as a powerful factor in keeping the public and medical profession tuberculosis conscious.

The Manitoba Tuberculosis Control Act as amended in 1948 defined the functions of the Sanatorium Board of Manitoba as follows: 'To operate the sanatorium at Ninette, the central tuberculosis clinic in Winnipeg, and the surveys; to coordinate and supervise the work of the King Edward Hospital in Winnipeg and the St Boniface Sanatorium in St Vital.'[4] The headquarters of the board was moved from Ninette, to Winnipeg, and Dr Ross became medical director and Mr Cunnings executive director.

The board continued its activities of educating the public and the profession, working closely with community surveys and annual Christmas Seal campaigns. Publication was started on the *News Bulletin*, which replaced the former *Messenger of Health*. It contained information and feature stories on various aspects of the Sanatorium Board's services as well as monthy reports on the tuberculosis situation.

Mr Cunnings, in assessing the role of voluntary associations in 1965, stated:

Voluntary health agencies have frequently sprung from the special interests of small groups of people in some particular health problem. Through the years the organizations have grown and multiplied. They have made a great and valuable contribution to the prevention and treatment of illness; they have organized rehabilitation services; developed patient care services; provided funds and stimulated interest in the field of research; supplemented and augmented the programs of official agencies; and stirred popular and governmental support in previously neglected areas of need ... They will function as a partner and an agent of government, with an increasing proportion of their operating funds coming from tax sources by way of government grant or purchase of services. This would permit the agency to spend less energy on fund raising and concentrate more on improving and developing its services.[5]

Looking to the future in 1965, the Sanatorium Board asked Dr G.J. Wherrett, executive director of the Canadian Tuberculosis Association, to assess the situation of the tuberculosis control program and report on his findings and recommendations. Dr Wherrett stated:

The place of the Sanatorium Board of Manitoba is unique in that it was the first semi-official body formed by a partnership of government officials and voluntary citizens, and given authority to conduct and direct the campaign against tuberculosis in a province. While many voluntary boards have built and directed the operation of institutions in Canada, this was the first time that a provincial grant was included in the function of a non-government body.

... The present status was clearly defined in the Tuberculosis Control Act as amended in 1948. This Act, with some minor amendments, is in effect the 'Charter for Tuberculosis Control in Manitoba.' This remarkable document constitutes the guiding principles which will determine the programme of the future.[6]

Dr Wherrett's report recommended the concentration of services for respiratory diseases in one medical centre in Winnipeg, which would include accommodation for tuberculous as well as non-tuberculous patients. It also recommended that the medical services be co-ordinated with the Department of Medicine of the University of Manitoba and that a program for undergraduate and graduate teaching for all chest diseases be undertaken.

Since 1965 there has been a complete change in the direction of the program in Manitoba. Dr Reuben Cherniack has become consultant to the Sanatorium Board and Dr Earl S. Hershfield was appointed medical director of the Central Clinic on the retirement of its first director, Dr D.M. Scott. The Department of Health has assumed full responsibility for the diagnosis and treatment of tuberculosis in the province. The Central Clinic has become the centre for a program that includes the diagnosis and treatment of all chest diseases.

Mr Cunnings retired as executive director of the Sanatorium Board in 1972 and was succeeded by Mr R.G. Birt. The board, relieved of its main task of diagnosis and treatment, now devotes much of its attention to education. It continues to conduct the Christmas Seal campaign and maintains its relations with the Canadian Tuberculosis and Respiratory Disease Association. It also supports the national and international committee of the Canadian association. Over the years Manitoba has made a great contribution to the control of tuberculosis in Canada. It is now in a position to assume leadership of the new program for the prevention and treatment of all chest diseases.

18

Ontario

Acceptance of responsibility in health matters by the province of Ontario was apparent shortly after Confederation. In 1873 the Ontario Health Act was passed establishing local boards of health. Five years later the select committee on public health appointed by the legislature reported that if impure air was eliminated the mortality rate among tuberculous patients could be cut by one-third, and that if sanitary measures were applied the disease would be greatly lessened. However, the report did not include plans for an antituberculosis program.[1]

In 1882 the Ontario Board of Health was established on a permanent basis, and Dr Peter Bryce was appointed secretary. The following year, the first public health exhibit was displayed in Toronto, and the legislature passed a comprehensive Public Health Act, based on information prepared by the board. This act, which still forms the basis of the present (1974) act, allowed the local health boards to appoint medical health officers, but such appointments were not made compulsory until 1911. In 1890 a public health laboratory, believed to be the first of its kind in North America, was established in Toronto by the Board of Health.

The National Sanitarium Association, the first voluntary association in Canada, was established in 1896, with the intention of building at Muskoka a sanatorium that would be large enough to take care of patients from Ontario, but this did not happen and sanatoria were built elsewhere. In 1897 the Muskoka Cottage Hospital opened with accommodation for thirty patients. In 1898 the Toronto Association for the Prevention and Treatment of Consumption and Other Forms of Tuberculosis was organized (it continued to meet annually until 1912). In 1900 the Ontario Association for the Prevention of Consumption and Other Forms of Tuberculosis was formed (it held only one meeting, however, because its founders felt its functions would overlap with those of the National Sanitarium Association and also because its founders became interested in the formation of the Canadian association). Other voluntary associations were started during the following years, and by 1906 the Hamilton Health Association began construction of the Mountain Sanatorium, which was eventually opened in 1910.

The efforts of most of the early associations were directed towards providing much-needed treatment beds, but those of the Toronto Association for the Prevention and Treatment of Consumption and Other Forms of Tuberculosis took a different direction, with emphasis on education and the principle of building municipal sanatoria. The members believed that it was necessary to have a sanatorium in each county or municipality so that it might act as an important local educator, and that patients would be more likely to take advantage of an institution if, in entering it, they did not have to change doctors or leave their families and friends. Also in 1906 the Ottawa Association for the Prevention of Tuberculosis attempted to help families with tuberculosis by 'the employment of a graduate nurse, whose effort in the way of education would be seconded by such means and in such ways as opened to the Executive.'[2]

The Ontario Board of Health was given a government grant of $1000 at this time for a tuberculosis exhibit. With further grants the Public Health Exhibit and 'moving picture show' travelled to various towns throughout the province. The public showed its interest by large attendance at the exhibit and lectures, and by requests for literature.

The Heather Club Chapter of the Imperial Order of the Daughters of the Empire was organized in Toronto in 1909 with the aim of helping all tuberculous children in their own homes, and of teaching their parents how to care for them and how to protect other children in the family. The club also provided proper nourishment and clothing for the children and helped send some away for a change, free of charge. A summer shack was planned on the ground of the Lakeside Hospital for treatment.[3]

The Samaritan Club of Toronto also did much valuable work from 1912 to 1971. Organized in 1912 with Mrs R.N. Burns as president and Margaret Burns as secretary, assisted by Miss Julia Stewart as visiting nurse, the club undertook it first efforts in social service. It was the first organization to interest itself in rehabilitation of the tuberculous and organized a similar club in Hamilton.

Typical of the early volunteers were wealthy and socially prominent men who had sufficient drive to enlist others to their cause and who used their influence to encourage the press to bring discussion of tuberculosis into the open, a necessary step in public education. All across the country were men and women who had full-time occupations to keep them busy but who somehow found time to devote to some local, provincial, or national tuberculosis association. They raised money or pushed programs. Most of the women were housewives, but the men's occupations covered a wide range.

In Toronto Sir William Gage's interest in tuberculosis began long before he was Sir William. As early as 1894 he was discussing with the Toronto Board of Trade what could be done, and to get something started in the way of treatment, he donated $25,000 towards the construction of a sanatorium. Two years passed and no building was started, which was hard on the patience of a man like Sir William. Just at that point Fred Victor Massey contracted tuberculosis. The anxious parents began to look for a hospital and found none. A friend suggested they contact Mr Gage, who was known to be interested, which they did. With that the building of the Muskoka Hospital at Gravenhurst was started, Canada's first sanatorium. Two years later it began to admit patients. It shortly appeared that far more accommodation was needed so a second hospital, the Muskoka Free Hospital, was built about a mile away in 1902. Even with the second hospital, all the patients from the Toronto area could not be admitted so Mr Gage bought the Dennis farm near Weston and founded what was to become the Weston Hospital in 1904. Then, in 1910, this very intelligent volunteer turned his attention to medical and nursing services. To encourage doctors to take an interest in specializing in tuberculosis, he offered five scholarships of $100 each to medical students who would make a special study of the disease. When he found out how important nursing was, and particularly how many patients remained in their own homes and needed the advice of a district nurse, he interested himself in the work of the Victorian Order of Nurses. When it became plain that a dispensary was needed where the disease could be diagnosed and to which patients not hospitalized could come for medical advice, Sir William gave the city a free dispensary in 1914, which later was named the Gage Institute. It is still operating on College Steet. Finally, to crown it all, in memory of King Edward VII, who as Prince of Wales had been in the vanguard of volunteers and had written a letter to the Earl of Minto, then governor general, suggesting that an association of volunteers be started, he created the Edward VII Memorial Fund of one million dollars. The funds were used to build the King Edward VII Hospital in 1907 and the Queen Mary Hospital for Children in 1913.

The stimulus which Sir William gave to the program in Toronto was supplied in London by Sir Adam Beck. Sir Adam and Lady Beck, on finding that their only child, Marion, had developed tuberculosis, were shocked to discover the lack of tuberculosis services. Marion recovered, which was considered a minor miracle, for which her parents in thankfulness devoted large sums of money to the building of sanatoria and an equally generous amount of their very considerable organizing ability and unflagging energy. Not only did they work hard themselves, they recruited others. Sir Adam persuaded twenty prominent men of the city to form the London Health Association, the aim of which was to muster financial backing for the Queen Alexandra Sanatorium, which was opened in 1910. While Sir Adam was organizing men to provide money, Lady Beck rallied the women of London to form a sanatorium auxiliary. They, too, devoted themselves to fund-raising. Like other auxiliaries of the period, they sponsored tag days and held whist drives, balls, ice cream socials, and rummage sales.

Volunteers of that day brought a degree of personal involvement and commitment which in this day of government services is all too rare. In addition to working for the sanatorium as an institution, Lady Beck, in a beautiful contralto voice, sang to the patients. In the first year that the sanatorium was open Sir Adam, who was chairman of the Ontario Hydro Commission, promised there would be electricity for Christmas. He spent the day riding up and down the lines encouraging the workers, and at six o'clock the lights went on. Learning one Sunday that the furnace was not working, he went to the sanatorium, examined the furnace, located the source of the trouble, and taking off his coat made the necessary repairs. Since, after the fashion of the time, the sanatorium was a considerable distance from the city, accommodation was needed for nurses. Sir Adam and Lady Beck donated $25,000 to pay for a residence, which opened in 1918 as the Marion Beck Nurses' Home. When Sir Adam, who was reading the opening address, became so choked with emotion that he could not continue, Lady Beck stepped forward and finished the speech.

By the time Sir Adam died in 1925 the Queen Alexandra Sanatorium was a million dollar institution, but still the founder was not satisfied. His deathbed wish was that a public appeal be made on behalf of the sanatorium. This was done and $500,000 was contributed. In 1941 the name of the sanatorium was changed to the Beck Memorial in his honour. Sir Adam had been president of the London Health Association, in which post he was succeeded by Colonel Ibbotson Leonard, who served for the next twenty-five years.

In Ottawa, Dr James Grant (later Sir James) campaigned with unflagging zeal. He combined medical practice with a career in politics, being elected to the House of Commons in Canada's first parliament in 1867. He was also one of the leading physicians in the city, including in his practice the governors general and their families. He was an eloquent speaker, whose gifts as an orator secured for him generous press coverage as he urged all and sundry to be up and doing in the struggle against tuberculosis.

There were also women who brought their wealth, enthusiasm, and social prominence to the cause. Their gifts of money were less imposing but they were still substantial and they brought in something else: the participation of a great number of other women. Conspicuous in this group were Mrs P.D. Crerar of Hamilton and Lady Gooderham of Toronto. They enlisted the help of the Imperial Order of the Daughters of the Empire, whose members were to do yeomen service for many years, particularly in programs for prevention and treatment of tuberculosis among children.

Mrs Crerar started a new chapter of the IODE, the St Elizabeth, whose duty it was to provide linen for the Mountain Sanatorium in Hamilton, which at that time (1906) consisted of a remodelled farmhouse and some tents. Mrs Crerar was an initiator of 'involvement,' which was to become the watchword of those promoting health and welfare causes later. For many years she was involved with the development of the Mountain Sanatorium.

Members of the Heather Club Chapter of the IODE came to Lady Gooderham in Toronto for her advice and help because they felt that a building was needed for care of children who had been exposed to tuberculosis but were thought not to have the disease. Lady Gooderham was much interested and stirred up enthusiasm in various chapters of the order. She and her husband made very large donations to the building and this money, along with that raised by the chapters, was sufficient to build the first 'preventorium' in North America, which opened in 1913 in Toronto. The first 'Rose Day' was also sponsored at Lady Gooderham's instigation.

By 1912 it was compulsory for physicians to report all cases of tuberculosis to the local medical officer of health. The government maintenance grant for patients in sanatoria was raised to $3.00 per patient per week. In the same year the Peterborough Health Association started its health work by hiring a nurse to work with the tuberculous.

The Fort William Anti-Tuberculosis Society reported to the Canadian Association for the Prevention of Tuberculosis in 1912 that they had set up a publicity committee, and that they had sent out a circular letter to the head of each fraternal, labour, commercial, and social association in the city, outlining the society's views and functions and requesting co operation in spreading knowledge of the association among those who needed its aid.[4]

Dr John W.S. McCullough, chief medical officer of Ontario, viewed the tuberculosis problem in Ontario in 1913:

To what then is the lessening of our death rate from consumption due? Principally to education. When the disease was thought to be directly due to heredity, there was a sort of fatalistic impression held respecting it. It was thought, and is still in the opinion of many people, that once tuberculosis is acquired death is a foregone conclusion. Steadily this idea is being dispelled. Following the knowledge of the germ, disease and its cause made available its prevention and cure: prevention, by the avoidance of close association with the consumptive, by living in pure air, the use of good food, good living conditions and lessened hours of labour: cure, by the same methods, including rest and avoidance of quack remedies and alcohol.

The facts contributing to the educative campaign have been public lectures, public health exhibits, the physician, the visiting nurse, the dispensary, the press and the sanatorium. The latter has become possible all over the Province by the government and municipal aid established within the last ten or twelve years.[5]

The Ontario Laennec Society was organized in 1916 to serve as the medical wing of the voluntary associations.

In 1923 the first school survey took place in the town of Dundas and the Township of West Flamboro, Wentworth County, under the auspices of the Canadian Tuberculosis Association. The following year the first provincial travelling clinic for diseases of the lungs began operation by visting Clinton and Hawkesbury. The clinic aimed to assist physicians who had no access to sanatoria or chest consultants and to educate the public in the importance of early diagnosis and treatment of pulmonary tuberculosis and the value of periodic check-ups by their family physician.[6] In 1925 it was reported that 'thirty-three city clinics report 65,352 persons examined last year. Eleven Ontario Red Cross Sanatorium Extension Clinics examined 614 people referred as suspicious by their family doctors.'[7]

In 1935 the Division of Tuberculosis Prevention was established in the Department of Health, with Dr George Clair Brink as director. Five travelling clinics for lung diseases were organized, based in Ottawa, Belleville, North Bay, Timmins, and Fort William. By 1940 they were conducting 131 clinics annually in 71 different centres.

The first course in health education for teachers was initiated in 1936. It was designed for elementary school teachers, and was sponsored by the Ontario Department of Health and Education. It attracted considerable attention in other parts of the country, as well as in the United States. The first year the enrolment stood at 45, the second year 55, the third 85, and 176 in the fourth. This obvious interest was highly gratifying to the voluntary and official agencies endeavouring to provide teaching material for the schools. The course was designed to teach positive concepts of health rather than negative ones of disease, and emphasized that children should develop good health habits at an early age and good attitudes towards life, as well as being allowed to develop their own individual personalities.

Dr Brink summarized the requirements for a future program in a paper on 'Influencing Factors in the Control of Tuberculosis in Ontario' issued in 1936 as follows:

1. More organized effort to control tuberculosis is necessary in most Ontario municipalities. In comparatively few centres are to be found records of known tuberculous cases and contacts. This is in part due to failure on the part of the attending physician to report his cases.
2. There is unnecessary delay in bringing about sanatorium treatment for patients from many municipalities, especially those in financial difficulties.
3. Sanatorium beds are urgently needed in eastern Ontario.
4. Many northern Ontario centres and some isolated centres in southern Ontario lack diagnostic facilities.
5. Discharge from sanatoria of patients who have received maximum benefit is being delayed due chiefly to lack of effort on the part of the municipal authorities to assume responsibility for after care.
6. It would appear that some strengthening of the Regulations for dealing with non-cooperative cases is indicated.
7. Greater cooperation is required between the local officer of health, the municipal council, the board of health and the attending physician.[8]

In 1938 new legislation concerning indigent patients came into effect, thus relieving the municipalities of the cost of their maintenance in sanatoria. Also more provincial funds than ever were devoted to preventive and curative work. Six travelling clinics, costing $85,000, conducted 152 local clinics, examining 13,591 persons and disclosing 707 new cases of tuberculosis.

In 1942 a law was passed providing for periodic medical examination of teachers. Following this there was a great impetus in x-ray surveys. Ottawa announced that 34,000 civil servants would be x-rayed at the expense of the Department of Pensions and National Health, the survey itself to be conducted by the Ontario Department of Health, Tuberculosis Prevention Branch. The Toronto *Globe and Mail* had the distinction of being the first Canadian newspaper to have its employees examined for tuberculosis. Some 9000 industrial workers in Hamilton were x-rayed and only two positive reactions were found.

The first survey of an entire community was conducted in the small town of Geraldton in 1943, situated in the Little Long Lac goldmining district. The local branch of the Canadian Red Cross Society sponsored the scheme, their volunteers making a house-to-house survey after the public had been acquainted with the reasons for the survey by the press and by lectures to various groups. The Kirkland Lake Lions Club purchased an x-ray machine which they turned over to the Township of Teck, thus making history by being the first community of its size to purchase its own machine and undertake its own antituberculosis campaign.

Until this time all the sanatoria in Ontario were run by the local organizations with the notable exception of the Calydor Sanatorium at Gravenhurst, founded by Dr C.D. Parfitt and Mr F. Deutch in 1916, which was privately owned and run until it was eventually closed in 1935. A successful province-wide association was needed to co-ordinate the work being done by so many individual agencies. In a letter dated 20 October 1943 Dr G.J. Wherrett, executive secretary of the Canadian Tuberculosis Association, suggested to Dr C.G. Shaver, chairman of the Ontario Sanatorium Superintendents Association:

I think this whole matter would be helped if we had an Ontario Tuberculosis Association, with a central office – say in Toronto – and a full-time officer, whose duties would be to coordinate all the work that is being done in the province. I think the Superintendents Association and the Laennec Society would work in very well with this organization. The Laennec Society would be the scientific group, the Superintendents Association would be the administrative group, and the provincial association would coordinate seal sale work and would help us in putting over a better educational programme. I was glad to see that there seemed to be a good deal of interest in this suggestion at the meeting and Dr. Brink and Dr. Crombie told me after the meeting that they thought it was a good idea.

I have already written to Mr. Ruddy and made the suggestion to him that this might be a good way to bring in the National Sanitarium Association, and suggested that they might be prepared to provide space for an office.[9]

At a meeting of the executive committee of the Canadian Tuberculosis Association in 1944 Dr D.A. Carmichael, Dr G.C. Brink, and Dr Wherrett agreed to draw up a constitution, setting out the aims and objectives of the proposed association. This was presented by Dr Wherrett to the Association of Sanatorium Superintendents at a meeting on 6 November 1944, and full approval was given for the formation of an Ontario association. Dr Wherrett assured the meeting that a grant would be available from the Canadian Life Insurance Officers' fund for the salary of an executive officer. On

10 February 1945 the Letters Patent were awarded the Ontario Tuberculosis Association: 'To promote and assist in providing adequate facilities for the prevention and control of tuberculosis,' Article 11 of the constitution outlined its objectives: to co-ordinate and assist in the work of all the province's local sanatorium associations, societies, and committees; to assist government, both provincial and local, in programs for prevention and control of the disease; to encourage the provision of adequate facilities for early diagnosis through sanatorium treatment to rehabilitation; to encourage the development of educational programs; and to constitute the co-ordinating link between the Canadian Tuberculosis Association and all local voluntary associations in Ontario. Mr E.J. O'Brien was appointed executive secretary on loan from the Department of Health.

The Department of Health had been devoting itself to the task of getting the machinery of the mass surveys into action. Because of the urgency of the matter, the service clubs were approached to help raise the money. Later, when it was found that the service club approach was inadequate, the county associations were developed by Mr O'Brien to raise funds. Regional reference clinics, staffed by regional sanatorium personnel, were set up to evaluate suspected cases found in the surveys. In the first four years of mass x-raying, a total of 304,521 active tuberculosis cases were discovered. By the end of 1946, eighty surveys had been conducted, thirty-five local tuberculosis committees formed, and a number of other organizations active in tuberculosis control were recognized by the Ontario Tuberculosis Association. Pembroke, the first city to institute mass chest x-ray surveys, was also the first to give routine chest examinations to all patients admitted to a general hospital. General hospitals soon followed the lead of the Pembroke Cottage Hospital, with the Brockville committee paying for equipment in two hospitals and financing the full cost of operation.

In 1948 the annual Federal Health Grants program to the provinces was established by the federal government. The grant to Ontario for the control of tuberculosis was used to administer free streptomycin and para-amino-salicyclic acid (PAS) to all sanatorium patients; to purchase x-ray equipment for use in clinics and hospitals, including the hospital admission program; to purchase a complete x-ray unit, including a bus, to be added to the division's mobile fleet; and to pay the expenses incurred by research programs.

At this time Ontario instituted a special immigration policy. All British immigrants wanting to come to Canada under the provincial government's air transportation plan were expected to be x-rayed first. Dr Brink went to London to inaugurate the scheme, taking x-ray equipment with him. Clinics were also planned for Glasgow.

In 1949 a committee consisting of Dr G.J. Wherrett, Dr S.A. Holling (assistant director of tuberculosis control), and Dr H.T. Ewart (medical superintendent, Mountain Sanatorium, Hamilton) was appointed to review and appraise the program of the Ontario Tuberculosis Association and its relation to the Department of Health. In their report to the department they stated:

The outstanding accomplishments have been the increase in local clinic facilities, the mass survey programme, which has been greatly extended, the hospital admission programme, which is well underway, and other local projects which have been undertaken.

... Programme planning becomes the most important problem of anti-tuberculosis effort in the province of Ontario. It should be studied together by all agencies and organizations, both official and voluntary, to exert the greatest pressure where it is most needed and so that each can carry out the tasks for which it is best suited.

... Consideration should be given to the appointment of a Medical Advisory Committee.

... There is need for intensifying the educational programme in the province. This includes not only education of the public, but also staff education projects such as post-graduate courses for doctors and nurses. It should also include affiliation courses for undergraduates. It seems evident that an additional staff member, trained in health education, should be added to the Ontario Tuberculosis Association staff. Such a person would enable the association to avail itself of all the avenues for health education and be a liaison officer with institutions, Departments of Health and Education, and also be in a position to assist local committees in organizing health education programmes. The preparation and distribution of health education material requires more attention. This applies to films, pamphlets and other educational aids. There is a dearth of such properly trained personnel in Canada and we believe someone should be adequately trained for the work. From our discussions so far with local committees, we believe that they appreciate these needs and would be prepared to assist financially in providing them.

The Executive Secretary has spent a very busy three years. He has had a great deal to do in organizing local committees, seal sale work, educational work, local clinics, mass surveys and the hospital admission programme. Much of this organization work is now in hand; the Department has taken over the hospital admission programme and the mass surveys and the Executive Secretary can, perhaps, spend more time on studying the constitution and strengthening the framework of the Association. More time should also be spent on local organization. Locals should have also a constitution or at least a working agreement with the provincial association. More uniformity in name and organization of local committees would perhaps make them feel more a part of the provincial association and wean them away from the present, perhaps exaggerated idea, of local autonomy and instil in them more responsibility in regard to the future unified provincial organization.[10]

Education of the public continued to be the voluntary agency's greatest challenge. If tuberculosis was to be eradicated, the public must be informed as to the cause, treatment, and prevention of the disease. An educated public would fully utilize the excellent diagnostic facilities in Ontario. In order to accomplish this, the service of a qualified health educator was deemed a necessity. Mrs May Dale was appointed in 1953 and in her first health education report for the Ontario Tuberculosis Association, she stated that, since education was so fundamental to every aspect of a tuberculosis association's activities, its reponsibility should not rest with the executive secretary but with executive council as a whole, and in particular with an education subcommittee.[11]

The tuberculosis scene was changing rapidly. Dr Brink reported that during 1953 the situation in sanatoria in Ontario had gone from a waiting list of 171 patients to 324 empty beds.[12] He also stated that the voluntary agencies in Ontario had contributed greatly to the control of tuberculosis, having taken a great part in the promotion and development of various services, particularly education, rehabilitation, and case-finding. The association that year had used the Christmas Seal funds to provide free clinic service in 181 of the 265 clinics in the province and to contribute towards the expenses of twenty-nine other clinics.

In 1959 the constitution of the Canadian Tuberculosis Association was changed to deal with all chest diseases. It was empowered to seek the prevention and control of tuberculosis and related contributory and similar diseases. In a review of the Ontario Tuberculosis Association, Dr C.W.L. Jeanes suggested that it revise its constitution in a similar manner for the purpose of promoting public health.

The Ontario Thoracic Society was formed in 1960 by amalgamation of the Ontario Laennec Society, which existed since 1916, and the medical section of the Ontario Tuberculosis Association.

The 1960s represented a period of rapid growth for the Ontario Tuberculosis Association. Its basic philosophy was to develop community understanding towards the betterment of the public's health, with particular regard to tuberculosis and other chest diseases. The desired goal was active participation in its various programs. The primary concern was to educate and encourage the full use of all facilities provided. It even went so far as to broaden its scope to an awareness of the problem on an international scale.

Being proud of Canada's success in the fight against tuberculosis was not enough, said Dr Matthew B. Dymond, minister of health for Ontario, in a luncheon address at the International Conference on Tuberculosis in September 1961, as 'no boundaries, be they race, of geography, or of creed can exist where the health and welfare of humanity is concerned ... There can never be too free exchange of information, collaboration in research, or rendering of all possible help while one race or nation experiences results less good than those of the most successful.'[13]

The most valuable contribution the developed countries could make to the internationl problem, he went on to say, would be to supply consulting services to assist emerging countries in organizing their voluntary associations, since these countries generally lacked the trained personnel to administer chemotherapy programs, even though they might have had enough money to supply the necessary drugs.[14] As Mr O'Brien said at the Eastern Region Meeting of the International Union against Tuberculosis in Bangkok, 19 January 1963: 'the basic goal of a voluntary tuberculosis association is to help develop community attitudes and knowledge so there will be improved *action* towards better health. We all know that neither law-making nor official policy-making can be successful without the understanding and support of an informed citizenry. It is this informed population that makes possible our TB programmes. By being knowledgeable, they demand better services and actively support financial needs.'[15]

Though the Ontario Tuberculosis Association's interest was broadening, it was not unaware of the necessity of continuing education at home. In September 1962 an Executive Secretary's Institute on Tuberculosis Education, in co-operation with the Extension Department and the School of Hygiene of the University of Toronto, was held at the university. This was the first time that a voluntary association had ever arranged an institute with a university.

In 1964 the Ontario Tuberculosis and Thoracic Research Foundation was organized to aid the established respiratory research units in university centres and to create new similar units. In November of the same year Supplementary Letters Patent were granted to the Ontario Tuberculosis Association in order that it might extend its activities to the field of 'tuberculosis and related, contributing and similar diseases for the purpose of promoting public health.' The basic philosophy continued to be the enlisting and training of public health workers.

Ontario is an example of a province that over the years has established an excellent program for the control of tuberculosis. The Division of Tuberculosis Control of the Department of Health has been well directed, first by

Dr G.C. Brink, then by Dr A.S. Holling, and now (1974) by Dr C.A. Rorabeck. The department covers all phases of control: diagnosis and case-finding, treatment, and prevention. Its rehabilitation program was excellent when such a program was essential, and the Division of Research and Statistics gives a complete picture of the disease from year to year.

The Ontario Tuberculosis Association, now the Ontario Tuberculosis and Respiratory Disease Association, has an excellent record over its 30 years of existence. The various scattered, large and small, local associations have been successfully co-ordinated into county associations. Its board of management is now drawn from the many competent members of the boards of the local associations. Since its inception in 1945 it has had a dedicated staff led by Mr O'Brien, ably assisted by Mrs Norma Lytle and Mr Trevor Pierce. Mr Fergus Kelly, who was in charge of the Christmas Seal campaign until 1974, gave outstanding service. The program of health education has been ably run by such people as Mr William Anderson, Mr John Keys, and Mr Les MacDonald. For over ten years Mr O'Brien has also been interested in the international field and has rendered excellent service to the Far East as consultant to the International Union against Tuberculosis.

The move into the wider field of respiratory diseases has been supported by the development of the Ontario Thoracic Society, which was directed by Dr Cameron Gray, an outstanding internist interested in chest diseases. On the retirement of Mr O'Brien from the Ontario Tuberculosis and Respiratory Disease Association in 1971, Dr Gray assumed the role of its executive director as well. He was also largely responsible for the development of the Research Foundation of the association.

With the accomplishments of the past, the present excellent organizations, and new programs, the Ontario organization, like those in the other provinces, is ready for a period of greater service in the future.

19

Quebec

At the turn of the century the government of the province of Quebec seems to have been fully conscious of the seriousness of the problem of tuberculosis. The interest of the citizens and the part they played in developing a national program are demonstrated in a masterly report submitted to the annual meeting of the Canadian Association for the Prevention of Tuberculosis in Ottawa, in 1905, by the Montreal League for the Prevention of Tuberculosis, on the subject of the 'Responsibility of the Federal Government in Relation to the Prevention of Tuberculosis' and 'Certain Measures Which Could be Taken to Aid in Its Prevention,' which analysed the tuberculosis problem in Canada and abroad.[1] Signed by Drs J. George Adami, J.E. Dubé, and A.J. Richer, it contained recommendations that set the pattern for the development of the campaign against tuberculosis in Canada.

Both French and English groups in Montreal and Quebec were active, the French in organizing the Bruchesi Institute in Montreal and the dispensary in Quebec City, both in 1912, and the English in organizing the Royal Edward Institute in Montreal, in 1909.

The first signs of an active tuberculosis conscience in Montreal appeared in 1901 when a public meeting was held on 29 November at the Art Gallery and steps were taken to form the Montreal League for the Prevention of Tuberculosis. The league's constitution declared its objectives to be the distribution of leaflets and pamphlets (which were published either by themselves, the provincial or municipal health authorities, or later the Canadian Association for the Prevention of Tuberculosis), the giving of lectures on the subject, and the use of all effective measures to educate the community, in particular the working classes, to the fact that tuberculosis was preventable and curable and by very simple methods could be deterred from spreading. The league was also to support and encourage the medical societies and the medical profession at large, and the provincial and municipal authorities; to establish sanatoria; and to contribute to the relief of indigent consumptives. The formation of the Montreal league led to the establishment of other local associations.

The first annual report of the Montreal League for the Prevention of Tuberculosis was given at the meeting of the Canadian Association for the Prevention of Tuberculosis in Ottawa in 1905. It stated that on 1 June 1903 the first reports on cases of consumption had been received, and on 7 November a dispensary had been opened with four doctors in attendance. Education and instruction had been given to the suffering, so that they could become acquainted with the disease and with the work being done to overcome it, and they also received 'sanitary cuspidors' and 'instructive literature.' The league was occupied, too, in doing relief work in providing food, clothing, and medical attention, and inspectors visited patients in their homes. The league's Committee for Publication and Education issued a series of six leaflets in French and English for general distribution. Large 'wall-cards' were also printed and prominently posted in institutions and factories.

The moving spirit of the antituberculosis campaign was Colonel Jeffrey Burland. He came of a wealthy family whose members took the unusual view that they had a responsibility to use their money for the benefit of the less fortunate. The first record of the family's interest in tuberculosis appeared in the annals of the organization of the Montreal league in 1902. Colonel Burland's father was among those who attended the public meeting called by the Earl of Minto to get the Canadian association started. The first task which the Montreal league took up was to open a clinic where people with tuberculosis could get help, but this was not easy since it had practically no money. The Colonel's father, Mr George B. Burland, offered an empty store, rent free and heated. The offer was, of course, accepted and Montreal's first clinic was opened at 11 Bleury Street. Two years later Colonel Burland was appointed to the board of directors of the league and his industry and enthusiasm very soon made him its moving spirit, the person to whom all looked for inspired guidance.

One facet of Colonel Burland's activity was as a member of an investigative committee set up by the league to gather statistical information about tuberculosis in Montreal. Working with this committee was Dr E.S. Harding. The committee's industry turned up much sobering information about the extent of the disease in the city, the result of which was the appointment of Dr Harding as medical officer of the Royal Edward Institute.

Colonel Burland was a tireless worker. On a trip to Boston he made a point of visiting tuberculosis headquarters there and was much impressed by the educational campaign which the local association was carrying on, aimed at acquainting persons with more than average risk with the facts of the disease. He returned to Montreal and, with the co-operation of Dr Harding and a great deal of hard work, managed to get the Emmanuel Church Tuberculosis Class started, which proved a sound venture in public health education.

On yet another ostensible holiday, this time in the British Isles, Colonel Burland visited Edinburgh, where pioneer efforts in coping with tuberculosis were attracting attention. In the Royal Victoria Dispensary he found the model for what was to be his most lasting contribution to the struggle against tuberculosis in his city: The Royal Edward Institute, later the Royal Edward Laurentian Hospital, Montreal Division, and now the Royal Edward Laurentian Chest Hospital. The building was the gift of Colonel Burland and his sisters to the city. Its opening provides a generation grown casual towards tuberculosis with some idea of how emotionally involved men and women were with it earlier in the century. It also demonstrates that Colonel Burland was far ahead of his time in the public relations field and knew the value of a touch of drama in capturing public attention to a cause. The Colonel had arranged 'the royal touch' for the opening. The audience was gathered at dusk in a marquee outside the building. Then, in England, more that 4000 miles away, King Edward VII pressed a switch and every window blazed with light and the royal standard was run up the flag staff. Not only to those present did this symbolize the wonders of a new era, but to all those who read the account in the press, which was lyrical in describing the ceremony, when the sovereign put out his hand and lit the windows across the Atlantic, anything seemed possible.

One of the most comprehensive and effective pieces of work of the old league was the organization of a tuberculosis exhibition in November 1908. Professor J.G. Adami served as chairman and Dr Frazer B. Gurd was secretary and organizer. The exhibition was open to the public for twelve days, and was visited by some 50,000 people, half of whom were students from various schools. The exhibition was planned to create interest in the different phases of work against the disease, and to stress its importance to all. There were eye-appealing charts, models, and photographs, which were supplemented by lectures and by practical explanations and demonstrations. Interesting articles were published by the press. Copies of *The Catechism on Tuberculosis* were distributed to the schools for study in class. With the founding of the Royal Edward Institute in 1909, the league became dormant.

The Royal Commission on Tuberculosis for the Province of Quebec of 1909–10 was an important landmark in Quebec as well as in the rest of Canada. In its reports it emphasized the serious nature of the disease and described the agencies that had been developed in other provinces for its prevention and treatment. It also made a number of recommendations: (a) that the laws regarding tuberculosis be applied more rigorously; (b) that instruction in elementary hygiene be given in all schools at all levels; (c) that the public be educated, under the direction of the Board of Health; (d) that all schools, shops, and factories undergo medical inspection; (e) that antituberculosis dispensaries be established and maintained in all principal cities; (f) that advanced cases among the poor be isolated; (g) that open-air schools for children prone to tuberculosis be established; (h) that curable cases receive treatment; (i) that legislation be passed to prohibit employment of young children; (j) that the hours of labour of adults in factories be investigated and controlled by legislation; (k) that there be further legislation against alcoholism and for the inspection of meat and control of milk sales.

Facilities for the treatment of tuberculosis in the province of Quebec were provided by the building of a number of sanatoria. The Laurentian Sanatorium at Ste Agathe (opened in 1908), the Grace Dart Home Hospital in Montreal (1922), and the Lake Edward Sanatorium (1922) were constructed for English-speaking patients. Laval Hospital in Quebec City and the Sacred Heart Hospital in Montreal provided much-needed beds for French-speaking patients. Later, sanatoria were built at Three Rivers, in 1928, and at Sherbrooke and Rosemount, a suburb of Montreal, in the 1930s. The final building program in the 1940s included sanatoria at Dorchester, Mont Joli, Gaspé, Roberval, and Noranda, which completed the quota of sanatorium beds required.

The Three Rivers Demonstration[2] was instituted in 1923 by the Canadian Tuberculosis Association and the Quebec Board of Health. In December, public health addresses were given to capacity audiences at two local theatres, and a morning and afternoon were devoted to clinical meetings of the city's medical men. At the end of the demonstration a cheque for $10,500 was presented to the Quebec Board of Health by the Canadian Tuberculosis Association on behalf of the federal government and the Sun Life Assurance Company. In 1924, after twelve months of operation, the results had proved gratifying: 2064 people had been examined and 382 had received a positive diagnosis. After a second year's work, 64 people had been hospitalized, 175 attended in their homes from the dispensary, and 422 cases of tuberculosis had been diagnosed in the demonstration area and surrounding districts. A summer camp had been opened for children, and a group of citizens had formed a corporation for the building of a fifty-bed sanatorium, towards which $75,000 had already been collected. Over $60,000 had been spent on the demonstration, but it caused a trebling of the city's health budget.

The Montreal Anti-Tuberculosis and General Health League was organized on 24 March 1924 as an expression of a desire to improve health conditions in Montreal. The league was directed by Dr Grant Fleming with the collaboration of Dr J.A. Baudouin. The league, financed mainly by a grant from Lord Atholston of the *Montreal Star*, strove to increase public interest, and so helped prepare the way for a health survey of Montreal. After the typhoid epidemic of 1925, the time seemed opportune for such a survey. A group of public-spirited men were asked to sponsor the survey, and to act as a health survey committee to consider its findings. The league offered its staff to help, and to defray expenses, with the understanding that the Committee on Administrative Practice of the American Public Health Association would be called in as consultants as a courtesy. The Metropolitan Life Insurance Company agreed to publish the report.

The Health Survey Committee recognized the need for public health instruction, and so recommended that there be a section of health education as well as an advisory committee on health education in the Health Department. The committee's recommendations for the tuberculosis problem were: that a conference of tuberculosis institutions be held to encourage the provision of the 350 beds required at that time, on the basis of one 'indigent bed per annual death'; that institutional care be provided for children; and that the school commissioners provide open-air classrooms for at least 1260 children needing such care.[3] The last recommendation indicates the importance given fresh air in the treatment of tuberculosis at that time.

The fourth annual report of the Montreal Anti-Tuberculosis and General Health League[4] outlined its activities under three headings: Social Hygiene Committee – Health Education; Surveys; and Demonstrations. The Social Hygiene Committee had been responsible for weekly press articles which appeared in 151 Canadian newspapers and reached a combined audience of 1,200,000; it had distributed almost 4000 copies, half in English and half in French, of *Health in the Home* as well as other literature; it had given health instruction to five groups of fifteen each, some in co-operation with the Junior Red Cross; it had also held public health nurses' camps at the Old Brewery Mission. The Surveys section had supervised tuberculosis home cases and contacts from the Bruchesi Institute, the Herzyl Dispensary, and the Royal Victoria Hospital Chest Clinic, as well as non-pulmonary cases of the Children's Memorial Hospital and a few from private physicians. The Demonstration Committee had continued clinic supervision with a moderate amount of home supervision in the Coursol Street area, had held clinics at both health centres for diphtheria immunization of children six years and younger, and had supervised the scarlet fever immunization. At the end of the demonstration (five years) the league disbanded as the facilities of the Bruchesi Institute and the Royal Edward Institute had been extended and their affiliation with the University of Montreal and McGill University, respectively, had been obtained.

The first county health units in Quebec were established in Beauce and Lac St Jean in 1926, and a year later travelling clinics for the diagnosis of tuberculosis were organized, the main result of which was public education. These were first financed by the Canadian Tuberculosis Association with grants from the Sun Life Insurance Company of Canada and the Health Committee of the Canadian Life Insurance Officers' Association.

In 1932 the first industrial surveys were organized by the Canadian Tuberculosis Association, the Montreal Department of Health, and the McGill University Faculty of Medicine using funds provided by the Canadian Life Insurance Officers' Association for the purpose of demonstrating and encouraging tuberculosis case-finding in industry.

The Quebec Tuberculosis Society, a medical group, was established in 1934 to bring together all chest specialists in the province. Its initial meeting was held on 13 October in Three Rivers, with Dr J.A. Jarry of Montreal in the chair and all the province's chest specialists as well as several from other parts of Canada in attendance. At the second annual meeting the proposed program for the coming year included the following: education of the public by giving lectures to both lay and professional people throughout the province; a general tuberculosis survey, commencing with colleges, convents, and orphanages, and including teachers and students; more general use of pneumothorax; making BCG vaccine available to all newborn babies; regular reporting and classification of the disease; and an increase in the number of sanatorium beds.

On 29 November 1937 representatives of all official and non-official agencies engaged in tuberculosis work in the province met at the Cercle Universitaire in Montreal to organize the Quebec Provincial Committee for the Prevention of Tuberculosis. This committee was to constitute a central advisory body in the antituberculosis campaign and to encourage and assist all agencies, official and non-official, and to be affiliated with, and serve as a branch association of, The Canadian Tuberculosis Association. It was also to study tuberculosis problems by co-operating in the collection of statistics and to organize committees to study special problems; and to carry out an educational program and disseminate information on the prevention and treatment of tuberculosis so that the public might by stimulated to take over greater measures in its control. The committee's campaign was launched on 27 May 1938 at a public meeting held at the Montcalm Palace in Quebec, when members of the government, clergy, and medical and education professions pledged their support. This organization was incorporated and is still in operation in the province.

In his report, to the Canadian Life Insurance Officers' Association, on the Quebec Provincial Committee for the Prevention of Tuberculosis in 1938, Dr G.J. Wherrett stated:

In acknowledging the help of the Canadian Life Insurance Officers Association in initiating the formation of this Committee, the Canadian Tuberculosis Association feels that this has been a signal advance in attacking the tuberculosis problem in the Province of Quebec.

Although the proposition as put forward to the Health Committee of the Canadian Life Insurance Officers Association referred only to a demonstration in the counties east of the St. Lawrence River, the interest of the Quebec Government was so stimulated that they have provided financial assistance which has made it possible to so organize that the Committee might be province wide in scope.

It is the intention of the Committee to survey the needs of the Province and stimulate interest by local groups in providing institutions where these are particularly needed.

There has been no provincial setup for the control of the disease. Facilities that exist have been provided by voluntary groups such as Religious Orders and such organizations as the Laurentian Sanatorium Association and the Federation of Jewish Philanthropies. These have served the cities of Montreal, Three Rivers and Quebec, but other parts of the Province have been singularly lacking in treatment beds.

Clinics have been operated by local Tuberculosis Leagues as in Quebec and Three Rivers and by the Royal Edward Institute and Bruchesi Institute in Montreal.[5]

The committee received its Letters Patent on 24 January 1938. The powers given the directors were much the same as those listed as their original objectives. The following year Dr Georges Grégoire, the executive secretary, reported that their program consisted of four main points: case-finding for tuberculosis, education of the public, hospitalization for the tuberculous, and the improvement of home sanitation. They also distributed thousands of pamphlets to physicians and school children. A letter describing the committee's work was sent to each of the 3000 doctors practising in the province. Lectures were given to medical societies, and a series of radio sketches were broadcast on the CBC. Fifteen daily newspapers and thirty-five weeklies published articles without charge that were estimated to be worth some $20,000. The Metropolitan Life Insurance Company contributed a brochure and booklet.

A post-graduate course in tuberculosis, modelled on the one given at the famous Trudeau School at Saranac Lake, New York, and organized by the staff of the Jewish General Hospital and the Mount Sinai Sanatorium, was given at that sanatorium at Prefontaine during the week of 14–21 June 1938. The purpose of the course was to give general practitioners and students an opportunity to familiarize themselves with modern methods and aids to the early diagnosis of the disease. Instruction in x-ray techniques, pathology, and new laboratory methods was given, as well as lectures.

In 1940 an educational radio program of eight weeks' duration was undertaken by the Quebec Provincial Committee for the Prevention of Tuberculosis with the object of pointing out the hazards of the disease and at the same time stimulating public interest in better facilities for treatment.

An act, known as the Perrier Law, was passed in 1941 to prevent the spread of tuberculosis in schools. It was decreed that no person could be engaged by a public school without producing a health certificate from a doctor stating him fit to teach and a certificate from a physiologist attesting that he had had a clinical and radiological pulmonary examination and had been found to be free of disease.[6]

In 1942 the two foremost English tuberculosis institutions in Quebec, the Laurentian Sanatorium at Ste Agathe and the Royal Edward Institute, merged under the name Royal Edward Laurentian Hospital, as a result of the work done by Mr Howard Murray, president of the Royal Edward Institute. On 1 March of the same year the Montreal Anti-Tuberculosis League, Inc., which had been founded the previous October, received its Letters Patent. Its first three objectives were: to help financially all established organizations, such as the Bruchesi Institute, the Royal Edward Laurentian Hospital, and other similar agencies; to organize an education campaign; and to carry on research in industry and other places where contamination prevailed. It issued a monthly publication called *Notes on Tuberculosis*.

Industrial surveys, particularly among war workers, received new impetus through the efforts of the Montreal Anti-Tuberculosis League, starting with an examination of employees of the St Paul l'Ermite plant of Canada War Munitions. Quebec City also started x-ray surveys for all industrial employees, college students, and school children, using equipment purchased jointly by the Junior Chamber of Commerce of the city, the provincial Department of Health, the city council, and the Shawinigan Falls Welfare Association.

In 1946 the Quebec legislature voted $10,000,000 towards combatting tuberculosis. Full credit for this progressive legislation should go to Dr J.A. Vidal, a member of the staff of the Sacred Heart Hospital at Cartierville, who had a keen interest in the disease and was a friend of and personal physician to Premier Maurice Duplessis. The bill was introduced by the minister of health, the Honourable Albiny Paquette, and stated primarily:

The government is authorized to adopt the measures it shall deem expedient to combat tuberculosis and more particularly it may, upon the recommendation of the Minister of Health, organize the detection of cases of tuberculosis, contribute to the cost of the enlargement, construction and equipment of sanatoria for consumptives, bear the cost of hospitalization of indigent consumptives, the training of specialists in the treatment of such disease and anti-tuberculosis educational campaigns and generally adopt any other proper method of securing the success of the fight against tuberculosis.

... The government is authorized to spend for such purposes, out of the consolidated revenue fund, in the manner, upon the conditions and at the time it deem expedient, during a period of not more than four years, as from the coming into force of this act, a sum not exceeding ten million dollars.[7]

In 1953 the Quebec Department of Health launched a BCG vaccination program in the schools, which entailed the vaccination of more than 100,-000 people a year throughout the province. At first only newborn babies in Montreal hospitals and children known to have been in contact with the disease were vaccinated but then all school children and pre-school children found to be tuberculin-negative were included in the program. In the first stages the district health officer called on school principals to explain the aims and objects of the program, and talked to teachers on the subject. Later, an address was given to parents outlining the vaccination procedure. Letters were also sent out to the churches to be read to the parishioners.

Although the topic of BCG has been treated in a separate chapter in this volume, special mention should be made here of the introduction of the vaccine to Canada by Dr J.A. Baudouin and Dr Armand Frappier. The first project was the vaccination of the contacts in the city of Montreal, under the direction of Dr Baudouin. This was a controlled study, supported by the National Research Council through the Associate Committee on Tuberculosis Research. The committee made a study of the project as reported by

Dr J.W. Hopkins, statistician for the council. On his return to Montreal from post-graduate study in Paris, Dr Frappier developed a laboratory for the production of the vaccine, from which it was provided for other provinces as well as Quebec.

In 1950, and for the following two years, the Quebec Provincial Committee for the Prevention of Tuberculosis resumed its seminars for physicians wanting instruction in chest diseases.

In 1958 Dr Wherrett prepared a memo on the Montreal Anti-Tuberculosis League, which stated:

The League was organized by the Canadian Tuberculosis Association and the Quebec Provincial Committee for the Prevention of Tuberculosis. The purpose of the League was to co-ordinate anti-tuberculosis efforts in Montreal and to co-operate with all provincial organizations and departments to improve the situation generally. We anticipated that all organizations in Montreal would receive assistance from the League and any services that were developed would be on a co-operative basis with good co-ordination by all concerned. The League was formed with high hopes and Mr. C.A. Monat was its first president.

... The League has developed only the mass survey programme. For this purpose it has set up a large organization which have made survey costs the highest in Canada. In order to expand the programme, it has withdrawn support from the Bruchesi and Royal Edward Laurentian Hospital dipensaries. It has branched out in twenty-two counties adjacent to Montreal, employs its own nurses and organizers, rather than developing community services or using those already in existence.

... The main source of revenue seems to be from Federal and Provincial grants, plus a direct charge to industries for work done. In addition, there is a subscription campaign which capitalizes on the publicity of the National Christmas Seal Campaign.

... On the credit side of the ledger, the League has developed a large volume of work accomplished by the mass survey, although costs are high and there is overlapping in the follow-up. No other phases of the campaign are covered by the League.

... Since the Montreal Anti-Tuberculosis League is not affiliated with either the provincial group or the Canadian Tuberculosis Association, we have no reports as to revenue received and expended on the work done, other than what appears in the press.[8]

Dr Herman Gauthier, as president, reviewed the development of the Quebec Provincial Committee for the Prevention of Tuberculosis in 1959, stating: 'The history of tuberculosis control in our Province can be divided into two distinct periods: the first period, extending from 1905 to 1944, featured the work of voluntary organizations. In 1938, the Provincial Commit-tee for the Prevention of Tuberculosis was founded; anti-tuberculosis leagues and clinics were strongholds in the war against tuberculosis. The outstanding feature of the period extending from 1945 to 1959 was the very active participation of government agencies in the control program.'9

In 1965 the Montreal League Tuberculosis Association, which included the Montreal Anti-Tuberculosis League, the tuberculosis clinics, the sanato-ria, and the Montreal Chapter of the Croix de Lorraine Association, was or-ganized for the purpose of encouraging rehabilitation of the tuberculous.

It will be seen that since the beginning of the century there has grown up an extensive organization in Quebec, both voluntary and official, for the prevention, diagnosis, and treatment of tuberculosis. The province has con-centrated on certain phases of the campaign, such as BCG vaccination, to a greater extent than other provinces. With the coming of the new drugs in 1948, there has been a rapid fall in the death rate from tuberculosis and in the need for sanatorium beds, many of which have been adapted to other uses. For more than ten years there has been an over-all case register that has utilized information from the local health departments and the tubercu-losis dispensaries and sanatoria. Although the campaign over the years has at times been somewhat disjointed, it has nevertheless been far-reaching, and with the advent of drug therapy it has been eminently successful.

20

New Brunswick

Prior to the formation of a provincial tuberculosis association there was a great deal of activity in regard to tuberculosis in New Brunswick. At the turn of the century the death rate from the disease in the province was still unknown but there were upwards of 100 deaths yearly in Saint John alone. Sanatoria were obviously needed, but it was not known who would establish or support them, though it was considered reasonable that everyone should contribute, as it was in everyone's best interest to do so.

In 1909 the Moncton Anti-Tuberculosis League and the Saint John Tuberculosis Association were formed, and the legislative assembly passed an act 'to assist in the prevention and cure of tuberculosis,' empowering the lieutenant-governor-in-council to appoint a commission to look into this. The commission's recommendation was that a sanatorium be built for incipient cases.

In 1913 the Jordan Memorial Sanatorium at River Glade, the former summer home of Mrs James C. Jordan, who had generously donated it for the purpose, was formally opened. As a young woman, then Jeanette Stiles, Mrs Jordan had gone to Boston to work in the Jordan & Marsh department store. There she met, and eventually married, one of the owners, James C. Jordan. She brought him back to her native New Brunswick and they built a beautiful summer home on an estate where they even made an artificial lake. Over the years Mrs Jordan made some twenty-four wills in which she always left $250,000 to the sanatorium for its work. Unfortunately, her twenty-fifth, and last, will omitted this bequest, but the family, realizing that the omission was inadvertent, saw to it that the sanatorium received the money, which was eventually used to build an extension opened in 1927.

The chairman of the Moncton Board of Health wrote a *Catechism and Primer for School Children* dealing with tuberculosis, which was published in 1911 in both English and French. It was financed jointly by the city and county councils of Moncton and Westmorland, and a supply was sent to each school teacher in the district for distribution to students.

The Saint John County Hospital, later the Saint John Tuberculosis Hospital, owned and maintained by the city and county of Saint John, was opened in 1915, with Dr H.A. Farris as medical superintendent (he served in that capacity until 1930).

New Brunswick created the first Ministry of Health in the British Commonwealth in 1917 under the Honourable William Flowers Roberts (a provincial board of health had been operating since 1887), and in 1918 the Public Health Act came into effect. Dr Roberts had a progressive outlook on the development of public health in the province and included in the program a plan to attack tuberculosis. In May 1924 he organized a public health conference in Fredericton, at which the disease was discussed. There were representatives from the Saint John Tuberculosis Hospital and the Jordan Memorial Sanatorium, and Dr Thaddeus Sienewicz came from Halifax. As the Saint John Anti-Tuberculosis Association was the only functioning lay organization in the province at that time, there was discussion about the organization of a provincial tuberculosis association. Dr Sienewicz remarked: 'To get efficient organization one must get a body of people who are really interested in the work, creation of fulltime tuberculosis physicians, who must have organizing ability and a good personality. A public health nurse or instructor is the best means of discovering unknown cases of tuberculosis in the homes. Educational methods must be extensively used. The public must find the means to finance this work. There is golden opportunity to attack tuberculosis in the school age – the problem there is largely one of under-nourishment.'[1]

Following this conference, Dr Roberts authorized the appointment of a travelling tuberculosis diagnostician, and the services of Dr George J. Wherrett of Fort Qu'Appelle Sanatorium were obtained. The developments during the next three years are outlined in a memorandum from Dr Wherrett to the New Brunswick Tuberculosis Association:

Somewhere along 1923 or 1924, a New Brunswick Tuberculosis Association was organized with Dr. L.G. Pinault of Campbellton as President, and Mr. H.M. Armstrong, Campbellton as Secretary. It was the Association that arranged for the first Tuberculosis Diagnostician. There was some confusion as to whom the Tuberculosis Diagnostician should report – whether the newly created Association or the Department of Health. The original plan was that he was to organize the New Brunswick Tuberculosis Association and that enough money to pay his salary would be forthcoming. Dr. Roberts arranged that the Tuberculosis Diagnostician became a member of the staff of the Department of Health. The Tuberculosis Diagnostician began to carry on clinics throughout the Province and no further progress was made on the New Brunswick Tuberculosis Association during 1924.

In 1926, it was realized that something should be done to stimulate the interest of the Province and a new Committee was formed for the prevention of tuberculosis with Mr. J.A. Murray of Sussex as Chairman: 2 or 3 informal meetings were held. The next development was that Dr. R.E. Wodehouse, then Executive Secretary of the Canadian Tuberculosis Association obtained $15,000 from the Canadian Life Insurance Officers' Association for an educational programme in the Maritime Provinces. The Maritime Tuberculosis Educational Committee was set up and from those funds we employed a second Diagnostician.[2]

As a preliminary survey of tuberculosis infection in the province, a survey of school children in Moncton and Rexton was undertaken. The universities of Mount Allison at Sackville and St Joseph at Memramcook were also surveyed in 1926. In every instance active infectious cases of tuberculosis were discovered. A child from Moncton public school was diagnosed and, although treated in the sanatorium, died within a year of admission. The surveys thus pointed up the presence of unknown spreaders of disease in the general population.

Dr Wherrett became medical director of the committee and divided his time between New Brunswick and Prince Edward Island. Dr Gordon McLean was appointed to his position with the Department of Health, thus providing two clinicians for the work in the two provinces. On Dr McLean's death and Dr Wherrett's departure for postgraduate training in London, England, in 1928, Dr C.W. MacMillan and Dr J.A. Melanson came to the Department of Health in the capacity of tuberculosis officers.

In 1931 Sir James H. Dunn gave his summer home and property near Bathurst to the Roman Catholic Bishop of Bathurst for the isolation of tuberculosis patients in the district. On this site was erected the sixty-bed sanatorium Notre-Dame de Lourdes, which was officially opened in 1932, thus increasing the provincial bed capacity to more than 400.

Also, in 1931, Dr Melanson prepared a script 'Public Enemy No.1,' in both English and French, for a film on tuberculosis, which was used in the province for many years, the first film of its kind in Canada.

The Letters Patent of the New Brunswick Anti-Tuberculosis Association came through on 30 January 1933. Its aims were: to promote the prevention and early treatment of tuberculosis; to educate the public in the knowledge of the real nature of the disease, and how to avoid it, prevent its spread, and cure it; to distribute literature; and to co-operate with the Canadian Tuberculosis Association and other tuberculosis organizations in their annual sale of Christmas Seals. From 1933 to 1948 the Seal money was administered by the chief medical officer of the province, Dr Charles W. MacMillan, who was also treasurer of the association. The money was spent on x-ray examinations for indigent patients, motion picture projectors for the showing of educational films, and small x-ray units for survey purposes.

By 1934 the New Brunswick Department of Health, under a minister, and a chief medical officer, maintained two especially trained travelling diagnosticians in a sub-department of tuberculosis. As well as providing diagnostic service, they also conducted school and college surveys and made arrangements for institutional treatment for indigent patients. County surveys had been under way for some time, and there were three sanatoria: the Saint John Tuberculosis Hospital, the Jordan Memorial Sanatorium at River Glade, and Our Lady of Lourdes at Bathurst. An important feature in the government's program was the support it gave to the New Brunswick Anti-Tuberculosis Association to carry on its Christmas Seal campaign throughout the province, except where local organizations did not require it, in the realization that the sale did much to bring the prevention of tuberculosis to the public's mind, though, of course, the association did much more in its efforts to educate the public.[3]

In 1936 the New Brunswick Department of Health and the New Brunswick Tuberculosis Association sponsored a tuberculosis survey and did educational work in Northumberland and Gloucester counties. In February of the following year the Speech from the Throne to the legislative assembly announced that the Department of Health would undertake a tuberculosis survey of the whole province 'to secure exact data as to its prevalence with a view to its control and ultimate eradication.' That was the year in which New Brunswick, along with its sister Maritime province Prince Edward Island, was able to declare that it was entirely free of bovine tuberculosis.

A tax, the first in Canada, was imposed on the retail price of tobacco in 1940; the proceeds went to the municipalities on the basis of $1.00 per patient per day for the treatment of tuberculosis. By the late 1940s mass surveys were well under way. Saint John had embarked on a survey of its working population. Just prior to this, in 1945, the provincial government announced that it would assume all responsibility for the cost of hospitalization of tuberculosis patients. The need for further treatment accommodation was taken care of by taking over the air force hospital at Moncton, which operated, together with an outdoor clinic, until after the effect of the new drugs became apparent and the hospital was no longer needed.

On 31 January 1946 representatives of the voluntary groups working on tuberculosis in New Brunswick held a special meeting to reorganize the New Brunswick Anti-Tuberculosis Association. These groups were the Saint John Tuberculosis Association and the Christmas Seal committees of the cities of Bathurst, Campbellton, Edmundston, Fredericton, Moncton, Saint John, and Woodstock. A planning committee was formed. It recommended that all members of the existing New Brunswick Anti-Tuberculosis Association and Christmas Seal committees be invited to become members of the reorganized New Brunswick Tuberculosis Association, and that an enlarged executive council be formed so that there would be one member for each county, as well as one each for Saint John, Moncton, and Fredericton, and two members-at-large.[4] The first full-time secretary, Mr John J. Arsenault, who was appointed at this meeting, was fully occupied for a time in re-establishing the association's program. The deputy minister of health and secretary-treasurer of the New Brunswick Tuberculosis Association, Dr J. Arthur Melanson, urged the association to push more strongly the program for early diagnosis and health education, advocating an increase in the Seal sale, the establishment of a full-time clinic (which had been curtailed during World War II), and the launching of mass surveys.[5] By 19 September 1946 Mr Arsenault was able to report that the reorganization of the association had made it truly provincial in scope.[6]

In 1947 Dr George Edward Maddison was appointed director of tuberculosis control with the responsibility for planning and supervising the anti-tuberculosis program as well as for co-ordinating the diagnostic treatment and educational services of all agencies, official and voluntary.

Also in 1947 the New Brunswick Tuberculosis Association purchased a mobile x-ray unit, complete with generator, and in 1948 the rehabilitation program was started. Mr Frank G. Baker was appointed rehabilitation director, to provide vocational counselling and training and placement guidance. With the reorganization of the association, the educational services throughout the province were expanded, and local committees increased their sales of Christmas Seals.

A new tuberculosis clinic in Saint John was officially opened on 17 November 1950 in a building purchased by the Saint John Anti-Tuberculosis Association assisted by the Christmas Seal fund. The cost of equipping the clinic was borne by grants from the federal government, and the New Brunswick Tuberculosis Association agreed to meet the operating expenses.

In his presidential address to the membership that year Mr G.L. Miller reported that the New Brunswick Tuberculosis Association was directing its time and resources to case-finding, education, and rehabilitation. The case-finding program, he said, was carried out satisfactorily in co-operation with the Department of Health. The policy of the association was to embark on new projects and, when they proved successful, to let the official agency take over, which was what had been done with the case-finding program. The department was slowly assuming responsibility for the mass x-ray programs and the permanent clinics, which allowed more money to be devoted to other programs. The educational program was carried out in conjunction with the x-ray surveys and the annual Seal sales. Rehabilitation was still a new aspect of the association's work, a director of rehabilitation having been appointed, with staff provided by the Department of Health.[7]

In 1951 the Department of Health arranged a one-day clinical session for some thirty doctors at the Jordan Memorial Sanatorium, as part of its plan to bring physicians together to consider new methods of planning the treatment of tuberculosis. In attendance were members of the departmental administrative staff, the medical superintendents of the five sanatoria and their medical staffs, and the district and federal medical health officers.

The New Brunswick Tuberculosis Association continued the usual work in connection with their educational program. Thousands of leaflets, pamphlets, and booklets concerned with various aspects of tuberculosis were distributed to hospitals, sanatoria, nurses' schools, clinics, teachers' colleges, public health nurses, schools, service clubs, and libraries. Films were distributed, and programs were featured in the newspapers and theatres and on radio and television stations. Meetings were organized, featuring speakers and films. Letters were sent throughout the province in connection with the Christmas Seal sale.

Allied with the provincial association were fourteen county, three city, and two area associations, which were almost exclusively fund-raising organizations, giving the proceeds of their Seal sales, in whole or in part, to the provincial association. Exceptions to this were the Moncton and Saint John associations, who organized their own local programs. The Saint John association had such an active program that there was usually no money left over to pass on, but, though Moncton was equally active, the association there often had funds left over.

The conclusion to the story of the campaign against tuberculosis in New Brunswick is indicated in the Annual Report of Tuberculosis Control in New Brunswick for 1972 by the director, Dr Maddison. Deaths had been reduced to nine, or 1.4 per 100,000 persons. The number of cases had fallen to the lowest ever recorded, 87 or 13.7 per 100,000, well below the national average. The five institutions, which in 1953 provided 930 beds (including the St Joseph Sanatorium of St Basile of 132 beds and the Moncton Tuberculosis Hospital of 153 beds, which had been taken over by the province from the federal Department of Defence), had been either closed or converted to other uses and actually had only thirty-five patients in residence at the end of the year.

21

Nova Scotia

Antituberculosis efforts in Nova Scotia began early in the century, when a number of local associations were organized, some of which are still in operation. Among the first was the Colchester Society for the Prevention of Tuberculosis, which began operation in January 1905. Local clergymen and physicians assisted the society with the preparation and circulation of pamphlets on the nature of tuberculosis and its prevention. The Anti-Tuberculosis Leagues of Nova Scotia, organized in 1908, carried out an educational program by distributing the booklet *Consumption, Its Cause and Cure*, financed by the sale of advertising space and small grants from county and town councils. The Tri-County Tuberculosis League, which included the counties of Antigonish, Guysboro, and Pictou, as well as Cape Breton, Inverness, Richmond, and Victoria, was organized by St Francis Xavier University and the medical members of the seven counties of eastern Nova Scotia.

The earliest *treatment* facility was the Highland View Sanatorium in Wolfville, opened in 1899. This private institution of eight beds closed in 1903. In 1904 the Nova Scotia Sanatorium at Kentville was built with a bed capacity of eighteen. Dr. A.F. Miller, an ex-patient of the sanatorium at Saranac Lake, New York, was appointed medical superintendent. His frail frame gave no hint of the determined spirit within or the long life of service he would give to the institution. His successor Dr. J. Earle Hiltz, appointed on his retirement in 1937, also gave distinguished service until his death in 1969.

The Halifax Tuberculosis League, formed in 1908, employed a nurse to make home visits to the tuberculous. As early as 1914 it became responsible for the maintenance of a house it had purchased for use as a sanatorium. The league also assisted the city of Halifax in the building of the 65-bed Halifax Tuberculosis Hospital which was opened in 1921.

The Massachusetts-Halifax Health Commission was set up in 1919 to supervise the money remaining from the generous donations made to assist victims of the Halifax disaster of 1917.* In fact, there was enough money for the commission to carry on other work until 1933. Its contribution to the tuberculosis cause was substantial. It included the provision of a diagnostic clinic, which was available to all physicians in the city for consultation, as well as assistance to the teaching program of Dalhousie Medical School, which was under the direction of Dr. T. Sieniewicz. It also made its personnel available to the Halifax Tuberculosis Hospital and provided public health nurses and visiting housekeepers for home instruction services under the guidance of the medical officers. In doing this it assumed the duties of the Halifax Anti-Tuberculosis League.

The tuberculosis service in the province was further strengthened in 1924 when the Dalhousie Public Health Clinic, which included a chest clinic, was built with assistance from the Rockefeller Foundation. This was also directed by Dr. Sieniewicz.

In 1926 the Nova Scotia Tuberculosis Commission was organized by the Canadian Tuberculosis Association with funds from the Canadian Life Insurance Officers' Association. A five-year demonstration was carried out with the continued support of the life insurance grant and thus helped to establish a firm foundation for the tuberculosis control movement, giving great impetus to public activities. Adequate permanent and travelling clinical, medical, and nursing services were established. The commission's campaign, under the direction of Mr Joseph Hayes, consisted of addresses with slides or moving pictures, and distribution of literature encouraging municipalities to assume their responsibilities and the provincial government to provide more services for the tuberculous.

In 1931 the Department of Public Health was formed with Dr George H. Murphy as minister of health and Dr Peter S. Campbell as deputy minister. The government voted $400,000 for tuberculosis control. Much of the program of the commission was assumed by the new department, including the travelling clinics and the building of tuberculosis annexes to the general hospitals in Sydney, Glace Bay, and Antigonish. In 1934 the Cape Breton Health Unit was set up under Dr C.J.W. Beckwith, who was also in charge of tuberculosis treatment in the hospital units in the area.

By this time the Nova Scotia Tuberculosis Commission's function had

---

* When a French steamer carrying TNT, explosive acid, and benzine collided in the harbour with a Norwegian steamer, the resulting explosion killing nearly 2000 people, seriously injuring an equal number, and devastating much of the north side of the city.

become an educational one. It assisted the staff of the tuberculosis hospital, the clinics, and public health nursing services by providing educational material, which included pamphlets for patients and booklets for undergraduate nurses and medical students. It also conducted the Christmas Seal sale in the rural areas of the province.

The mass survey program was started in 1938, and by 1942 there was routine x-raying of all school teachers. The need for assistance in this work was increasing, however, and in 1946 the commission was reorganized and renamed the Nova Scotia Tuberculosis Association. The objectives of the new association were to assist in the prevention and control of tuberculosis in the province; to co-ordinate and assist in the work of the local agencies in the sale of Christmas Seals; to assist the provincial and regional health services in their programs of early diagnosis, education, and rehabilitation; and to form the connecting link between the Canadian Tuberculosis Association and the various voluntary groups in the province. Mr Frank G. Willard was named executive secretary and became the first full-time paid worker employed in Nova Scotia to direct the voluntary antituberculosis campaign.

In 1946 Dr Frank R. Davis, minister of health, announced there would be free treatment for tuberculosis in Nova Scotia.

The Department of Health acquired two defence hospitals to complete the requirement of sanatorium beds in the late 1940s: the Roseway Hospital in 1946, of which 130 beds were used for tuberculosis, and the Point Edward Hospital, near Sydney, in 1949, which provided 187 beds.

In 1948 a mass miniature x-ray unit was purchased and placed in operation by the Nova Scotia Tuberculosis Association.

In 1947 Dr Charles Beckwith, then medical superintendent of the Tuberculosis Hospital in Halifax, in a report to the association summarized the tuberculosis control program for the previous year. An addition to the hospital had been opened, a portable x-ray unit had been acquired to speed up case-finding, a tuberculosis register had been set up, mass surveys had been started, and attempts at vocational training and rehabilitation had been made.

Rehabilitation began to receive more emphasis in 1949. The *Canadian Tuberculosis Association Bulletin* reported that the program afforded 'a fine example of the manner in which voluntary and official efforts have worked together for the common good of the tuberculosis patient. The Department of Health employs the supervisors who have charge of the program in the sanatoria, but the over-all direction is in the hands of Mr. Fred G. Barrett who is employed by the Nova Scotia Tuberculosis Association.'[1]

The program progressed successfully for many years. In 1963 Mr Ralph Ricketts, then executive secretary of the Nova Scotia Tuberculosis Association, reported recent changes in the association. On the invitation of the Halifax County Tuberculosis League the association had taken over its program. The association had also assumed the supervision and direction of the programs of all the local associations in the province and all their records had been transferred to the association's office in Halifax.

Also in 1963 a provincial conference on the subject 'Rethinking Tuberculosis in Nova Scotia' was held. Medical health officers, public health nurses, medical and nursing staff of sanatoria, and representatives of the Nova Scotia Tuberculosis Association considered all aspects of the problem. The importance of furnishing *Tuberculosis Abstracts* to fourth-year medical students through the *Nova Scotia Medical Bulletin* to physicians was stressed. Teachers and teachers-in-training were also supplied with educational material.

In 1965 the Nova Scotia Tuberculosis Association acquired a building of its own, and in 1969 it became the Nova Scotia Tuberculosis and Respiratory Disease Association.

The tuberculosis cause has been well served in Nova Scotia by such men as Dr A.F. Miller and Dr Charles J.W. Beckwith. It is fitting that this section close with a tribute to Dr J. Earle Hiltz, who had succeeded Dr Miller on his retirement from the Kentville Sanatorium in 1937, and had then served as administrator of tuberculosis for the province from 1956 until his untimely death in 1969. Following his death, a colleague, Dr J.J. Quinlan, said:

His formal duties were only a part of the tremendous effort he put forth throughout all his professional life. The Nova Scotia Tuberculosis Association knew him well, he organized the Nova Scotia Thoracic Society, he was President of the Canadian Tuberculosis Association, and had a great deal to do with the formation of the Canadian Thoracic Society. He was a very active member of the International Union Against Tuberculosis and his biennial vacations were busman's holidays to wherever in the world the meeting of the International Union was being held.

Few committees having to do with the subject of tuberculosis or respiratory diseases did not count Earle Hiltz either as chairman or a prominent member, were they provincial, national, or international. Yet he found time to lecture to the affiliate student nurses at the Sanatorium, the medical students at Dalhousie University, to the students of the Dalhousie School of Nursing, and he did not neglect research. His contributions to the medical literature, provincial, national, and international, totalled at the time of his death some sixty scientific articles. He was certified in Internal Medicine by the Royal College of Physicians and Surgeons of Canada, he was a Fellow of the American College of Chest Physicians, and a member and past director of the American Thoracic Society.

22

Prince Edward Island

The story of the tuberculosis crusade in Prince Edward Island goes back to the turn of the century. In 1906 the Summerside or Prince County Association for the Prevention of Consumption and Other Forms of Tuberculosis reported that the prospect of erecting a sanatorium in Prince Edward Island at that time was still a matter of conjecture. The work in Summerside was then of an educational nature, carried out through a legislative and press committee and school and visiting committees.

In the same year, the first annual report of the Provincial Association for the Prevention of Consumption, in Charlottetown, was issued. It listed the work accomplished to date, which involved arranging the proper ventilation of schoolhouses and the disinfection of all houses where consumptive persons had died, making provision for a district nurse to give special attention to the instruction of consumptive patients, and the encouragement of city physicians to report all cases of tuberculosis.

In 1907 the Western Association of Prince Edward Island was engaged in educating the public. It arranged lectures; placed conspicuous posters in schools, halls, and other places; distributed pamphlets to school children; and arranged for articles in the press. It was also actively involved in securing legislation for the prevention of the disease and endeavouring to secure reports of all tuberculosis cases. It was enlisting the support and interest of the public in its work, as well as instructing patients in the proper methods of dealing with sputum and distributing sanitary cups and holders free to the needy.[1]

The Dalton Sanatorium was built in 1913 about fifteen miles north of Charlottetown, at North Wiltshire, a gift to the provincial government from Sir Charles Dalton, who made a fortune from fox farming at a time when a breeding pair of foxes sold for fifteen to twenty thousand dollars. Sir

Charles had been distressed by the sickness and death from tuberculosis of a close relative, and he appreciated the need for proper care and treatment for the tuberculous. The sanatorium, its twenty-five beds and equipment, and the almost fifty acres of land cost Sir Charles $53,000. At first it was doubtful whether the site was a wise one, as great difficulties were encountered when an attempt was made to dig a well for water. However, by November 1914 the main buildings and pavilions had been erected, and the sanatorium opened in March 1915, with Dr W. Miles Garrison as superintendent. In 1917, in an agreement with the board of the sanatorium, the provincial government, which defrayed the institution's expenditures, and the federal Military Hospitals Commission transferred the sanatorium to the commission for the duration of the war and for some time after, with the stipulation that it would eventually be restored to the province in good condition. The commission enlarged and extended the facilities, and in 1920 returned the institution to its donors. However, the province felt that it was completely beyond its powers to run the greatly enlarged sanatorium, and so never opened it for civilian use. It was suggested that the federal government should operate it, or make a yearly grant for its maintenance, but these suggestions were turned down. The federal government suggested instead that the province be paid a sum of money as a final compensation, but this offer was refused. Finally the property was returned to its generous donor, on a tax-free basis as long as it was put to some charitable purpose and not more than three acres were used for farming. A newspaper editorial from Charlottetown commented: 'It would not be too much to say that in the whole Dominion of Canada if indeed anywhere in the world a similar instance of ingratitude or political animus could be found.'[2] Sir Charles was understandably annoyed with this turn of affairs, and he gave permission to the Roman Catholic Bishop of Charlottetown, Bishop O'Leary, to tear the sanatorium down and use the materials, furniture, and equipment to reconstruct the Charlottetown Hospital, which had been gutted by fire some time before. For years, all that remained at North Wiltshire was the smokestack and the doctors' residence, an unhappy memorial to the arrest of progress in antituberculosis work in Prince Edward Island.

Eventually, the early local antituberculosis leagues, many of them originally organized by Dr George Porter, secretary of the Canadian Association for the Prevention of Tuberculosis (1908–21), became dormant, except in Charlottetown where the league conducted some relief and welfare work among the families of the tuberculous.

In 1925 Dr Robert E. Wodehouse, executive secretary of the Canadian Tuberculosis Association, obtained the services of Dr G. Clair Brink of the

Ontario Department of Health to conduct an x-ray survey in the province during the month of July, using a portable x-ray unit. Some 100 cases of active tuberculosis were discovered. The patients were treated at home, often under the supervision of a Red Cross nurse.

In 1926 Dr Wodehouse obtained a grant from the Canadian Life Insurance Officers' Association to encourage tuberculosis surveys in the Maritime Provinces. It was then that the Maritime Tuberculosis Educational Committee was set up, with Dr George Jasper Wherrett as medical director. He was loaned for a month by the New Brunswick Department of Health to conduct clinics in Prince Edward Island, and he visited every physician in the province in an endeavour to diagnose and locate as many cases of the disease as possible. The clinics had been arranged by the Red Cross Society, who also had their nurses assist in the supervision of home treatment of the patients.

In 1928 a five-year demonstration was set up for the island, paid for by a grant of $15,000 from each of the Canadian Life Insurance Officers' Association, the provincial government, and the Prince Edward Island branch of the Red Cross Society. An agreement was made between the Canadian Tuberculosis Association and the provincial government whereby a department of health would be established. Dr Prescott A. Creelman became the first health officer and tuberculosis officer for the province, and his appointment led to the establishment of the provincial Department of Health in 1931. The three Red Cross nurses were then transferred to the department, with Miss Mona Wilson as director of nursing.

In 1929 Dr Benjamin C. Keeping was sent to Toronto for training in public health. On his return he became chief health officer and later deputy minister of health for the province. Dr Creelman became director of tuberculosis control and later director of the new sixty-bed Provincial Sanatorium at Charlottetown, which was opened in 1931. The sickest of the 325 afflicted persons in the province were immediately admitted. By 1938 there were ninety beds, but there was still a long waiting list of sick people who undoubtedly spread the disease within their families while awaiting admission. By 1945 there were 135 beds and the long list of patients receiving home treatment was finally erased; the reservoir of tubercle bacillus thus became diluted as fewer and fewer new cases were detected. Because of the expanded program of case-finding and prevention, and the use of the new 'wonder drugs,' by 1955 the number of tuberculosis patients requiring treatment became so small that thirty beds in the Provincial Sanatorium were made available for the treatment of other diseases. This part of the sanatorium became known as the Rehabilitation Centre. Later, in 1962, another sixteen beds were given over, and by 1972 only fifteen beds, out of a total of 105, were being used for chest cases.

The Prince Edward Island Tuberculosis League was organized in 1936, with Mr F.A. Stewart Jones as president. It was sponsored by the Gyro Club of Charlottetown and some of the women's institutes. At that time, the annual death rate in the province from tuberculosis was 64.1 per 100,000. The league was incorporated in 1942, and two years later the first executive director, Mr Alfred Doucette, was appointed. During the 1930s and 1940s the league provided the services of a full-time visiting nurse. In 1945 the league purchased a $20,000 mobile x-ray unit for a survey which was to include the whole of the population. In conjunction with this, an education and tuberculin testing program was carried on. From 1945 to 1955 mass chest x-ray surveys were conducted throughout the province, and from 1956 to 1966 community-wide tuberculosis testing and x-ray surveys were carried out. Over 300 cases of tuberculosis, as well as many non-tuberculous chest conditions, were discovered through these surveys, but the annual yield became extremely low and they were terminated in 1966.

Dr Eric MacLean Found, who succeeded Dr Creelman as director of tuberculosis control in 1942, intensified the case-finding program, and also organized the Prince Edward Island branch of the Canadian Thoracic Society in 1963, the same year that he was chosen as the Rotary Club's 'Islander of the Year' by an almost unanimous vote of the club's judges and the public: patients, former patients, and those who were just generally thankful for his leadership in the campaign against tuberculosis and his constant kindness to patients in his care.[3]

From 1942 on the Prince Edward Island Tuberculosis League continued its effective methods of public education by encouraging participation in its work and by organizing meetings to teach about the disease, its detection and prevention, and the reasons for tuberculin testing. Practical up-to-date information concerning chest disease was continuously sent out to the doctors of the province, and pertinent material was supplied to the press, radio, and television, and to school teachers as well as various organizations. The over-all program of the league included mass chest x-ray surveys and the establishment of outpatient clinics in Alberton, Souris, and Montague general hospitals and at the Health Centre in Summerside and the Provincial Sanatorium in Charlottetown. Dr Found assumed direction of these clinics after retiring as director of the Provincial Sanatorium in 1970. Through these clinics Dr Found established a rapport with family doctors.

The Prince Island Tuberculosis League's program proved so successful that since 1970 there have been no deaths in the province due to tuberculosis. This can be compared to 1925, when there were over 100 deaths per year, the highest rate in Canada at that time.

23

Newfoundland and Labrador

In no other province are the results of the campaign against tuberculosis in Canada more dramatic than in Newfoundland and Labrador.

Although this province did not enter Confederation until 1949, efforts to deal with the problem, as in the rest of the country, go back to the turn of the century. As a result of a growing consciousness of the need for an anti-tuberculosis program in Newfoundland, a tuberculosis commission was formed in 1906 by the Honourable John Harvey, with the assistance of the Honourable M.P. Gibbs and Dr Herbert Rendell. A district nurse was appointed, public meetings were held, and literature distributed throughout Newfoundland. Soon after its formation in 1911, the local chapter of the Imperial Order of the Daughters of the Empire collected money to build a camp, near the head of Mundey Pond, for the open-air treatment of incipient tuberculosis. The first summer produced fine results, and the nurse visited the patients in their homes the following winter. During the second season, the chapter ran out of operating funds, and the government had to come to its aid when the patients refused to leave. The results of this camp were so striking that the government was finally convinced it should take a hand in the matter, and so bought Bowcock's Farm, Topsail Road in St John's, and converted the buildings into a sanatorium.[1]

In 1911 Dr Rendell was appointed to head the Tuberculosis Public Service with the assistance of Miss Ella Campbell, RN. They carried out the first educational campaign throughout Newfoundland to enlighten the public on the true nature of tuberculosis and its prevention and treatment. In 1912 Dr Rendell inaugurated a tuberculosis clinic in the Renouf Building in St John's, and in 1917, when the government opened the 52-bed sanatorium at Topsail Road, he became its first medical superintendent. His successor (from 1930), Dr Raymond Bennett, was to see the sanatorium reach a capacity of 365 beds after the adjacent Royal Canadian Navy Hospital was acquired from the Canadian government after World War II.

In 1917, on his return from war service, Dr Cluny MacPherson, then director of medical services, 'asked the Government to provide accommodation for the many Newfoundland soldiers who ... were in Sanatoria in Great Britain. Escazoni, which was seized enemy property, was fitted up and Jensen Camp built, which filled the gap while the two large wards were built running south from the original Sanatorium building bringing total beds of Sanatorium to 111 by 1921 when Escazoni and Jensen Camp were closed.'[2]

The Honourable Dr James McGrath has summarized the steps that led to the development of a very active program in Newfoundland:

In looking backward the most striking fact – and striking it certainly is – is that in the year 1930 deathrate from tuberculosis in Newfoundland was 208 [per 100,000] – or TWO THOUSAND percent higher than it is today.

I do not think any more impressive statement could be made to illustrate the progress that has been made in tuberculosis in Newfoundland since then.

The seven years between 1930 and 1937 were essentially years of stagnation in which very little progressive work was being done in the field of tuberculosis. This, however, was but the dark hour before the dawn, because in 1937 was commenced an effort that has never since been relaxed and that has achieved a high degree of control of this disease.

In that year the first serious field study of tuberculosis was made by a group headed by Dr. Chester Stewart ... and the late Dr. Raymond Bennett.

As a result of their report the Commission Government established in 1938 the beginning of an organization for the control of tuberculosis. The Avalon Health Unit was established at Harbour Grace with full clinical facilities for diagnosis and a travelling x-ray unit that was able, in time, to survey the whole Avalon Peninsula. Just as the Avalon Health Unit itself was established as the result of the Stewart-Bennett survey, so the facts and figures produced by the work of the Unit convinced Government of the seriousness of the problem and the need for action.

A new Sanatorium was planned, though it was not started until 1947 and completed in 1951.

None of the people concerned with this effort at the time would have believed it possible that the death rate from tuberculosis could be reduced to what it is today in so comparatively short a time; nor could they have conceived that by 1963 approximately half the tuberculosis beds in the Province would be redundant and converted to other uses.[3]

There are no accurate data on the incidence of tuberculosis in New-foundland in the 1940s. The survey in the Avalon Peninsula had revealed an incidence of four to five per cent active tuberculosis among the population. For many years the only treatment facilities on the island were at Twillingate, the Grenfell Mission, and the St John's Sanatorium. Greater results in tuberculosis control were achieved after confederation with Canada in 1949.

The whole of the Northern Peninsula and Labrador were in a different administration area than the island proper. It was here that Sir Wilfred Grenfell had developed the Grenfell Mission under the Grenfell Association, which was financed from American, British, and Canadian sources. This medical service was operated quite apart from the official one in Newfoundland. Further, the economy of the area, depending mostly on fishing, was subject to great variations, with periods of exceedingly low incomes. Within its boundaries were Indians and Eskimos as well as the fishermen, all characterized by an extremely high incidence of, and mortality from, tuberculosis. In northern Labrador, Dr H. Paddon, who began his work with the Grenfell Mission shortly before World War I, and his son Dr W.A. (Tony) Paddon merit mention. A report by the son in May 1957 outlines the historical background of the area and the development of the program.[4] The observations made by these very competent observers on the epidemiology in the population of this area carry considerable weight. It was their conclusion that racial predisposition, as applied to Indians and Eskimos, is minor compared with environmental factors such as overcrowding, poverty, wretched hygiene, periodic or chronic malnutrition, and complete lack of tuberculosis control measures. The relation between close contact and massive infection is demonstrated by the marked improvement that followed the gradual application of all measures for early diagnosis, treatment, and isolation in the facilities of the Grenfell Mission at North West River and St Anthony and again after the introduction of the new drugs. In the Mission's program BCG vaccine was used with striking benefit and some valuable observations were made concerning its long-range use. Later on, when local epidemics were noted as vigilance in case-finding was relaxed, they were successfully controlled by vigorous reapplication of the control program. The report from these excellent observers is so valuable that it is regretted that the full text cannot be included here; it should be studied in its entirety by anyone interested in the problem of tuberculosis among the native peoples of Canada.

In assessing the effects of the depression on Newfoundland, none could be more poignant than the description given by the Honourable Joseph E. Smallwood in a paragraph in his book *I Chose Canada:*

In the United States, across Canada, and in Newfoundland, the same word was employed to describe the amount of unemployment, poverty, disease, and hunger there was in each country: depression. But it was totally incongruous to use the same work to describe the widely different conditions in the three countries. In Newfoundland, depression meant hunger, real hunger; hunger for over half the population; hunger that left people hungry day after day, for months, for years; hunger that so weakened families that their resistance to disease was reduced close to the minimum. Many of the men who were fortunate enough to get jobs in the pulp and paper companies' logging camps came in ravenously hungry and had to eat for two and three weeks before they put enough flesh on their bones to be able to swing a bucksaw again. The report of the Canadian medical team that investigated the state of people's health in superbly beautiful Bonne Bay shocked us all. We were all frightened of tuberculosis, suspicious of neighbours and friends – and relatives – afraid to get x-ray photographs of our lungs, and afraid not to. We had the highest incidence of tuberculosis to be found anywhere north of the Mexican border. We also had the highest rates of infant mortality, maternal mortality (deaths of mothers in childbirth), and contagious, infectious, and otherwise communicable disease in North America. The one-third of our people who were on the six cents a day, $1.80 a month, dole deteriorated visibly in health for the dole was simply not enough to sustain life.[5]

It was not until 1937 that x-ray facilities were made available at the sanatorium in St John's and at the Grenfell Mission at St Anthony. Despite extensive surveys numerous communities were still denied the advantages of the x-ray, however, because of the paucity of roads and the isolation along the rugged sea coast. In 1944, through the efforts of the St John's Rotary Club, the Newfoundland Tuberculosis Association was formed. A group of public-spirited citizens, stimulated by the writings of Mr Edward (Ted) Meaney, who suffered from tuberculosis, were the prime organizers. During its development outstanding leadership was given by Mr Gordon Higgins and Mr James Ewing, both long-time presidents, and the present executive secretary, Mr Edgar C. House, a former teacher and rehabilitation officer for the association. The association was fully organized by Mr Walter Davis, who took over after World War II. An inspired and successful school teacher, he threw himself into the work of the newly created association and made it successful in both case-finding and fund-raising. In this he was assisted by the National Association of New York. Mr Davis also developed a dual program of rehabilitation with the Newfoundland Department of Health, as well as a successful voluntary health education program for the province. After an unsuccessful and highly frustrating attempt at politics, he left the association and served for a time in Ceylon with the Foreign Aid Program in the fields of mental health and leprosy. Eventually he returned to Canada and, after spending some time with the Ontario Tuberculosis Association, became executive officer of the newly organized Tuberculosis and Respiratory Disease Association of Toronto and York County.

In 1945 an independent team of British tuberculosis experts, Drs D'Arcy Hart and T.O. Garland, investigated the problem of the disease in Newfoundland. Their recommendation was that the relief allowance to the sick poor be increased, since tuberculosis was a long-term disease that was only aggravated by any lowering of the standards of living. They also recommended that the dispensary and diagnostic services be extended and the number of treatment beds increased.

Also in 1945, in appreciation of the many kindnesses they had received from the Newfoundlanders during the war years, the Canadian naval ratings stationed in Newfoundland donated $10,000 out of their canteen funds to the association to help in the campaign against tuberculosis which was being launched.

In 1947 the Newfoundland Tuberculosis Association, as a result of Mr Walter Davis's efforts, acquired the flagship of the US Navy in Newfoundland during World War II, raised funds to equip it with an x-ray unit, and provided for maintenance and salaries of the crew. This floating unit made it possible to check large numbers of people in the remote corners of Newfoundland. As the result of a province-wide contest among school children and sanatorium patients, the boat was rechristened MV *The Christmas Seal.* The gleaming white vessel visited outports, distributing literature, arranging rallies, showing health films, and generally educating the people infected with the disease and their contacts. Also the Newfoundland Railway made a car available for x-ray service.

In 1949 Newfoundland joined Canada and the Newfoundland Tuberculosis Association became affiliated with the Canadian Tuberculosis Association. In 1948 federal grants for tuberculosis work had become available to all provinces and so, in 1949, they were extended to Newfoundland. A report to the Department of National Health and Welfare made by Dr G.J. Wherrett in 1949 outlined the program in Newfoundland and the assistance which the health grants had provided.

During the next thirty years remarkable progress was made – much more than could have seemed possible in the late 1940s. There were four major contributing factors: (1) the great increase in facilities for diagnosis and treatment that were quickly developed; (2) the founding of the Newfoundland Tuberculosis Association in 1944; (3) the implementation of a program for the elimination of bovine tuberculosis; and (4) the marked improvement in the financial and economic picture in Newfoundland and Labrador, as a result of the war and Confederation, which made available to Newfoundlanders generally the social legislation available to other Canadians, such as increased veterans' benefits, family allowances, old age pensions, and the Federal Health Grants for the public health program, including tuberculosis.

The great increase in treatment facilities came at the same time as the new drugs, which meant that drugs were able to exert their greatest effect on tuberculosis patients. This in no small measure contributed to the astounding decline in the mortality rate in Newfoundland following their introduction.

1951 saw the opening of the West Coast Sanatorium in Corner Brook, with 270 beds. In the new year, the Newfoundland Department of Health, in co-operation with the Newfoundland Tuberculosis Association, extended BCG vaccination services to all parts of the province; 14,000 school children in St John's were among the first to take part in this extended program.

Rehabilitation began to receive more emphasis in 1951. The association had one rehabilitation officer, and two were appointed to the St John's Sanatorium and one to the West Coast Sanatorium. At the same time, the association became concerned about the need for a greater and more concentrated educational program, and so set up a committee to formulate one. The program was financed by a grant from the Canadian Life Insurance Officers' Association.

In 1955 the Newfoundland Tuberculosis Association conducted a program of teachers' training in health education, consisting of talks on the different phases of the disease, and on nutrition, sanitation, and general health. Guest speakers were doctors, nurses, health officers, and prominent community leaders. The object was to give teachers enough information to enable them to help to improve the health conditions in the communities where they lived and worked, since they were generally considered community leaders.

Changes were being made in the rehabilitation procedures. In the sanatoria stress was moving away from occupational and pastime activities to educational and vocational courses. More attention was being paid to academic work, correspondence courses, and commercial courses. By 1965, 1702 job placements had been made, with peak years 1954 and 1962.

In 1962 the MV *The Christmas Seal* extended its work beyond the area of tuberculosis and began administering oral Sabin polio vaccine, and in 1963 it conducted a survey of physically handicapped children on the south coast in addition to continuing other services to the communities it served. The vessel was the symbol of good health in Newfoundland and Labrador. It was phased out in 1974.

It was not until the fall of 1964 that a director of tuberculosis control, Dr E.S. Peters, was appointed in the provincial Department of Health.

As Dr G.A. Frecker, minister of education, stated in a paper read at a health education institute in Avondale in 1958:

A great deal has already been achieved in the matter of promoting better health standards and one of the most successful activities in the field of health education has been the health institute one of which is being held today in Avondale. One of the reasons for the success of these institutes is that they bring together in a close and friendly partnership the officials of the Department of Health, the staff of the Newfoundland Tuberculosis Association and the teachers, and thus lay the groundwork for future positive collaboration when the teacher carries the message of the institute back into the classrooms.[6]

For the amazing strides made in the campaign against tuberculosis in Newfoundland great credit must go to the Department of Health under the Honourable Dr James McGrath and the deputy minister, Dr L.A. Miller, and to the Newfoundland Tuberculosis Association under the present executive secretary, Mr Edgar C. House, who assisted and co-operated with the department throughout. The reduction in the mortality rate from tuberculosis has been phenomenal, dropping from 308 per 100,000 in 1906 to 208 in 1930 and 3.1 in 1971.

24

Yukon and Northwest Territories

Voluntary effort was lacking in the Yukon and Northwest Territories until relatively recently. What health and medical services existed were provided by the federal government, assisted by the churches of the area. Some efforts at education in regard to tuberculosis were made as early as 1912, as shown by a letter from Isaac O. Stringer,[1] Anglican Bishop of the Yukon, to Professor G.N. Wrong, University of Toronto, requesting educational slides to demonstrate tuberculosis germs and healthy and unhealthy dwellings.

A fair amount of tuberculosis control work was carried on in Mayo, Dawson City, and Whitehorse for some years before 1953, when an effort was made to have the program of the British Columbia Tuberculosis Society extended to the Yukon. In a letter to Dr G.J. Wherrett of the Canadian Tuberculosis Association, Dr Gordon F. Kincade, director of tuberculosis control in British Columbia,[2] had suggested the possibility of this development. The society felt that the first step should be a meeting of the Christmas Seal committees of the Yukon Territory, adding that it would be happy to assist in the setting up of a system of broad coverage by mail, similar to the one used in British Columbia; it also offered to lend the services of its Health Education Department and community x-ray organizer.

The Yukon Tuberculosis and Health Association was formed on 25 September 1964 at Whitehorse, with representatives present from Watson Lake, Elso, Dawson City, Keno Hill, Mayo, and Whitehorse. This was a historical occasion in the field of public health in the North, and Dr C.W.L. Jeanes, executive secretary of the Canadian Tuberculosis Association, made the journey to be present. Also present were Dr Matthew Matas, regional superintendent of Medical Services, Department of National Health and Welfare; Dr D.R. Kinloch, Yukon-zone superintendent for the Department of National Health and Welfare, who agreed to act as medical advisor to the new association; Mr Douglas Geekie, executive secretary of the British Columbia Tuberculosis and Christmas Seal Society; and Mr J.M. McKenzie, executive secretary of the Alberta Tuberculosis Association. This association now carries on a program in co-operation with the government services.

There is no tuberculosis association in the Northwest Territories. As early as 1944–45 Dr G.J. Wherrett carried out a survey of health and hospitals in the area for the Social Science Research Council of Canada and the Northwest Territories Council. His report recommended more full-time medical services and the development of a tuberculosis service using the hospitals already in the Territories, which would carry out x-ray surveys of the schools and nutritional studies.[3] This service was largely implemented after World War II and the Northwest Territories hospitals along with the Charles Camsell Hospital in Edmonton were utilized for the treatment of tuberculous patients from the western Arctic.

The medical patrol of the Medical Services of the Department of National Health and Welfare was extended to cover the eastern and central Arctic in 1947, and x-ray services by air were developed. After 1950 tuberculosis patients were evacuated to hospitals in Hamilton, Toronto, and Moose Factory as well as in Manitoba. A very complete program of treatment was instituted. Later a fuller use of domiciliary drug treatment was organized by the Northern Region Medical Services and a satisfactory reduction in the incidence of tuberculosis was noted in the area. By the 1970s deaths from the disease had fallen to zero in the eastern Arctic although the yearly incidence of the disease remains high.

APPENDICES

APPENDIX 1
A Tale of Two Cities, Mortality Rate for Tuberculosis, 1880–1970

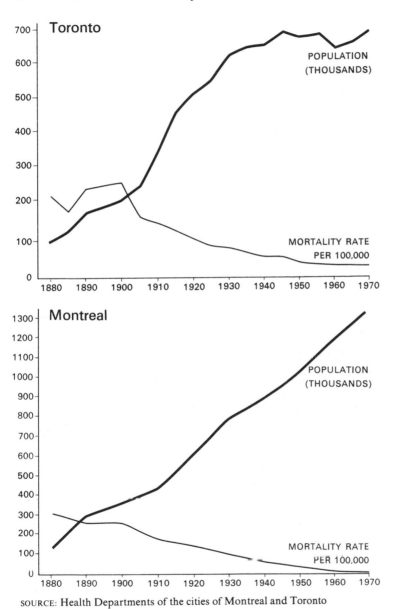

SOURCE: Health Departments of the cities of Montreal and Toronto

APPENDIX 2
Ups and Downs in Mortality Rate for Tuberculosis in Ontario, 1880–1970

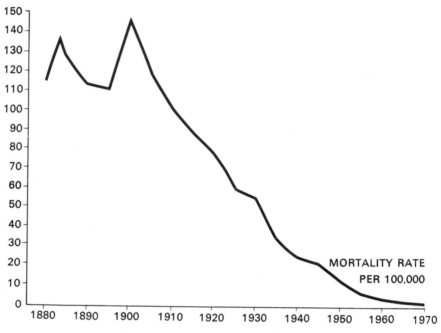

SOURCE: Information obtained from the Ontario Ministry of Health

It is to be noted that in a paper on 'The Death Throes of Tradition: Change in a Tuberculosis Sanatorium,' published in *Social Science and Medicine*, volume 5 (1971), J. Ivan Williams, Eileen N. Healey, and Christina Gow append the following note to a table of tuberculosis deaths in Ontario, 1901–60, on page 548: 'Until 1922 more females than males died of tuberculosis. Between 1922 and 1929 the mortality rate of females was greater in 5 of the 7 years. Beginning in 1929 the mortality was greater in males than in females, 994 males to 719 females. The rate in males has continued to be in excess of that in females. In 1960 there were 157 tuberculosis deaths, 109 in males and 48 in females, roughly 7 males to 3 females.'

251

APPENDIX 3
Deaths from Tuberculosis in Canada, 1921–71

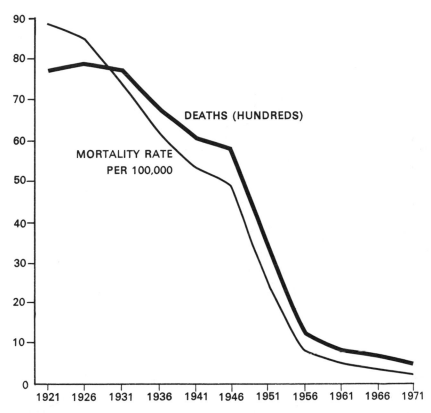

SOURCE: Information obtained from Statistics Canada

APPENDIX 4
Deaths from Tuberculosis among Canadian Indians, 1930–65

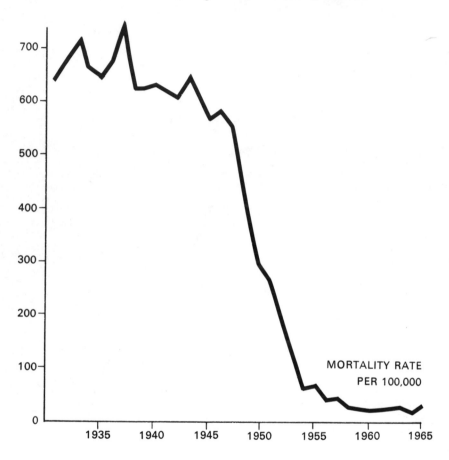

MORTALITY RATE
PER 100,000

SOURCE: Information obtained from Statistics Canada

APPENDIX 5
Deaths from Tuberculosis (all forms) in the Provinces, 1921–71

Year	Canada	Nfld	PEI	NS	NB	Que	Ont	Man	Sask	Alta	BC	Yuk	NWT
1921	7698		128	702	413	2909	2083	420	322	313	408		
1922	7664		112	·695	418	2923	1979	376	342	312	507		
1923	7847		93	652	439	3029	1989	402	352	366	525		
1924	7675		100	665	419	3025	1823	388	363	365	527		
1925	7469		86	580	405	2937	1842	383	344	354	538		
1926	7929		90	644	417	3277	1835	387	382	365	532		
1927	7814		72	643	412	3145	1803	369	391	396	551	6	26
1928	7914		100	571	403	3206	1832	399	378	338	633	6	48
1929	7808		75	522	379	3286	1703	424	377	391	615	8	28
1930	8149		103	548	392	3350	1791	456	407	408	620	15	59
1931	7645		68	524	339	3178	1728	429	326	382	642	11	18
1932	7198		88	519	328	2983	1604	397	281	401	565	13	19
1933	6983		72	478	352	2927	1465	414	297	390	544	15	29
1934	6474		93	467	285	2680	1337	389	293	318	569	11	32
1935	6664		60	488	335	2813	1303	432	272	329	565	22	45
1936	6846		61	485	357	2890	1327	420	279	382	562	33	50
1937	6728		65	461	388	2769	1315	426	303	340	602	12	47
1938	6172		81	415	342	2616	1237	349	271	280	535	17	29
1939	6044		63	428	286	2680	1085	367	233	283	552	18	49
1940	5845		56	415	295	2503	1011	369	241	321	578	4	52
1941	6157		70	429	314	2685	1100	328	284	329	533	11	74
1942	6061		43	379	330	2719	1093	336	251	271	558	18	63
1943	6263		42	417	225	2842	1101	384	250	294	613	14	81
1944	5853		58	357	238	2624	1068	348	223	291	517	27	102
1945	5694		42	338	266	2555	1015	315	227	263	525	21	127
1946	5941		55	382	277	2628	1054	324	223	302	576	19	101
1947	5577		63	309	261	2436	1042	308	231	263	536	18	110
1948	4887		37	247	230	2216	825	288	229	259	442	13	101
1949	4382	285	22	184	195	1897	686	224	185	211	406	16	71
1950	3679	247	29	176	159	1571	585	179	153	171	313	15	81
1951	3481	256	17	126	134	1553	579	158	156	146	292	9	55
1952	2538	175	24	94	100	1108	398	115	104	125	214	5	76
1953	1861	111	13	72	69	844	311	89	87	68	146	5	46
1954	1593	105	10	76	51	714	307	71	42	63	123	2	29
1955	1403	82	6	48	43	608	242	72	57	81	143	3	18

Year	Canada	Nfld	PEI	NS	NB	Que	Ont	Man	Sask	Alta	BC	Yuk	NWT
1956	1256	82	4	44	45	572	221	61	46	43	110	–	28
1957	1183	82	11	45	32	513	221	70	31	68	86	1	123
1958	1027	64	5	36	35	504	186	42	23	44	70	–	18
1959	959	54	4	28	44	485	166	41	27	44	54	1	11
1960	823	41	3	33	20	389	157	39	34	34	63	1	9
1961	769	34	6	28	32	366	137	39	25	32	59	1	10
1962	785	47	3	28	25	362	164	34	30	30	48	–	14
1963	756	27	2	28	21	368	158	39	19	37	48	–	9
1964	670	27	2	29	16	301	146	34	22	32	56	–	5
1965	697	15	4	26	14	334	148	35	27	31	53	–	10
1966	669	30	3	20	14	340	132	28	10	33	55	–	4
1967	658	16	–	33	24	309	144	33	21	33	39	–	6
1968	630	15	1	27	13	315	129	31	25	24	48	–	2
1969	526	10	1	23	13	283	96	24	19	20	30	–	7
1970	527	14	1	23	11	273	102	24	20	13	43	–	3
1971	447	16	–	17	9	222	85	19	10	24	41	–	4

SOURCE: Information obtained from Statistics Canada

255

APPENDIX 6
Mortality Rates per 100,000 Population for Tuberculosis (all forms) by Province, 1921–71

Year	Canada	Nfld	PEI	NS	NB	Que	Ont	Man	Sask	Alta	BC	Yuk	NWT
1921	87.7		144.4	134.0	106.4	123.2	71.0	68.8	42.5	53.2	77.8		
1922	86.0		125.8	133.1	107.5	121.3	66.4	61.0	44.5	52.7	93.7		
1923	87.2		106.9	125.9	112.9	123.8	66.0	64.9	45.2	61.7	94.6		
1924	84.1		116.3	128.9	107.2	121.2	59.6	62.1	45.9	61.1	92.3		
1925	80.5		100.0	112.6	103.1	115.2	59.2	60.6	42.7	58.8	91.5		
1926	84.0		103.4	125.0	105.3	125.9	58.0	60.6	46.5	60.0	87.8		
1927	81.1		82.8	124.9	103.5	118.4	56.0	56.7	46.5	62.6	88.4	150.0	288.9
1928	80.5		113.6	110.9	100.5	118.1	55.9	60.1	43.9	51.4	98.8	150.0	533.3
1929	77.9		85.2	101.4	93.8	118.5	51.1	62.6	42.7	57.2	93.3	200.0	311.1
1930	79.8		117.0	106.6	96.6	118.6	52.9	66.2	45.1	57.6	91.7	375.0	655.6
1931	73.7		77.3	102.2	83.0	110.6	50.4	61.3	35.4	52.2	92.5	275.0	200.0
1932	68.5		98.9	100.0	79.2	102.0	46.2	56.3	30.4	54.2	79.9	325.0	190.0
1933	65.7		80.0	91.0	84.0	98.5	41.7	58.5	32.1	52.0	75.9	375.0	290.0
1934	60.3		102.2	87.9	67.4	88.9	37.7	54.9	31.6	42.0	78.3	275.0	320.0
1935	61.4		65.2	91.0	78.3	92.0	36.4	60.8	29.2	43.0	76.8	440.0	409.1
1936	62.5		65.6	89.3	82.4	93.3	36.8	59.1	30.0	49.4	75.4	660.0	454.5
1937	60.9		69.9	84.0	88.8	88.2	36.2	59.6	32.9	43.8	79.3	240.0	427.3
1938	55.3		86.2	74.8	77.4	82.2	33.7	48.5	29.6	35.9	69.0	340.0	263.6
1939	53.6		67.0	76.3	64.0	83.0	29.3	50.6	25.7	36.0	69.7	360.0	408.3
1940	51.4		58.9	72.9	65.3	76.4	27.0	50.7	26.8	40.6	71.8	80.0	433.3
1941	53.5		73.6	74.2	68.6	80.6	29.0	44.9	31.7	41.3	65.2	220.0	616.7
1942	52.0		47.8	64.1	71.1	80.2	28.1	46.4	29.6	34.9	64.1	360.0	525.0
1943	53.1		46.2	68.8	48.6	82.2	28.1	53.1	29.8	37.5	68.1	280.0	675.0
1944	49.0		63.7	58.4	51.6	75.0	26.9	47.9	26.7	36.0	55.5	540.0	850.0
1945	47.2		45.7	54.6	57.0	71.8	25.4	43.3	27.3	32.5	55.3	420.0	1058.3
1946	48.3		58.5	62.8	57.9	72.4	25.8	44.6	26.8	37.6	57.4	237.5	631.3
1947	44.4		67.0	50.2	53.5	65.7	25.0	41.7	27.6	31.9	51.3	225.0	687.5
1948	38.1		39.8	39.5	46.2	58.5	19.3	38.6	27.3	30.3	40.9	162.5	631.3
1949	32.6	82.6	23.4	29.3	38.4	48.9	15.7	29.6	22.2	23.8	36.5	200.0	443.8
1950	26.8	70.4	30.2	27.6	31.1	39.6	13.1	23.3	18.4	18.7	27.5	187.5	506.3
1951	24.8	70.9	17.3	19.6	26.0	38.3	12.6	20.4	18.8	15.5	25.1	100.0	343.8
1952	17.6	46.8	24.0	14.4	19.0	26.5	8.3	14.4	12.3	12.8	17.8	55.6	475.0
1953	12.5	29.0	12.9	10.9	12.9	19.8	6.3	11.0	10.1	6.7	11.7	55.6	287.5
1954	10.4	26.6	9.9	11.3	9.4	16.3	6.0	8.6	4.8	6.0	9.5	20.0	170.6
1955	8.9	20.2	6.0	7.0	7.9	13.5	4.6	8.6	6.5	7.4	10.7	27.3	100.0

Year	Canada	Nfld	PEI	NS	NB	Que	Ont	Man	Sask	Alta	BC	Yuk	NWT
1956	7.8	19.8	4.0	6.3	8.1	12.4	4.1	7.2	5.2	3.8	7.9	–	147.4
1957	7.1	19.3	11.1	6.4	5.7	10.8	3.9	8.1	3.5	5.8	5.8	8.3	121.1
1958	6.0	14.8	5.0	5.1	6.1	10.3	3.2	4.8	2.6	3.6	4.6	–	90.0
1959	5.5	12.2	4.0	3.9	7.6	9.7	2.8	4.6	3.0	3.5	3.4	7.7	52.4
1960	4.6	9.2	2.9	4.5	3.4	7.6	2.6	4.3	3.7	2.6	3.9	7.1	40.9
1961	4.2	7.4	5.7	3.8	5.4	7.0	2.2	4.2	2.7	2.4	3.6	6.8	43.5
1962	4.2	10.0	2.8	3.8	4.1	6.7	2.6	3.6	3.2	2.2	2.9	–	56.0
1963	4.0	5.7	1.9	3.7	3.4	6.7	2.4	4.1	2.0	2.6	2.8	–	34.6
1964	3.5	5.6	1.8	3.8	2.6	5.4	2.2	3.5	2.3	2.2	3.2	–	18.5
1965	3.5	3.1	3.7	3.4	2.3	5.9	2.2	3.6	2.8	2.1	2.9	–	37.0
1966	3.2	6.1	2.8	2.6	2.3	5.9	1.9	2.9	1.0	2.3	2.9	–	13.9
1967	3.2	3.2	–	4.4	3.9	5.3	2.0	3.4	2.2	2.2	2.0	–	20.7
1968	3.0	3.0	0.9	3.6	2.1	5.3	1.8	3.2	2.6	1.6	2.4	–	6.5
1969	2.5	1.9	0.9	3.0	2.1	4.7	1.3	2.5	2.0	1.3	1.5	–	21.9
1970	2.5	2.7	0.9	3.0	1.8	4.5	1.3	2.4	2.1	0.8	2.0	–	9.1
1971	2.1	3.1	–	2.2	1.4	3.7	1.1	1.9	1.1	1.5	1.9	–	11.5

SOURCE: Information obtained from Statistics Canada

Notes

PART I

Chapter 1: Historical Background

1 G.M. Wrong, *The Canadians: The Story of a People* (Toronto: Macmillan, 1938):
   62
2 Department of Agriculture, Report, 1879: xxvii
3 Peter Bryce, Chief Medical Officer for Department of the Interior, Report,
   1903–4; 169
4 As quoted in J.B. Brebner, *Canada: A Modern History* (Ann Arbor: University of
   Michigan Press, 1960): 356
5 Empire Club of Canada, Addresses, 1907: 196 – 7
6 Peter Bryce, Chief Medical Officer for Department of the Interior, Report,
   1906–7
7 As quoted in J.J. Heagerty, *Four Centuries of Medical History and a Sketch of the
   Medical History of Newfoundland* (Toronto: Macmillan, 1928), 1: 359
8 Goldwin Smith in *The Week*, 24 April 1884: 324
9 *Canadian Monthly*, III (1879): 407
10 *Queen's Quarterly*, III (July 1895): 22
11 R.H. Hubbard, 'Viceregal Influences on Canadian Society,' in W.L. Morton
   (ed.), *The Shield of Achilles* (Toronto and Montreal: McClelland and Stewart,
   1968): 270
12 *Sanitary Journal*, II (1876): 274
13 Ibid.
14 Canadian Medical Association, *Transactions*, 1877: 25
15 Ibid., 26
16 Ibid., 27
17 Provincial Board of Health of Ontario, Report, 1901: 6

18 'Ventilation and Health,' *Sanitary Journal*, IV (1879): 123
19 'Air Vitiated by Exhalation from the Lungs, Skin, and Its Effect upon Health,' *Sanitary Journal*, IV (1879): 76
20 As quoted in S.D. Clark, *Social Development of Canada: An Introductory Study with Select Documents* (Toronto: University of Toronto Press, 1942): 402
21 Ibid., 254–5
22 Ibid., 400
23 Canada, Commission on Conservation, Committee on Public Health, 'Before Collection and Disposal': 6 – 7
24 *Sanitary Journal*, IV (1879): 78
25 'Tuberculosis Insurance,' *Canadian Journal of Medicine and Surgery*, 1899: 309–14
26 Daniel Clark, 'Medical Manias,' *Canadian Monthly Magazine*, 3 (1879): 256
27 G.C. Brink, *Across the Years; Tuberculosis in Ontario* (Willowdale, Ont.: Ontario Tuberculosis Association, 1965)
28 J.H. Elliott, 'The Present Status of Antituberculosis Work in Canada – 1908,' a paper prepared for the Canadian Committee of the International Congress on Tuberculosis for presentation at the Washington Meeting, September 1908, typewritten ms. pp. 1 and 2. In Records of the Canadian Association for the Prevention of Tuberculosis, PAC
29 G.D. Porter, *Crusading against Tuberculosis. The memoirs of George Dana Porter* (Ottawa: Canadian Tuberculosis Association, 1953): 5–6
30 Brink, *Across the Years ...*

Chapter 2: Canadian Tuberculosis Association

1 Canadian Association for the Prevention of Consumption and Other Forms of Tuberculosis, Transactions of the Second Annual Convention held at Ottawa on Thursday, April 17th, and Friday, April 18th, 1902: 17
2 CTA Records, PAC
3 Canadian Association for the Prevention of Tuberculosis, Transactions of the Second Annual Convention, Ottawa, 20 April 1904, Report of the Education Committee: 55–7
4 CTA Records, PAC
5 Ibid.
6 Canadian Association for the Prevention of Tuberculosis, Transactions of the Fifth Annual Meeting, held at Ottawa on Wednesday, March 15, 1905: 7
7 Canadian Association for the Prevention of Tuberculosis, Minutes of the Meeting, Ottawa, 4 November 1908.
8 'A Tribute to Dr George D. Porter,' *Canadian Tuberculosis Association Bulletin*, 19/1 (Sept. 1940): 3

9 George D. Porter, *Crusading against Tuberculosis – Memoirs* (Ottawa: Canadian Tuberculosis Association, 1953): 7
10 CTA Records, PAC
11 Porter, *Crusading against Tuberculosis*: 3, 5
12 Letter to Dr Porter, 27 October 1913. In CTA Records, PAC
13 'Canadian Tuberculosis Association Educational Facilities,' *Canadian Tuberculosis Association Bulletin*, 1/1 (Sept. 1922): 7

Chapter 3: Medical Care of the Tuberculous

1 A.D. Lapp, 'Treating Tuberculosis in Dry Climate Belt,' *Canadian Medical Association Journal*, 15 (Aug. 1925): 819–22
2 New York and Chicago: Fleming H. Kenell Co., 1922
3 Philadelphia and London: J.B. Lippincott, 1917
4 G.J. Wherrett, 'Follow-up Information on 2031 Tuberculosis Patients One to Thirteen Years after Discharge from Sanatoria,' *American Review of Tuberculosis*, 31/1 (Jan. 1935): 62–73

Chapter 6: Tuberculosis Nursing

1 Ottawa Association for the Prevention of Tuberculosis, Annual Report, 1906, Appendix no. 3: 50
2 Annual Report to Canadian Association for Prevention of Tuberculosis, 1919
3 Ibid., 1914
4 John Murray Gibbon, *Three Centuries of Canadian Nursing*, in collaboration with Mary S. Mathewson (Toronto: Macmillan Co. of Canada, 1947): 319
5 Sir William Osler, in *Medical News*, 12 December 1903
6 *Landmarks of Progress* (New York: National Tuberculosis Association, 1932): 10
7 Canadian Association for the Prevention of Tuberculosis, 8th Annual Meeting, 1908: 44–5
8 Canadian Nurses Association Bulletin, 1944
9 Gibbon, *Three Centuries of Canadian Nursing*: 438–9
10 G.F. Kincade, 'Domiciliary Treatment of Tuberculosis,' *Canadian Medical Association Journal*, 95 (1966): 818–20

Chapter 7: Tuberculosis in Native Races

1 Except where indicated otherwise the quotations are from Annual Reports of the Department of Indian Affairs, 1880–1928
2 In *Canada, Department of Indian Affairs, Annual Report*, 1920: 7
3 Quoted in *Canada, Department of Indian Affairs, Annual Report*, 1926: 8

4 CTA Records, PAC
5 Ibid.
6 Ibid.

Chapter 8: War and Tuberculosis

1 G.C. Brink, *Across the Years: Tuberculosis in Ontario* (Willowdale, Ont.: Ontario Tuberculosis Association, 1965): 73, figure 11
2 'The Tuberculous Soldier,' *Canadian Medical Association Journal*, old series 45, new series 6 (1916): 922–3
3 In Records of the Department of Veterans Administration and the CTA, PAC
4 In Records of the Department of Veterans Affairs and the CTA, PAC
5 Canada, House of Commons, Special Committee to Consider Questions Relating to Pensions, Insurance and Re-establishment of Returned Soldiers, and Any Amendments to the Existing Laws in Relation Thereto, Proceedings, no. 11, Wednesday, April 13th, 1921: 262–3
6 Day and month unknown
7 David A. Stewart, 'Tuberculosis Problems of Today – Doctrines, Conditions and Needs,' *American Review of Tuberculosis*, 4/1 (Mar. 1920): reprinted article, 8
8 Canadian Association for the Prevention of Tuberculosis, Seventeenth Annual Report, 1917: 17
9 Canada, House of Commons, Special Committee ... Proceedings, no. 11, Wednesday, April 13th, 1921: 262
10 Stewart, 'Tuberculosis Problems of Today': 11
11 CTA Records, PAC
12 F.S. Burke, 'Deaths among War Pensioners,' *Canadian Medical Association Journal*, 41 (1939): 457–65
13 J. Adamson and others, 'Tuberculosis in the Canadian Army 1929 to 1944,' *Canadian Medical Association Journal*, 52 (1945): 123–7
14 'Pulheems: A system of medical classification for recording the physical and mental states of recruits in the British armed services, representing: P, physical capacity; U, upper limbs; L, lower limbs; H, hearing (acuity); EE, eyesight (visual acuity); M, mental capacity; S, stability (emotional).' *Dorland's Illustrated Medical Dictionary*, 25th ed. (Philadelphia: Saunders, 1974): 1286
15 From G.J. Wherrett to Colonel W. Warner, in CTA Records, PAC
16 Report to Dr W.P. Warner by Dr G.J. Wherrett and Dr R.A. Benson on Sanatorium Needs in Province of Quebec, October 19, 1946, in CTA Records, PAC

Chapter 9: The Effect of Immigration on Tuberculosis

1 P.H. Bryce, 'Tuberculosis in Canada as Affected by Immigration,' *British Journal of Tuberculosis*, 2 (1908): 264–7
2 Ibid., 267

3 C.F. Bennett, 'Tuberculosis in Recent Immigrants,' *Canadian Journal of Public Health*, 31/11 (Nov. 1940): 515–30
4 Annual Report of the Tuberculosis Division, Ministry of Health, Ontario, 1953
5 Ibid., for 1961 and 1971

Chapter 10: Bovine Tuberculosis

1 J.H. Elliott, 'Bovine Tuberculosis in Man,' in *Canadian Association for the Prevention of Tuberculosis, Annual Report*, 1914: 91
2 Letter to R.S. Weir from Dr Wm Moore, 12 November 1904. In CTA Records, PAC
3 Ibid.
4 Mazyck P. Ravenel, 'Animal Tuberculoses and Their Relation to Human Health,' in *Canadian Association for the Prevention of Tuberculosis, Annual Report*, 1904: 39
5 International Commission on the Control of Bovine Tuberculosis, Report ... presented for the consideration of the Dominion Public Health Conference, a meeting of dominion and provincial public health representatives with the members of the Committee on Public Health of the Commission of Conservation ... October 12th, 1910 ... (Ottawa, 1910): 5
6 Ibid., 3
7 F. Torrance, 'Bovine Tuberculosis and the Federal Department of Agriculture,' in *Canadian Tuberculosis Association, Annual Report*, 1924: 79
8 'Control of Bovine Tuberculosis,' in *Canadian Tuberculosis Association, Bulletin*, December 1925: 6
9 Ibid.
10 Great Britain Royal Commission on Tuberculosis (Human and Bovine), Final Report ... Part 1, Report Presented to Both Houses of Parliament by Command of His Majesty (London: HMSO, 1911): iii
11 A. Stanley Griffith, 'Bovine Tuberculosis in Man,' *Tubercle*, Sept. 1937: 529–43
12 'The Final Report of the Royal Commission on Tuberculosis – Editorial,' *Canadian Journal of Public Health*, 11 (1911): 427
13 Ibid.
14 Ibid., 428
15 International Commission on the Control of Bovine Tuberculosis, Report ...: 18
16 Ottawa: Government Printing Bureau
17 Federal Department of Agriculture, Health of Animals Branch. Cited in *Canadian Tuberculosis Association, Annual Report*, 1924: 20
18 Elliott, 'Bovine Tuberculosis in Man': 90
19 'Control of Bovine Tuberculosis': 7
20 Personal letter to G.J. Wherrett from R.J. McClenaghan, Director, Contagious Diseases Division, Canada Department of Agriculture, 30 November 1972

21 *Canadian Tuberculosis Association Bulletin*, March 1925: 5
22 G.C. Brink, *Across the Years: Tuberculosis in Ontario* (Willowdale, Ont: Ontario Tuberculosis Association, 1965): 23
23 Ibid.
24 Adelard Groulx, 'Pasteurization in the Province of Quebec, with Special Reference to Montreal,' in *Canadian Journal of Public Health*, 37 (Jan. 1946): 18
25 Ibid., 20
26 'The Canadian Public Health Association and Pasteurization,' *Canadian Journal for Public Health*, 29 (1938): 309

Chapter 11: The International Picture

1 S.A. Knopf, *Tuberculosis as a Disease of the Masses and How to Combat It*, 1st Amer. ed. (New York: M. Finesback, 1901)
2 J.H. Elliott, 'The Present Status of Antituberculosis Work in Canada – 1908,' prepared for the Canadian Committee of the International Congress on Tuberculosis, Washington, September 1908
3 J.O. Leclerc, 'Essay on the Organization of Anti-tuberculosis Campaign' (Report of Paris Meeting of International Union against Tuberculosis), referred to in 21st Annual Report of the Canadian Association for the Prevention of Tuberculosis, May 21, 1921: 13
4 Frederick D. Hopkins, *International Tuberculosis Conferences and Congresses*, 2nd ed. (New York: National Tuberculosis Association, Historical Series No. 10): 20
5 Ibid., 29–30
6 Ibid., 53
7 J. Holm, *Fifty Years of the Union* (International Union against Tuberculosis, Jan. 1971): 15

PART II

Introduction

1 H.M. Biggs, Report of New York City Board of Health, 1912

Chapter 14: British Columbia

1 C.J. Fagan, 'Report of the British Columbia Association for the Prevention and Treatment of Consumption,' *Transactions of the Sixth Annual Meeting of the Canadian Association for the Prevention of Tuberculosis*, held in Ottawa, March 28th and 29th, 1906: 79

2 W.H. Hatfield, *A History of Tuberculosis in British Columbia* (Vancouver: Department of Health and Welfare, 1952): 9
3 British Columbia Tuberculosis – Christmas Seal Society Constitution and By-Laws, 5 May 1949, and amendments up to and including 28 May 1964
4 'British Columbia Tuberculosis – Christmas Seal Society,' Sixty-fifth Annual Report of the Canadian Tuberculosis Association, Ottawa, 1965: 18

Chapter 15: Alberta

1 Copy of Petition, Calgary, *Transactions of the Seventh Annual Meeting of the Canadian Association for the Prevention of Tuberculosis*, held in Ottawa, 13 and 14 March, 1907

Chapter 16: Saskatchewan

1 A.B. Cook et al., *Report of the Saskatchewan Anti-Tuberculosis Commission* (Regina: J.W. Reid, King's Printer, 1922): 58
2 *Canadian Tuberculosis Association Bulletin*, 3/2 (Dec. 1924): 7
3 'Research in Saskatchewan – Under National Research Assistance,' *Canadian Tuberculosis Association Bulletin*, 5/3 (Mar. 1927): 4
4 'Real Public Health,' *Canadian Tuberculosis Association Bulletin*, 11/1 (Dec. 1932): 5
5 R.G. Ferguson, 'Activities in a Province-Wide Programme for the Control of Tuberculosis,' *Canadian Public Health Journal*, 26/3 (Mar. 1935): 130
6 G.J. Wherrett and S. Grzybowski, *Report and Recommendations on Tuberculosis Control in Saskatchewan* (Ottawa: Department of National Health and Welfare, 1966): 4
7 Ibid., 7–8
8 CTA Records, PAC
9 *The Saskatchewan Anti-Tuberculosis League News Quarterly*, 4/2 (summer 1973): 1, 4

Chapter 17: Manitoba

1 Dedication and Unveiling of Dr David A. Stewart Memorial, Manitoba Sanatorium, Ninette, 24 July 1940: 12. In CTA Records, PAC
2 Ibid., 9–10
3 D.A. Stewart papers, CTRDA Records, PAC
4 Manitoba, the Tuberculosis Control Act, chap. 274, RSM., c222, s.1, as amended in 1948
5 T.A.J. Cunnings, 'The Voluntary Agency – Reflections on the Current Scene,' *Canadian Journal of Public Health*, 56/10 (Oct. 1965): 418–19

6 G.J. Wherrett, *Report and Recommendations on the Tuberculosis Programme in Manitoba* (Jan. 1965), 3–4. G.J. Wherrett's personal files in CTA Records, PAC

Chapter 18: Ontario

1 G.C. Brink, *Across the Years* (Willowdale: Ontario Tuberculosis Association, 1964): 17–18
2 Ottawa Association for the Prevention of Tuberculosis, 1st Annual Report, 1906: 77
3 'First Annual Report of the Heather Club,' in Canadian Association for the Prevention of Tuberculosis, Annual Report, 1909: 60
4 'Report of Fort William Anti-Tuberculosis Society,' in Canadian Association for the Prevention of Tuberculosis, Annual Report, 1912: 61
5 J.W.S. McCullough, 'The Tuberculosis Problem in Ontario,' in Canadian Association for the Prevention of Tuberculosis, Annual Report, 1913: 95
6 G.C. Brink, 'The Travelling Diagnostic Chest Clinic,' *Canadian Public Health Journal*, 22/4 (April 1931): 163
7 Revised Directory, in *Canadian Tuberculosis Association Bulletin*, 3/3 (Mar. 1925): 3
8 G.C. Brink, 'Influencing Factors in the Control of Tuberculosis in Ontario,' *Canadian Public Health Journal*, 27/10 (Oct. 1936): 488
9 CTA Records, PAC
10 G.J. Wherrett, Preliminary Report of the Provincial Committee on Tuberculosis Problems in the Province of Ontario, Toronto, May 1949, ms. As quoted in Floris Ethia King, 'Historical Study of the Voluntary Tuberculosis Community Health Program in Canada, with Projective Emphasis,' PH D thesis, University of North Carolina, Chapel Hill, 1967: 287–8
11 May Dale, 'Community Tuberculosis Education,' A Presentation to District Meetings in Ontario, 1953–1954. In Records of Ontario Tuberculosis Association
12 G.C. Brink, 'Tuberculosis in Ontario,' *Canadian Journal of Public Health*, 45/5 (May 1954): 201
13 Records of Ontario Tuberculosis Association
14 Ibid.
15 E.J. O'Brien, 'Voluntary Associations,' presentation made to the Asian Conference, International Union against Tuberculosis, Bangkok, Thailand, November 1962

Chapter 19: Quebec

1 Report of the Montreal Anti-Tuberculosis League to the Annual Meeting of the Canadian Association for the Prevention of Tuberculosis, 1905
2 'Three Rivers Demonstration,' *Canadian Tuberculosis Association Bulletin*, 3/2 (Dec. 1924): 3

3 'The Recommendations of the Montreal Health Survey Report,' *Canadian Public Health Journal*, 20/4 (Apr. 1929): 182–3

4 A.G. Fleming, 'Montreal Anti-Tuberculosis and General Health League,' *Canadian Public Health Journal*, 19/6 (June 1928): 263–8

5 G.J. Wherrett, 'Report of the Quebec Committee for the Prevention of Tuberculosis,' Quebec, 1938: 1ff. Ms in Canadian Tuberculosis and Respiratory Disease Association's archives.

6 'Must Prove Health,' *Canadian Tuberculosis Association Bulletin*, 20/1 (Sept. 1941): 8

7 'Quebec May Vote $10,000,000 to Fight Tuberculosis,' *Canadian Tuberculosis Association Bulletin*, 24/3 (Mar.-Apr. 1946): 3

8 G.J. Wherrett, Montreal Anti-Tuberculosis League, 1958. In personal file of Dr G.J. Wherrett, CTA Records, PAC

9 Herman Gauthier, 'Provincial Committee for the Prevention of Tuberculosis,' Annual Report, Canadian Tuberculosis Association, 1959

Chapter 20: New Brunswick

1 Public Health Conference, Health Centre, Fredericton, NB, 27 May 1924

2 Memorandum re Voluntary Tuberculosis Association in the Province of New Brunswick, 26 September 1952. In personal file of Dr G.J. Wherrett

3 R.J. Collins, 'Anti-Tuberculosis Activities in New Brunswick,' *Canadian Public Health Journal*, 24/7 (July 1934): 326–8

4 Minutes of a Special Meeting of the New Brunswick Tuberculosis Association, Saint John, NB, 31 January 1946

5 'New Brunswick Plans More Active Campaign,' *Canadian Tuberculosis Association Bulletin*, 24/3 (March-April 1946): 5

6 J.J. Arsenault, 'Report of the Executive Secretary,' read at the Annual Meeting of the New Brunswick Tuberculosis Association, Moncton, 19 September 1946

7 G.L. Miller, 'President's Address,' New Brunswick Tuberculosis Association Annual Report, 1950: 13–14

Chapter 21: Nova Scotia

1 'Progress in Nova Scotia,' *Canadian Tuberculosis Association Bulletin*, 28/2 (Dec. 1949): 5

Chapter 22: Prince Edward Island

1 'The Second Annual Report of the Western Association of Prince Edward Island for the Prevention of Tuberculosis,' Annual Report, Canadian Association for the Prevention of Tuberculosis, 1907

2 A clipping from a newspaper, possibly an editorial, in the files of the Prince Edward Island Archives, no source or date indicated

3 'Dr Eric Found – Islander of the Year,' *Canadian Tuberculosis Association Bulletin*, 41/3 (Mar.-Apr. 1963): 7

Chapter 23: Newfoundland and Labrador

1 '1900–1930 (The Late Dr. Cluny MacPherson Recalls),' *The Northern Light*, October 1969: 14
2 Ibid.
3 '1930–1943 (Dr. James McGrath Recalls),' *The Northern Light*, October 1969: 15
4 W.A. Paddon, 'Tuberculosis Control in Northern Labrador,' typewritten ms., May 1957: 42. In CTA Records, PAC
5 J.R. Smallwood, *I Chose Canada: The Memoirs of the Honourable Joseph R. Smallwood* (Toronto: Macmillan Co. of Canada, 1973): 194
6 G.A. Frecker, 'Message to Teachers, Doctors, Nurses, etc. at Health Education Jubilee,' paper presented at Avondale, Newfoundland, 25 April 1958. In CTA Records, PAC

Chapter 24: Yukon and Northwest Territories

1 Letter from Isaac O. Stringer, Bishop of Yukon, Dawson, 10 April 1912. In CTA Records, PAC
2 Letter from G.F. Kincade, Division of Tuberculosis Control, Vancouver, BC, 22 October 1953. In CTA Records, PAC
3 G.J. Wherrett, 'Arctic Survey: Survey of Health Conditions and Medical and Hospital Services in the North West Territories,' *Canadian Journal of Economics and Political Science*, 11/1 (Feb. 1945): 49–60

A Bibliography of
Tuberculosis in Canada

The following bibliography contains a list of selected articles and books which may be of interest to the reader who wishes to pursue further the subject of the history of tuberculosis in Canada. It will be noted that most of the references are more than twenty years old. Once tuberculosis became a controllable disease its interest as a topic for publication dropped. The newer articles tend to describe an unexpected outbreak, conditions among the Indians and Eskimos, or recent basic research work in biochemistry or immunology. The older ones expressed general concern, and considered how to cope with the disease, how to conquer it, and how to treat the sufferers in and out of the sanatoria.

It will also be noted that many of the journal articles appeared in *The Canadian Journal of Public Health* (or under its former names *The Public Health Journal* and *The Canadian Public Health Journal)* and *The Canadian Medical Association Journal.* There are many more in these two important journals. Also, no references from the publications of the Canadian Tuberculosis and Respiratory Diseases Association (formerly the Canadian Association for the Prevention of Tuberculosis, 1901–21, and the Canadian Tuberculosis Association, 1922–68) have been listed. Its *Annual Reports with Transactions, Bulletins,* and *Medical Papers* are full of interesting and important papers and articles, but to list them all here would make this bibliography too cumbersome by far. Several items have been referred to in the text, however, and exact bibliographical information will be found in the notes at the ends of individual chapters.

Since this book is a social history of the disease, we have not included any purely medical publications. The list also excludes many publications on BCG since the article on BCG contains an extensive reference list on the subject, prepared by Dr Armand Frappier.

Adamson, J.D., and others. Tuberculosis in the Canadian army 1939-1944. *Canadian Medical Association Journal,* 52/2 (Feb. 1945): 123-7

Allen, E.A., M. Stewart, and P. Jeney. The efficiency of post-sanatorium management of tuberculosis. A study of one thousand tuberculosis patients discharged from sanatoria in Ontario. *Canadian Journal of Public Health,* 55/8 (Aug. 1964): 323-33

The anti-tuberculosis demonstration in Nova Scotia. *Canadian Public Health Journal,* 23/4 (Apr. 1932): 182

Arneil, A.S., and J. Batterskill. A mini-epidemic of tuberculosis in the Upper Fraser Valley Health Unit. *Canadian Journal of Public Health,* 64/5 (Sept.-Oct. 1973): 497-9

Ashley, M.J., T.W. Anderson, and W.H. LeRiche. The influence of immigration on tuberculosis in Ontario. *American Review of Respiratory Disease,* 110 (Aug. 1974): 137-45

Baker, F.J. Rehabilitation of the tuberculous patient. *Canadian Public Health Journal,* 44/8 (Aug. 1953): 281-4

Barrick, E.J. How to deal with the consumptive poor. *Canadian Journal of Medicine and Surgery,* 6/3 (Sept. 1899): 254-61

Baudouin, J.A. Vaccination against tuberculosis with BCG vaccine. *Canadian Public Health Journal,* 27/1 (Jan. 1936): 20-6

–   Vaccination against tuberculosis with BCG vaccine. *Canadian Public Health Journal,* 31/8 (Aug. 1940): 362-6

Beckwith, C.J.W. The tuberculosis control program in Halifax. *Canadian Journal of Public Health,* 37/12 (Dec. 1946): 481-7

Bennett, C.F. Tuberculosis in recent immigrants. *Canadian Public Health Journal,* 31/11 (Nov. 1940): 515-30

Berenstein, D.H. Home treatment of the tuberculous. *Canadian Medical Association Journal,* 18/1 (Jan. 1918): 38-48

Bernard, M. The Christmas seal. *Imperial Oil Review,* 47/6 (Dec. 1963): 8-11

Botsford, M.E., comp. Conference on tuberculosis nursing. *Canadian Nurse,* 41 (Jan. 1945): 39-43

Brien, F.S. Tuberculosis: a challenge to the general practitioner. *Canadian Medical Association Journal,* 87/25 (1962): 1326-31

Brink, G.C. Influencing factors in the control of tuberculosis in Ontario. *Canadian Public Health Journal,* 27/10 (Oct. 1936): 482-8

–   The travelling diagnostic chest clinic. *Canadian Public Health Journal,* 22/4 (Apr. 1941): 163-8

–   Recent advances in tuberculosis control in Ontario. *Canadian Journal of Public Health,* 32/10 (Oct. 1941): 502-8

–   Tuberculosis control. *Canadian Journal of Public Health,* 37/1 (Jan. 1946): 1-6

–   Tuberculosis in Ontario. *Canadian Journal of Public Health,* 45/5 (May 1954): 195-201

– *Across the Years: Tuberculosis in Ontario.* Willowdale, Ont.: Ontario Tuberculosis Association, 1965

Bruce, O. Pulmonary tuberculosis. *Canadian Medical Association Journal,* 2/3 (Mar. 1912): 181-99

Bryce, P.H. A dominion health service: its necessity and practicability. *Public Health Journal of Canada,* 1/8 (1910): 393-4

– Tuberculosis in Canada as affected by immigration. *British Journal of Tuberculosis,* 2/4 (Oct. 1908): 264-7

– The History of American Indians in Relation to Health. *Ontario* (1914): 128-41

Burke, F.S. Deaths among war pensioners. *Canadian Medical Association Journal,* 41/5 (Nov. 1939): 457-65

Cameron, A.E. The prevalence and extent of bovine tuberculosis in Canada. *Canadian Public Health Journal,* 20/1 (1929): 1-5

– Bovine tuberculosis in Canada. *Canadian Public Health Journal,* 29/6 (June 1938): 262-5

Campbell, A. Nursing opportunities in the tuberculosis control program. *Canadian Nurse,* 47 (Nov. 1951): 787-8

Campbell, M.F. *Holbrook of the San.* Toronto: Ryerson, 1953

Canada, Bureau of Statistics. *Tuberculosis among Indians and Eskimos, 1950-1952.* Ottawa: Queen's Printer, 1956

– *Tuberculosis Statistics Handbook.* 2nd rev. ed. Ottawa: Queen's Printer, 1958

Canada, Department of National Health and Welfare. *Report on Health Conditions in the Northwest Territories 1963-1966.* 4 vols. Ottawa, 1964-7 (Northern Health Service Report)

– *Incidence of Tuberculosis.* Ottawa: issued monthly from vol. 1, no. 1, 1961

Canada, Department of National Health and Welfare, Epidemiology Division. *Trends in Tuberculosis Incidence and Control; Report of a Committee of the Department ... April 1955.* Ottawa, 1956

Canada, Department of National Health and Welfare, Research Division. *Tuberculosis Services in Canada.* Ottawa, 1955 (General Series, Memorandum 11, mimeo.)

Canadian Tuberculosis and Respiratory Disease Association. *Canadian Tuberculosis Standards for Use in General and Special Hospitals.* Ottawa, 1972

Casselman, E. Public health nursing services for Indians. *Canadian Journal of Public Health,* 58/11 (Dec. 1967): 543-6

Cassidy, J.J. The duty of the physician in preventing tuberculosis; an editorial *Canadian Journal of Medicine and Surgery,* 4/1 (July 1898): 41-4

Chaisson, J.D. *Irregular Discharges from Ontario Sanatoria; Study Covering the Period July 1, 1957-July 1, 1958.* Toronto: Ontario Tuberculosis Association, 1958

Clarke, A.M. Tuberculosis control in New Brunswick. *Canadian Public Health Journal*, 29/3 (Mar. 1938): 103-8

Collins, R.J. Anti-tuberculosis activities in New Brunswick. *Canadian Public Health Journal*, 24/7 (July 1934): 326-8

- After-care and rehabilitation of the tuberculous. *Canadian Public Health Journal*, 31/5 (May 1940): 209-15

Collins, R.J. and C.W. MacMillan. Tuberculosis and the student nurse. *Canadian Public Health Journal*, 31/12 (Dec. 1940): 579-83

Craig, D.A. Tuberculosis problems from a public health standpoint. *Public Health Journal*, 6/7 (July 1915): 330-2

Crombie, D.W. The present anti-tuberculosis problem in Ontario. *Canadian Public Health Journal*, 26/10 (Oct. 1935): 486-93

Cruikshank, H.C. The problem of tuberculosis among Toronto children. *Public Health Journal*, 16/2 (Feb. 1925): 71-5

Cunnings, T.A.J. Rehabilitation of the tuberculous patient – the Manitoba program. *Canadian Journal of Public Health*, 35/4 (Apr. 1944): 137-43

- The voluntary agency – reflections on the current scene. *Canadian Journal of Public Health*, 56/10 (Oct. 1965): 418-20

Currie, Sir A.W. Montreal Anti-Tuberculosis and General Health League. *Public Health Journal*, 19/6 (June 1928): 261-2

Dalhousie University, Department of Preventive Medicine. *Tuberculosis Services, Present and Future, Nova Scotia 1972*. A report to the Nova Scotia Council of Health. Dalhousie, NS, 1972

Davidson, Miss. Control of the tuberculosis contact. *Canadian Public Health Journal*, 22/5 (May 1931): 258-61

Davis, J.W. BCG vaccination – its place in Canada. *Canadian Journal of Public Health*, 56/6 (June 1965): 244-52

- Epidemics of tuberculosis in Canada in the sixties. *Canadian Medical Association Journal*, 96/16 (Apr. 22, 1967): 1156-60

Defries, R.D. The Montreal health survey. *Canadian Public Health Journal*, 20/4 (Apr. 1929):196-7

Dixon, W.G. Integration of social welfare in tuberculosis control programs. *Canadian Journal of Public Health*, 49/6 (June 1958): 240-7

Dobbie, W.J. A provincial program for the control of tuberculosis. *Canadian Journal of Public Health*, 26/10 (Oct. 1935): 494-505

Dyke, E.H. Tuberculosis in Toronto. *Public Health Journal*, 14/7 (July 1913): 402-4

Eidus, L., and others. La chimiothérapie intermittente de la tuberculose: une étude des problèmes impliqués et compte rendu des contributions faites récemment au Canada. *L'Union médicale du Canada*, 103/7 (July 1974): 1271-4

Elliott, J.H. *The Present Status of Anti-tuberculosis Work in Canada – 1908*. Prepared for the Canadian Committee of the International Congress on Tuberculosis for presentation at the Washington meeting, September 1908. Ottawa: Canadian Association for the Prevention of Tuberculosis, 1909

- The anti-tuberculosis movement in Canada. *British Journal of Tuberculosis,* 4/2 (Apr. 1910): 73-89
- The prevention of tuberculosis. *Public Health Journal,* 13/1 (Jan. 1913): 28-30
- How Canada is meeting the tuberculosis war problem. *American Review of Tuberculosis,* 2/7 (Sept. 1918): 400-8

Fenton, A.E. The public health nurse in the tuberculosis hospital. *Canadian Journal of Public Health,* 39/5 (May 1948): 187-91

Ferguson, R.G. The most important agencies in a provincial campaign against tuberculosis. *Canadian Medical Association Journal,* 15/8 (Aug. 1925): 799-803

- *Tuberculosis among the Indians of the Great Canadian Plains.* Preliminary report of an investigation being carried out by the National Research Council of Canada. London: Adlard and Son, 1929
- The Indian tuberculosis problem and some preventive measures. *Canadian Medical Association Journal,* 30/5 (May 1934): 544-7
- Activities in a province-wide program for the control of tuberculosis. *Canadian Public Health Journal,* 26/3 (Mar. 1935): 130-7
- Some fundamentals in tuberculosis prevention. *Canadian Public Health Journal,* 29/5 (May 1938): 203-12
- Recent advances in tuberculosis control. *Canadian Journal of Public Health,* 35/3 (Mar. 1944): 109-12
- BCG vaccination in hospitals and sanatoria of Saskatchewan. *Canadian Journal of Public Health,* 37/11 (Nov. 1946): 435-51
- Provisions for the prevention and care of tuberculosis in Canada. *Canadian Medical Association Journal,* 62/2 (Feb. 1950): 131-5
- *Studies in Tuberculosis.* Toronto: University of Toronto Press, 1955

Fleming, A.G. Montreal Anti-Tuberculosis and General Health League. *Public Health Journal,* 19/6 (June 1928): 263-9

Foley, A.R., J.O. Roy, and R. Desjardins. BCG vaccination as a public health measure in the province of Quebec. *Canadian Journal of Public Health,* 43/2 (Feb. 1952): 43-6

Found, E.M. The role of the public health nurse in tuberculosis case finding. *Canadian Journal of Public Health,* 53/3 (Mar. 1962): 126-7

Gale, G.L. Tuberculosis in Canada today. *Applied Therapeutics,* 12/6 (June 1970): 8-10

Gale, G.L., and N.C. Delarue. Surgical history of pulmonary tuberculosis: the rise and fall of various technical procedures. *Canadian Journal of Surgery,* 12/4 (Oct. 1969): 381-8

Garland, T.O., and P. D'A. Hart. *Tuberculosis in Newfoundland 1945,* n.p.: Trade Printers and Publishers, 1946

Gooderham, Mrs A. What the Daughters of the Empire are doing towards the prevention of tuberculosis. *Public Health Journal,* 4/4 (Apr. 1913): 190-4

Graham, D. Educational opportunities for undergraduates through sanatorium residence during the vacation period. In Papers on tuberculosis, printed and distributed by the Canadian Tuberculosis Association, Ottawa, following the annual meeting, Ottawa, April 8, 9 and 10, 1924: 38-64

Graham-Cummings, G. The health of the original Canadians 1867-1967. *Medical Services Journal,* 23/2 (Feb. 1967): 115-66

Grant, A. Health education at the local level. *Canadian Journal of Public Health,* 42/6 (June 1951): 254-6

– The voluntary health association and the prevention of illness. *Canadian Journal of Public Health,* 54/1 (Jan. 1963): 24-6

Grant, Sir J. Our race and consumption. *Montreal Medical Journal,* 29/1 (Jan. 1900): 673-9

– Tuberculosis and public health. *Public Health Journal,* 3/6 (June 1912): 321-2

– Tuberculosis and the bacteriology of every day life. *Public Health Journal,* 6/10 (Oct. 1915): 497-9

Grenier, E. The anti-tuberculosis campaign – a social campaign – the role of the government – the role of private effort. *Canadian Medical Association Journal,* 10/8 (Aug. 1920): 729-32

Hall, O. Progress of tuberculosis eradication in Canada. *Canadian Journal of Comparative Medicine,* 3/2 (Feb. 1939): 47-50

– Present status of tuberculosis eradication in Canada. *Canadian Journal of Comparative Medicine,* 5/3 (Mar. 1941): 75-7

– Tuberculosis eradication in Canada. *Canadian Journal of Comparative Medicine,* 6/2 (Feb. 1942): 55-7

Hatfield, W.H. Progress in tuberculosis control in British Columbia. *Canadian Public Health Journal,* 27/7 (July 1936): 360-2

– *Handbook on Tuberculosis.* Victoria: Provincial Board of Health of the Province of British Columbia, 1944

– Some thoughts on tuberculosis control in Canada. *Canadian Journal of Public Health,* 35/11 (Nov. 1944): 423-30

Hiltz, J.E. Emerging patterns and trends in tuberculosis treatment. *Canadian Journal of Public Health,* 56/3 (Mar. 1965): 100-2

– Length of stay in Canadian tuberculosis hospitals. *Canadian Journal of Public Health,* 58/4 (Apr. 1967): 167-71

Holling, S.A. A tuberculosis survey among Ottawa federal civil servants. *Canadian Journal of Public Health,* 36/7 (July 1945): 261-7

- Tuberculosis case-finding techniques in the province of Ontario. *Canadian Journal of Public Health,* 40/1 (Jan. 1949): 1-6
- The tuberculosis situation in Ontario 1955. *Canadian Journal of Public Health,* 48/1 (Jan. 1957): 7-11

Hunter, J. Pulmonary tuberculosis. *Canadian Journal of Medicine and Surgery,* 4/5 (1898): 285-8
- Tuberculosis and insurance. *Canadian Journal of Medicine and Surgery,* 6/5 (1899): 309-14

Hutton, S.K. *Health Conditions and Disease Incidence among the Eskimos of Labrador.* Poole, England: Wessex Press, 1925?

International Commission on the Control of Bovine Tuberculosis. *Report ... Presented for the Consideration of the Dominion Public Health Conference, Held at Ottawa, Oct. 12, 1910.* Ottawa: Copeland-Chatterson-Crain Ltd., 1910; and Ottawa: Government Printing Bureau, 1911 (for the Department of Agriculture, Health of Animals Branch).
- *Tuberculosis; a Plain Statement of Facts Regarding the Disease; Prepared Especially for Farmers and Others Interested in Live Stock.* Ottawa: Government Printing Bureau, 1911

Keeping, B.C. The development of public health in Prince Edward Island. *Canadian Public Health Journal,* 26/1 (Jan. 1935): 9-14

Kincade, G.F. Domiciliary treatment of tuberculosis. *Canadian Medical Association Journal,* 95 (Oct. 15, 1966): 818-20

King, D.M. What the federal government might do to assist in the control of tuberculosis. *Public Health Journal,* 3/7 (July 1912): 383-7
- *The Battle with Tuberculosis and How to Win It. A Book for the Patient and His Friends.* Philadelphia and London: J.B. Lippincott, 1917

King, F.E. The past and the future of the Canadian voluntary tuberculosis associations. *Canadian Journal of Public Health,* 59/3 (1968): 123-5

King, W.L.M. Introduction to *Nerves and Personal Power; Some Principles of Psychology as Applied to Conduct and Health,* by D.M. King. New York and Chicago: Fleming H. Kevell Co., 1922

Kirby, R.W. Discovery of cases of active tuberculosis amongst ex-patients in a rural province. *Canadian Public Health Journal,* 28/1 (Jan. 1937): 10-12

Laberge, L. Detection of tuberculosis in school teachers in the Province of Quebec. *Canadian Journal of Public Health,* 34/3 (Mar. 1943): 121-9

Ladouceur, L. The fight against tuberculosis in Montreal. *Canadian Journal of Public Health,* 36/1 (Jan. 1945): 22-6

Leboeuf, A. The prevention of tuberculosis through travelling clinics. *Canadian Public Health Journal,* 25/11 (Nov. 1934): 544-7

Lee, J.H. The decrease in the length of stay of patients in sanatoria. *Canadian Journal of Public Health,* 39/9 (Sept. 1948): 375-80

Lewis H.W., and G.J. Wherrett. An x-ray survey of Eskimos. *Canadian Medical Association Journal,* 57/4 (Oct. 1947): 357-9

Looking at the tuberculosis problem: a symposium. *Canadian Journal of Public Health,* 48/12 (Dec. 1957): 495-504 (contains the following papers: 'The tuberculosis officer,' by J.E. Hiltz; 'The health officer,' by S. Murray; 'The general practitioner,' by E.C. McCoy; 'The volunteer worker,' by T.A. Saul)

McCurdy, D.G. The recalcitrant tuberculosis patient. *Canadian Journal of Public Health,* 45/8 (Aug. 1954): 350-2

McHugh, W.P. Trends in the tuberculosis field. *Canadian Journal of Public Health,* 56/1 (Jan. 1965): 7-10

Mahood, C.S. Tuberculosis and its control. *Public Health Journal,* 5/7 (July 1914): 439-43

Marshall, M. My personal experience of tuberculosis. *Public Health Journal,* 4/9 (Sept. 1913): 491-8

Massachusetts-Halifax Health Commission. *Final Report ... with Appendices. October 1919 to October 1929.* Halifax, 1932

Medical examination of inhabitants of James Bay and Hudson Bay. *The Polar Record,* 6/46 (July 1953): 798

Middleton, F.C. Evolution of tuberculosis control in Saskatchewan. *Canadian Public Health Journal,* 24/11 (1933): 505-13

Minister's Conference on Tuberculosis, Toronto, 1962. *Proceedings.* Toronto: Department of Health, 1962

Minns, F.S. The method of dealing with tuberculosis in the public schools of Toronto. *Canadian Medical Association Journal,* 5/10 (Oct. 1915): 902-8

- The method of dealing with tuberculosis in the public schools of Toronto. *Public Health Journal,* 7/3 (Mar. 1916): 145-8

Moore, P.E. No longer captain: a history of tuberculosis and its control amongst Canadian Indians. *Canadian Medical Association Journal,* 84/18 (May 6, 1961): 1012-16

- Puvalluttuq: an epidemic of tuberculosis at Eskimo Point, Northwest Territories. *Canadian Medical Association Journal,* 90/21 (May 23, 1964): 1193-1202

Morris, W. Survey of tuberculosis patients in the home, Vancouver, BC, 1936. *Canadian Public Health Journal,* 29/4 (Apr. 1938): 166-70

Nadeau, E. The Grancher system, as applied in the Province of Quebec, for the protection of childhood against tuberculosis. *Canadian Public Health Journal,* 21/8 (Aug. 1930): 382-6

Nadeau, G. A TB'S progress; the story of Norman Bethune. *Bulletin of the History of Medicine,* 8/8 (Oct. 1940): 1135-71

National Research Council of Canada. *Abstracts on Protective Inoculation with B.C.G.* Ottawa, 1931

Nutrition and health of James Bay Indians. *Arctic Circular,* 2/4 (Apr. 1949): 43-5

Ogden, W.E. Factors frequently overlooked in the early diagnosis of pulmonary tuberculosis. *Canadian Medical Association Journal,* 2/11 (Nov. 1912): 999-1009

Ontario Department of Health, Division of Tuberculosis Prevention. *Tuberculosis Prevention as an Economic Factor in the Province of Ontario and Statistical Tables and Graphs Covering the Period 1930-1939.* Toronto 1941

– *Report of Tuberculosis Survey of Ottawa Federal Civil Servants.* Toronto, 1944

– *The Organization of Community Mass X-Ray Surveys.* Prepared by the Division ... in conjunction with the Ontario Tuberculosis Association. Toronto, 1945

– *The Organization and Maintenance of a Tuberculosis Case Register.* Prepared by the Division. Toronto 1945

Ontario, Department of Health, Division of Medical Statistics. *Study of Deaths in which Tuberculosis Was Mentioned on the Medical Certificate of Death, Ontario, 1960.* Toronto, 1962 (Special Report no. 17)

Osler, Sir W. The home in its relation to the tuberculosis problem. *Medical News,* 1903: 1105-10; *Sanatorian,* 1904: 322-36; *Canada Lancet,* 1904-5: 600-12; *Revue internationale de la tuberculose,* 1905: 403-13

– Bibliography ... relating to tuberculosis. *American Review of Tuberculosis,* 3/12 (Feb. 1920): 748-9

Parfitt, C.D. Our present attitude towards tuberculosis. *Canadian Medical Association Journal,* 2/6 (June 1912): 477-86

– An address before the Canadian Tuberculosis Association. *Canadian Medical Association Journal,* 14/7 (July 1924): 573-9

– Osler's influence in the war against tuberculosis. *Canadian Medical Association Journal,* 47/4 (Oct. 1942): 293-304

Paulson, E. The scope and challenge of tuberculosis nursing. *Canadian Nurse,* 42 (Jan. 1946): 29-31

Peirce, C.B., and G. Jarry. The incidence of pulmonary tuberculosis in the Royal Canadian Naval Service. *Canadian Medical Association Journal,* 51/1 (July 1944): 46-51

Phipps, W.J. Why a student experience in tuberculosis? *Nursing Outlook,* 13/12 (Dec. 1965): 30-1

Porter, G.D. Tuberculosis and the public. *Public Health Journal,* 3/10 (Oct. 1912): 561-3

– The tuberculosis problem in Canada. *Public Health Journal,* 12/1 (Jan. 1921): 1-5

– Pioneers in tuberculosis work in Canada. *Canadian Public Health Journal,* 31/8 (Aug. 1940): 367-9

– *Crusading against Tuberculosis The Memoirs of George Dana Porter.* Ottawa. Canadian Tuberculosis Association, 1953

Porth, F.J. Tuberculosis control among Indians of Saskatchewan. *Canadian Journal of Public Health,* 59/3 (Mar. 1968): 111-14

Progress in tuberculosis control *Canadian Journal of Public Health,* 29/4 (Apr. 1938): 188-90

Quebec (Province), Ministry of Health. *The Application of Tuberculin and Cuti-BCG Test in Tuberculosis.* Quebec, n.d.

Quebec, Royal Commission on Tuberculosis. *Report.* n.p., 1909-10

Race, J. Milk supply in relation to tuberculosis in Ontario. *Public Health Journal,* 6/8 (Aug. 1915): 378-83

Reid, A.P. Sanatorial treatment of tuberculosis. *Public Health Journal,* 2/7 (July 1911): 309-16

Riches, J.V. An experiment in tuberculosis control. *Canadian Journal of Public Health,* 34/10 (Oct.1943): 470-1

Riddell, A.R. Tuberculosis in industry. *Canadian Public Health Journal,* 30/3 (Mar. 1939): 156-60

Robertson, J.S. A tuberculosis survey in Bridgetown, Nova Scotia. *Canadian Public Health Journal,* 31/4 (Apr. 1940):194-7

Ross, E.L. Tuberculosis in nurses; a study of the disease in sixty nurses admitted to the Manitoba Sanatorium. *Canadian Medical Association Journal,* 22/3 (Mar. 1930): 347-54

– The control of tuberculosis in Manitoba. *Canadian Medical Association Journal,* 49/2 (Aug. 1943): 82-5

Ross, E.L. and A.L. Paine. A tuberculosis survey of Manitoba Indians. *Canadian Medical Association Journal,* 41/2 (Aug. 1939): 180-4

Ross, M.A. Tuberculosis mortality in Ontario. *Canadian Public Health Journal,* 25/2 (Feb. 1936): 73-86

Rousseau, A. Mémoire sur les conditions achielles de la butte anti-tuberculouse dans la province de Québec. *Le Bulletin médical de Québec,* 27 (Nov. 1926): 329-34

Rousselière, G.M. A few comments on the health services in the Arctic. *Eskimo,* 59 (June-Sept. 1961): 6-7

Saul, T.A. The volunteer worker. *Canadian Journal of Public Health,* 48/12 (Dec. 1957): 502-4

Savard, E.M. Anti-tuberculosis leagues in the districts of sanitary inspection. *Canadian Medical Association Journal,* 9/9 (Sept. 1919): 823-9

Schaeffer, O. Medical observations and other problems in the Canadian Arctic, I. *Canadian Medical Association Journal,* 81/4 (Aug. 15, 1959): 248-53

– Medical observations and other problems in the Canadian Arctic, II. *Canadian Medical Association Journal,* 81/5 (Sept. 1, 1959): 386-93

Schroeder, E.C. The relation of bovine tuberculosis to public health. *Public Health Journal,* 2/6 (June 1911): 263-72

Shaver, C.G. A basis for the control of tuberculosis in a defined area. *Canadian Public Health Journal,* 26/7 (July 1935): 329-34

Shortt, Mrs A. Some social aspects of tuberculosis. *Public Health Journal*, 3/6 (June 1912): 307-12

Smith, G.M., M. McLellan, and J.E. Hiltz. An outbreak of pulmonary tuberculosis in a public school. *Canadian Journal of Public Health*, 41/2 (Feb. 1950): 60-5

Somerville, A. Tuberculin testing of high school pupils in the Foothills Health District, Alberta. *Canadian Public Health Journal*, 29/11 (Nov. 1938): 573-4

Stalker, H.S., W.J. Nichol, and E. Paulson. A tuberculosis hospital minimal care unit. *Nursing Outlook*, 8/11 (Nov. 1960): 620

Stewart C.B., and C.J.W. Beckwith. Hazards of tuberculosis in the general hospital. *Canadian Journal of Public Health*, 40/12 (Dec. 1949): 483-90

Stewart, D.A. *The Social Ramifications of Tuberculosis.* Winnipeg: Veteran Pr. Ltd., 1920?

- Tuberculosis problems of today, doctrines, conditions and needs. *American Review of Tuberculosis*, 4/1 (Mar. 1920): 1-11

- Anti-tuberculosis measures in rural districts. *Canadian Medical Association Journal*, 19/6 (Dec. 1928): 669-74

- *Travel Notes, as Jotted down by David Alexander Stewart ... with a Foreword by T.B. Macauley.* European tour of Canadian doctors associated with tuberculosis sanatoria and clinics, September-October 1928, organized by the Canadian Tuberculosis Association, assisted financially by the Sun Life Assurance Company of Canada. n.p., 1929

- What is new in tuberculosis? *Canadian Medical Association Journal*, 26/1 (Jan. 1932): 34-40

- The challenge of tuberculosis. *Canadian Public Health Journal*, 23/3 (Mar. 1932): 109-17

- Tuberculosis among nurses. *American Journal of Nursing*, 32/11 (Nov. 1932): 1-4

- When a province tackles tuberculosis. *Canadian Public Health Journal*, 24/6 (June 1953): 269-75

Stone, E.L. Tuberculosis among Indians of the Norway House Agency. *Public Health Journal*, 16/2 (Feb. 1925): 76-81

Suk, V. *On Occurrence of Syphilis and Tuberculosis amongst Eskimos and Mixed Breeds of the North Coast of Labrador* (a contribution to the question of the extermination of aboriginal races). Brno: Prirodovedeska Fakulta, 1927 (Publications of the Faculty of Sciences, Masaryk University, 84)

Symposium on Tuberculosis. *Canadian Public Health Journal*, 28/5 (May 1937): 209-22 (contains the following papers: '1. The extent of the public health problem in Ontario,' by N.E. McKinnon; '2. The early diagnosis of tuberculosis,' by D.W. Crombie; '3. The provincial tuberculosis program in Ontario,' by G.C. Brink; 'Discussion,' by W.J. Dobbie)

Thomas, G.W. Pulmonary tuberculosis in northern Newfoundland and Labrador. *New England Journal of Medicine*, 251/10 (Sept. 1954): 374-7

– The decline and fall of pulmonary tuberculosis in northern Newfoundland and Labrador. *Among the Deep Sea Fishers,* 60/1 (Apr. 1962): 3-4

Thomson, J.J. The early diagnosis of pulmonary tuberculosis. *Canadian Medical Association Journal,* 1/1 (Jan. 1911): 47-52

Trout, F. Tuberculosis affiliation course. *Canadian Nurse,* 41 (June 1945): 451-4

Tuberculosis and the medical officer of health. *Canadian Public Health Journal,* 27/10 (Oct. 1936): 511

Tuberculosis mortality in the United States, Canada and Western Europe. *Metropolitan Life Insurance Company, Statistical Bulletin,* 52 (Sept. 1951): 2-5

Tuberculosis returns to the fold. *Canadian Medical Association Journal,* 105/7 (Oct. 9, 1971): 685-7

The tuberculosis services of the Massachusetts-Halifax Health Commission, June 30, 1921 – July 1, 1922. *Public Health Journal,* 13/8 (Aug. 1922): 372-5

Tuberculosis survey: James and Hudson bays, 1950. *Arctic Circular,* 4/3 (Mar. 1951): 45-7

Wherrett, G.J. Follow-up information on 2,031 tuberculosis patients one to thirteen years after discharge from sanatoria. *American Review of Tuberculosis,* 31/1 (Jan. 1935): 62-73

– The need for uniformity in tuberculosis records and statistics. *Canadian Public Health Journal,* 28/2 (Feb. 1937): 75-81

– Brief presented to the Rowell Commission. *Canadian Tuberculosis Association, Bulletin,* 16/3 (Mar. 1938): 2-4

– The tuberculosis problem in Canada. *Canadian Medical Association Journal,* 44/3 (1941): 295-9

– Progress in tuberculosis control in Canada. *Canadian Public Health Journal,* 32/6 (June 1941): 287-92

– The control of tuberculosis in wartime. *Canadian Public Health Journal,* 33/9 (Sept. 1942): 438-45

– Newer drugs in the treatment of tuberculosis. *Nova Scotia Medical Bulletin,* 31/12 (Dec. 1942): 277-8

– Memorandum on tuberculosis presented to House of Commons committee. *Canadian Tuberculosis Association, Bulletin,* 21/4 (June 1943): 1-3

– The tuberculosis problem in the western hemisphere. *National Tuberculosis Association, 50th Anniversary Meeting, 1944, Transactions,* 84-90

– Survey of health conditions and medical and hospital services in the North West Territories. *Canadian Journal of Economics and Political Science,* 11/1 (Feb. 1945): 49-60 (Arctic Survey, 1)

– Industrial medicine and respiratory diseases. *Canadian Medical Association Journal,* 52/3 (Mar. 1945): 271-5

– First aid in tuberculosis. *Canadian First Aid,* 1/2 (Apr. 1945): 6-7

- Recent developments in Canada's tuberculosis services. *Canadian Journal of Public Health*, 46/3 (Mar. 1955): 93-9
- The rehabilitation of the tuberculosis casualty. *Canadian Medical Association Journal*, 73/5 (Sept. 1, 1955): 376-9
- Health programs of the future. *Canadian Journal of Public Health*, 47/11 (Nov. 1956): 457-61
- The effect of new treatments on the organization of the fight against tuberculosis in Canada. *International Union against Tuberculosis, 13th Conference* (New Delhi, 1957), *Libro de actos*, 1082-8
- Trends in tuberculosis. *Canadian Medical Association Journal*, 76 (1957): 121-6
- A tuberculosis control programme. *Indian Journal of Tuberculosis*, 4/2 (Mar. 1957): 47-56
- Changing views on tuberculosis as a national and international problem. *Canadian Journal of Public Health*, 50/5 (May 1959): 201-5
- The role of health education in the anti-tuberculosis campaign. *International Union against Tuberculosis, Bulletin*, 29/4 (July-Oct. 1959): 878-81 (volume of reports, xvth International Tuberculosis Conference, Istanbul, Sept. 1959)
- Present tuberculosis problems. *Canadian Journal of Public Health*, 51/7 (July 1960): 264-7
- Let us now praise dauntless men. *Canadian Journal of Public Health*, 51/12 (Dec. 1960): 469-73
- The diamond jubilee of the Canadian Tuberculosis Association. *Canadian Medical Association Journal*, 84/2 (Jan. 14, 1961): 99-101
- *Tuberculosis – A World Problem.* Ann Arbor: University of Michigan, 1963 (The 1963 Baker Lecture, delivered before the School of Public Health, University of Michigan, December 9, 1963, under the auspices of the Michigan Tuberculosis and Respiratory Disease Association)
- *Tuberculosis in Canada.* Ottawa: Queen's Printer, 1965 (for Royal Commission on Health Services)
- Emerging patterns and trends in tuberculosis. *Canadian Journal of Public Health*, 56/3 (Mar. 1965): 97-9
- World tuberculosis – a task of Sisyphus? *Archives of Environmental Health*, 11/1 (July 1965): 98-102
- Tuberculosis. *Encyclopedia Canadiana*, 10 (1966 cd.): 154-6
- Standard techniques and methods of tuberculin testing and B.C.G. vaccination applicable to public health programs. *Medical Services Journal Canada*, 22/10 (Nov. 1966): 918-21
- The tuberculosis problem – international and national. *Medical Services Journal Canada*, 23/10 (Nov. 1966): 847-51
- Tuberculosis services: a problem of integration. *Canadian Medical Association Journal*, 95 (Dec. 24 and 31, 1966): 1375-6

- The Arctic – the Eskimo and tuberculosis. *Valley Echo,* 49/6 (Dec. 1968): 1-4
- A study of tuberculosis in the eastern Arctic. *Canadian Journal of Public Health,* 60/1 (Jan. 1969): 7-14
- An epidemiological study of non-tuberculous respiratory diseases in the eastern Arctic. *Canadian Journal of Public Health,* 61/2 (Mar.-Apr. 1970): 137-40
Wicks, C.A. The post-sanatorium care of tuberculous patients in Ontario. *Canadian Public Health Journal,* 31/6 (June 1940): 259-70
- Sanatorium treatment of tuberculous patients in Ontario. *Canadian Medical Association Journal,* 67/5 (Nov. 1952): 446-50
- Tuberculosis mortality and morbidity – age and sex trends. *Canadian Journal of Public Health,* 48/4 (Apr. 1957): 146-52
- Comments on tuberculosis control. *Canadian Journal of Public Health,* 54/10 (Oct. 1963): 447-54
Wigle, W.D., and others. Bovine tuberculosis in humans in Ontario; the epidemiologic features of 31 active cases occurring between 1964 and 1970. *American Review of Respiratory Disease,* 106/4 (Oct. 1972): 528-34
Williams, J.I., E.N. Healey, and C. Gow. The death throes of tradition: change in a tuberculosis sanatorium. *Social Science and Medicine,* 5/6 (Dec. 1971): 545-59
Willis, J.S. Disease and death in Canada's north. *Canadian Medical Services Journal,* 19/9 (1963): 747-68
Wilson, H. The role of the public health nurse in tuberculosis control. *Canadian Journal of Public Health,* 56/1 (Jan. 1965): 11-16
Wodehouse, R.E. The public health nurse in the control of tuberculosis. *Canadian Public Health Journal,* 22/1 (Jan. 1931): 28-32
- How sanatoria can help in the prevention and control of tuberculosis. *Canadian Medical Association Journal,* 23/3 (Mar. 1931): 668-71
- Observations on tuberculosis statistics in Canada, 1921 and 1931. *Canadian Public Health Journal,* 24/9 (Sept. 1933): 433-9
Wright, J.S. The sociologic and economic aspects of tuberculosis. *Canadian Medical Association Journal,* 8/9 (Sept. 1918): 791-6
Young, W.A. Consumption now a communicable disease; an editorial. *Canadian Journal of Medicine and Surgery,* 1/3 (Mar. 1897): 129-32

Index